The
Brain
Warrior's Way
Cookbook

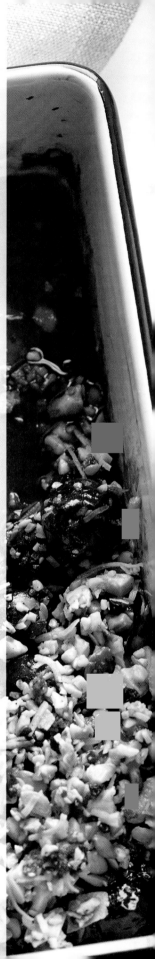

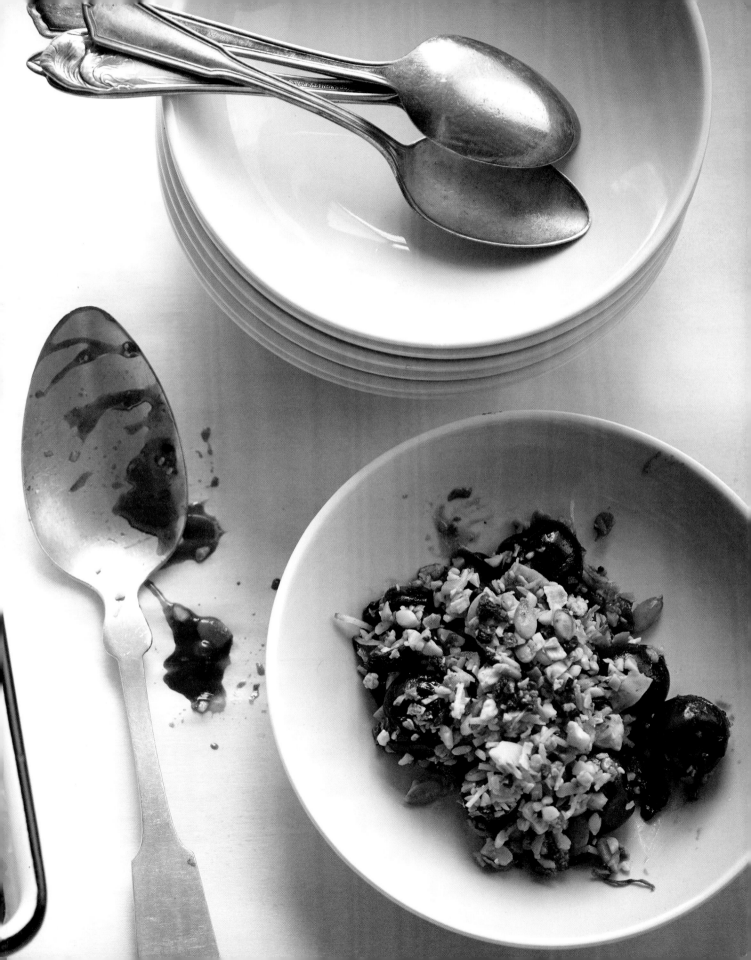

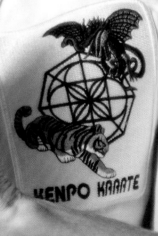

"Become a warrior for your brain and body."

The
Brain
Warrior's Way
Cookbook

Over 100 Recipes to Ignite Your Energy and Focus, Attack Illness and Aging, Transform Pain into Purpose

TANA AMEN, BSN, RN

DANIEL G. AMEN, MD

New American Library

New York

NEW AMERICAN LIBRARY
Published by Berkley
An imprint of Penguin Random House LLC
375 Hudson Street, New York, New York 10014

All text photographs used by permission of Amen Clinics except the following: p. 10 by Brent Hofacker/Shutterstock.com; pp. 15–16 by Africa Studio/Shutterstock.com; p. 20 by iravgustin/Shutterstock.com; p. 58 by Alexussk/Shutterstock.com; pp. 89–90 by Magdalena Kucova/Shutterstock.com; and p. 270 by Wiktory/Shutterstock.com

New American Library and the NAL colophon are registered trademarks of Penguin Random House LLC.

Library of Congress Cataloging-in-Publication Data

Names: Amen, Tana, author. | Amen, Daniel G., author.
Title: The brain warrior's way cookbook: over 100 recipes to ignite your energy and focus, attack illness and aging, transform pain into purpose/Tana Amen, BSN, RN, Daniel G. Amen, MD.
Description: First edition. | New York: National American Library, 2016.
Identifiers: LCCN 2016026861 (print) | LCCN 2016029901 (ebook) | ISBN 9781101988503 (paperback) | ISBN 9781101988510 (ebook)
Subjects: LCSH: Mental illness—Nutritional aspects. | Nutrition—Psychological aspects. | Cooking. | Cookbooks. lcgft | BISAC: COOKING/Health & Healing/General. | HEALTH & FITNESS/Diseases/Nervous System (incl. Brain).
Classification: LCC RC455.4.N8 A44 2016 (print) | LCC RC455.4.N8 (ebook) | DDC 641.5/63—dc23
LC record available at https://lccn.loc.gov/2016026861

First Edition: November 2016

Printed in the United States of America
1 3 5 7 9 10 8 6 4 2

Cover photographs used by permission of Amen Clinics
Cover design by Steve Meditz
Book design by Pauline Neuwirth

The recipes contained in this book are to be followed exactly as written. The publisher is not responsible for your specific health or allergy needs that may require medical supervision. The publisher is not responsible for any adverse reactions to the recipes contained in this book.

While the author has made every effort to provide accurate telephone numbers, Internet addresses and other contact information at the time of publication, neither the publisher nor the author assumes any responsibility for errors, or for changes that occur after publication. Further, publisher does not have any control over and does not assume any responsibility for author or third-party websites or their content.

MEDICAL DISCLAIMER

The information presented in this book is the result of years of practice experience and clinical research by the authors. The information in this book, by necessity, is of a general nature and not a substitute for an evaluation or treatment by a competent medical specialist. If you believe you are in need of medical interventions, please see a medical practitioner as soon as possible. The stories in this book are true. The names and circumstances of the stories have been changed to protect the anonymity of patients.

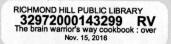

To Chloe, Eli, Emmy, Liam, and Louie, and the rest of our tribe, our reasons to be Brain Warriors.

"You CAN optimize your health by doing better today than you did yesterday."

Contents

■

SECTION 8:

Meat, Lamb, and Pork 161

SECTION 9:

Staples, Not Sides 181

SECTION 10:

Snacks 207

SECTION 11:

Sauces, Spreads, and Condiments 231

SECTION 12:
Bakery 261

SECTION 13:
Brain Warrior Holiday Meal Plan 297

SECTION 14:
Brain Warrior Herbs and Spices 307

SECTION 15:
Rations for Brain Warriors on the Road 317

SECTION 16:
Junior Brain Warriors 329

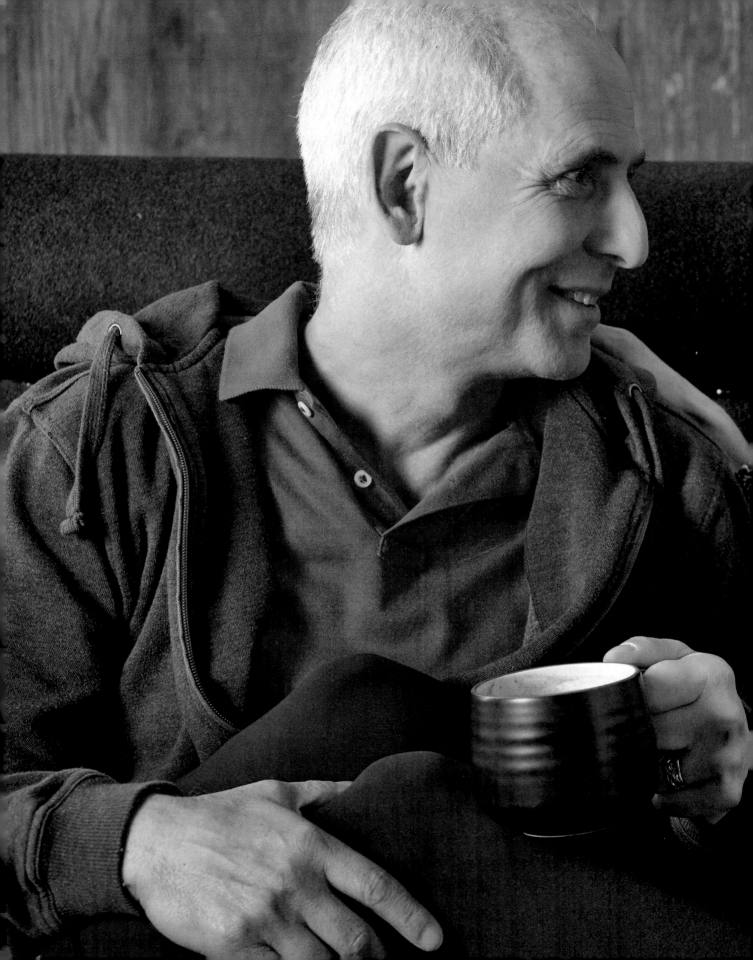

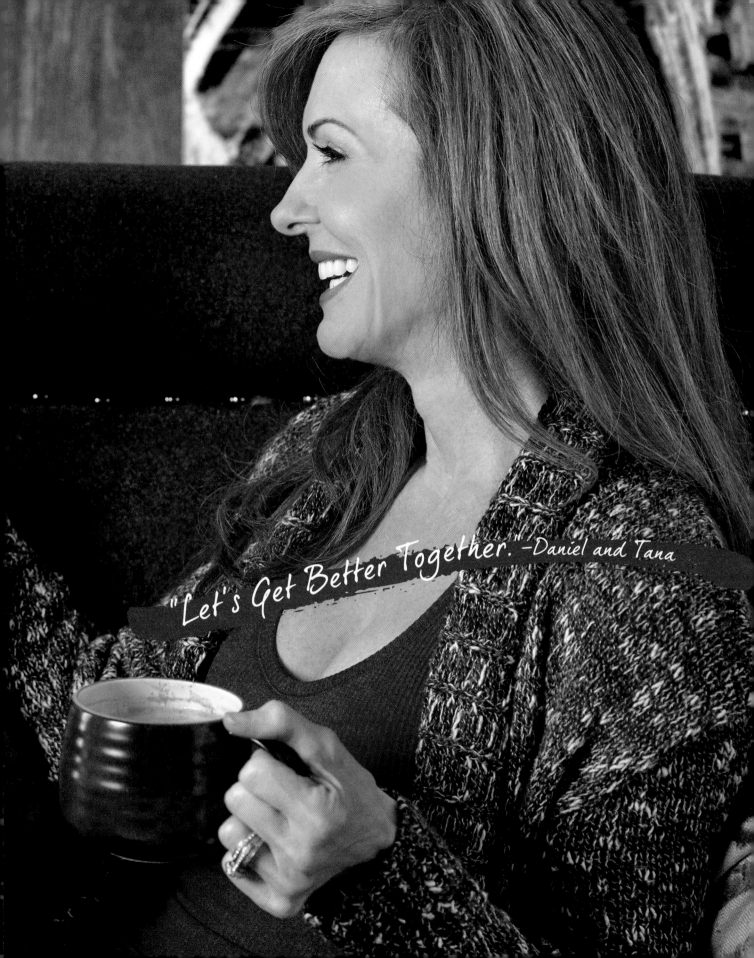

"Let's Get Better Together." –Daniel and Tana

The Brain Warrior's Way Cookbook

Over 100 Recipes to Ignite Your Energy and Focus, Attack Illness and Aging, Transform Pain into Purpose

■

> Warriors are not born or made.
>
> Warriors create themselves
>
> through trial and error,
>
> pain and suffering
>
> and their ability to
>
> conquer their own faults.
>
> —UNKNOWN

If you or a family member have ever suffered from chronic illness or cared for a child with special needs, you know you are in a war for the health of your brain and body! But it's a war you can win. In fact, winning the war for the health of your brain and body is easier and more delicious than you can imagine. It starts with making a few good decisions, especially about nutrition. A vibrant, victorious life is about abundance! It's never about deprivation. In this cookbook we'll give you simple, delicious recipes, tips, and tools for ultimate success.

Food is a major part of our daily lives. Food matters. In fact, it matters so much that food manufacturers and advertisers have noticed, exploiting consumers every day for the sake of their bottom lines and feeding us lies about what to eat and where to buy food. Food is as healing as medicine or as toxic as poison. We're surrounded by opportunities to make food choices that will fuel success or, sadly, drive failure every day. The war for health is one that the food industry and advertisers have been winning for far too long. They have advanced technology and strategies that have been hijacking your taste buds, your brain, and your body for decades, causing you to be a prisoner of war to their technology, addictive concoctions, and foodlike substances. This war has been literally stealing the health, wealth, and happiness of Americans (and people in other nations who have adopted the standard American diet) for far too long. The good news is that you can break these chains, starting today, and it's easier than you think! *It's not brain surgery; it's brain science!*

In *The Brain Warrior's Way* we give you the detailed program and simple science to teach you how to live the life of a Brain Warrior, including ways to decrease inflammation, increase focus and energy, reverse illnesses caused by lifestyle factors, and fight the war against chronic pain, diabetes, heart disease, ADHD, depression, and Alzheimer's disease. Now, in the companion cookbook, we're going to take that one step further and help you eat like a Brain Warrior! This is the fun part, because once you understand it, you realize the power and delight of real food. You will feel stronger and happier; your mind will be sharper and your waistline smaller.

After working with tens of thousands of patients from around the world, we know that for you to truly think and eat like a Brain Warrior, we have to give you the winning formula. Brain Warriors have specific nutrition needs. The diet of a Brain Warrior must:

▶ Be delicious
▶ Be simple to prepare
▶ Be easily packed for "road rations"
▶ Be healing
▶ Build strength
▶ Improve brain function and focus

Additionally, as a Brain Warrior, your nutrition will be focused on ten simple nutrition principles that will guide your journey. All of the recipes are created according to these principles. These guiding principles, in addition to this cookbook, will help you make smart food decisions at home, work, and school, and when you travel or eat in restaurants.

TEN BRAIN WARRIOR NUTRITION PRINCIPLES

1. Think high-quality calories.
2. Drink plenty of water, not your calories.
3. Eat high-quality protein in small doses throughout the day.
4. Eat smart carbohydrates (low glycemic, high fiber).
5. Focus your diet on healthy fats.
6. Eat from the rainbow.
7. Cook with brain-healthy herbs and spices to boost your brain.

8. Make sure your food is as clean as possible.

9. If you're having trouble with your mood, energy, memory, weight, blood sugar, blood pressure or skin, eliminate any foods that might be causing trouble, especially wheat and any other gluten-containing grain or food, dairy, soy, and corn.

10. Focus on brain-healthy eating throughout the day, but fast for at least twelve hours between dinner and breakfast.

You can find more information about these principles and more in *The Brain Warrior's Way*.

We will always be surrounded by companies and individuals who stand to gain from our weakness and suffering by pushing food products that make us sick. Many people who come to us for help feel outraged when they come to understand that it's often with full knowledge and intent that companies add toxic amounts of sugar and chemicals to food in order to keep them addicted. We want you to use that outrage as a signal to take personal responsibility for your health. Responsibility means the ability to respond and make choices. Yes, this is war, but the best way to fight back is to be armed with knowledge and a plan to win back your health. Ultimately, your health is your responsibility. You must be your own health advocate for yourself and your loved ones if you want to win this war.

We want you to be victorious and join us in the journey to better memory, focus, energy, weight and mood! Become a Brain Warrior starting today!

—Tana and Daniel Amen, 2016

Inspiring Success Stories

Meet Brain Warriors Bobby, Inez, and Aitana

After hearing about your program, my wife and I decided to give it a try. We knew we had to make some changes for our family. My wife has Hashimoto's disease. My daughter has polycystic ovarian syndrome, and I had not felt great about myself in a long time.

I admit we struggled with cravings for the first few days. If it hadn't been for my wife pushing us, I would have quit. It would have been easy to say, "Let's try something else or try it later." But we made a commitment as a family to do what you said and give it two weeks.

After one week the cravings were gone! In fact, real food started to taste delicious. I was surprised how much the flavor was magnified in a carrot. I never noticed before. After two weeks on the program we couldn't have been happier. We all felt fantastic and had each lost between ten and twelve pounds and no longer thought about quitting. Each week on the program gets better and better, and we feel more energetic than ever! In fact, I can't remember the last time I have ever felt this wonderful. I lost twenty pounds after four weeks. People tell me that my skin looks great. I am more confident, more energetic, and I sleep so much better. I actually like what I see when I look in the mirror now.

Now we are all mentoring our family and friends to live this way. Both my wife and daughter had struggled with weight loss in the past in spite of exercising twice a day at times. My wife struggled as a result of her thyroid issues. She has now lost twenty-four pounds since she started eating this way, and people tell her that her skin is more vibrant. My eighteen-year-old daughter Aitana has PCOS, which makes weight loss difficult. She also struggled with acne and moodiness. She has lost twenty-two pounds and rarely has breakouts now. She feels happier and much more confident about her appearance. As soon as they started eating according to these food rules, they were able to exercise a fraction of the time and get more results. What you eat matters!

One of the amazing things we've noticed is how many other people ask us for help after seeing our family transformation. My mother, who lives with us after suffering several strokes, is now eating this way. Her moods and energy are much better. She is more social and no longer isolates herself to her room as much. My mother-in-law, who suffers from fibromyalgia, also reports less pain and is able to walk more easily. Even our two younger sons, who don't seem to have much interest in learning about our new lifestyle yet, are eating better without even realizing it

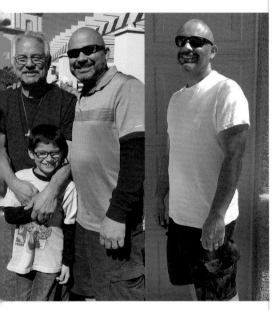

BEFORE   AFTER

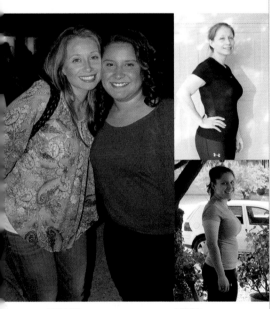

BEFORE   AFTER

because we no longer have junk food in the house. We know this will have a long-term effect on their health. As a family we are healthier and happier.

Even several of my coworkers noticed the changes and have started the program. Now they are asking me a ton of questions. When you feel good, you look better. I even walk differently and I think people notice. It's hard not to share what you learn when the changes are so obvious.

My family and I can't thank you enough!

—*Bobby Lucero*

Meet Brain Warrior Mary (Tana's Mom)

I was a sixteen-year-old runaway who became a single mom early in life. By the time I was twenty-one I also became the primary caretaker for a diabetic mother, a quadriplegic father, and a brother with a heroin addiction. Between working hard and taking care of others, taking care of myself was the last thing I had time for, and I paid the price with my health.

My daughter, Tana, can be a force to be reckoned with when she wants someone she loves to get healthy. But when I realized I was really hurting her by not putting my health first, I got serious. I'm very close to my family and I realized that I would not be around to see my granddaughter grow up if I didn't make changes. I have used these principles to change my life and my body!

BEFORE:

- ▶ Twenty pounds overweight
- ▶ Always tired
- ▶ Cared for others but not self
- ▶ ADD
- ▶ History of multiple concussions and brain injury
- ▶ Brain surgery
- ▶ Trouble focusing
- ▶ Moody
- ▶ History of fibroid tumors
- ▶ Digestive problems
- ▶ Hormonal imbalances
- ▶ Migraines

AFTER:

I was always too busy taking care of others to take care of myself. I never realized how much it was affecting the health of my brain. My focus, energy, mood, and weight are better than they have ever been. I got serious after seeing my brain scan. I knew I needed to become a Brain Warrior!

—*Mary Meeks*

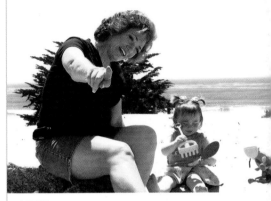

AGE 50

AGE 69

- ▶ Lost twenty pounds
- ▶ Improved relationships
- ▶ Improved focus
- ▶ Improved business
- ▶ More energy
- ▶ Enjoying taking care of myself

Meet Brain Warriors John and Bill

Master John Sepulveda is a ninth-degree black belt in Kenpo karate. He's a karate legend, highly respected in the karate world and loved by his students and fellow martial artists. Daniel and I had the honor and privilege of assisting Mr. Sepulveda to achieve his weight loss goals before attending a very special event where many of his longtime karate friends would be in attendance. Mr. Sepulveda wanted to lose twenty-four pounds in three months, which is a safe and realistic goal. Using the same food principles spelled out in this book we walked him through the program.

Mr. Sepulveda reached out to us two and a half months later, informing us he had lost seventeen pounds quite easily, but was struggling with the last seven pounds. He seemed to have hit a plateau. This is not uncommon, but he really wanted to lose those last few pounds before the event. We suggested he take a serious assessment of his food to see if he was slipping, increase his water intake, and increase weight lifting (if necessary). We made some fine-tuning adjustments to his food program by decreasing the starchy carbohydrates that had crept in, a common problem that occurs over time without close attention.

We became concerned a few days before the event when we hadn't heard a word from him. Usually this is an indication that people have gone off the program and are avoiding us. I reached out to him to nudge him a bit. However, I was delighted by the very matter-of-fact Brain Warrior response I received in return. Mr. Sepulveda had lost over seven pounds in a week. I asked if he was struggling with the program. He said, "Why would I struggle? You told me what to eat. I'm eating that and I'm not eating the other stuff." He just did exactly what we had told him to do. That is the focus and dedication of a Brain Warrior. Mr. Sepulveda lost the additional weight he wanted to lose over the next week and has kept the weight off for over three years.

Last August we received a message from Mr. Sepulveda letting us know he had gotten his brother to join him in becoming a Brain Warrior. His brother Bill started out weighing 277 pounds at that time. By Christmas he had lost forty-seven pounds. Like Mr. Sepulveda, he just did everything his brother coached him to do. However, like many people, he relaxed his program during the holidays. He was unaware that he was diabetic—a

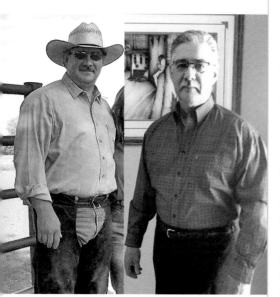

BEFORE   AFTER

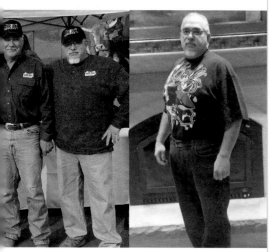

BEFORE   AFTER

condition that had likely gone undiagnosed for a long time; the holiday food he indulged in led to a very scary hospital visit. His doctors put him on medicine to control his blood sugar. Upon learning he was diabetic, he got serious and got back on the program. Within three months, his blood sugar was stable enough as a result of his new lifestyle changes that the doctor discontinued his medication and he is vigilantly sticking to the program.

Meet Brain Warrior Rob

Through the program I fell in love with my brain! I lost thirty-nine pounds and my memory, creativity, and mood have all been boosted. At work, in a meeting recently, I was able to remember the name of a client I had not seen in twelve years. Thank you!

—*Rob*

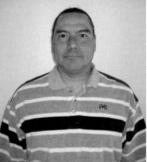

BEFORE

AFTER

Meet Brain Warrior John

(John learned about being a Brain Warrior while attending an addiction recovery center where we planted our program.)

When I took my intake picture I looked all bloated from drinking. Now people don't recognize me as the same person. I think I lost weight because I stopped drinking, eating sugar, and I eat a lot healthier in the program. I don't even think about drinking much. I feel really great about myself. My self-esteem is the highest it's ever been. I just feel a lot better. Thank you, God!

—*John*

BEFORE:
- ▶ Addiction ruined my life
- ▶ Bloated and overweight
- ▶ Brain fog
- ▶ Lack of motivation
- ▶ No confidence
- ▶ Lacked hope for the future

AFTER:
- ▶ Gained control over cravings
- ▶ Understanding of how food affects cravings
- ▶ Lost thirty-eight pounds
- ▶ Hope for the future
- ▶ Brain fog cleared
- ▶ New confidence in myself

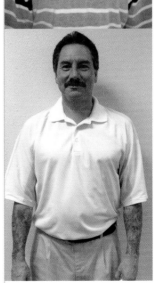

BEFORE

AFTER

"You can't start training on fight day and expect to win, especially with the fight for your health. You must train and prepare every day, and hopefully avoid the fight altogether!"

—Tana

Brain Warrior Basics

Getting Ready for Massive Change

■

*Moderation? It's mediocrity, fear, and confusion in disguise.
It's the devil's dilemma. It's neither doing nor not doing.
It's the wobbling compromise that makes no one happy.
Moderation is for the bland, the apologetic, for the
fence-sitters of the world afraid to take a stand. It's for
those afraid to laugh or cry, for those afraid to live or die.
Moderation . . . is lukewarm tea, the devil's own brew!*

—DAN MILLMAN, *WAY OF THE PEACEFUL WARRIOR*

Purge and Prepare Your Pantry

If you've been eating the standard American diet, it's likely your kitchen contains foods that are sabotaging the health of your brain and body. Now that you're a Brain Warrior, it's time to do a clean sweep of your entire kitchen and toss out all the foods that don't serve you and your family. Not having garbage food in the house also helps prevent impulsive, mindless snacking as you change your eating patterns. As Daniel and I like to say: make one decision to get rid of it instead of thirty decisions over time not to eat it in a weak moment!

We frequently hear patients parry this initial step with phrases like "everything in moderation." Moderation of things that are not addictive and destructive to your health may be all right. However, moderation of things that cause addiction, inflammation, and ultimately disease simply doesn't work. We have seen people fight this concept repeatedly, slide back into illness, brain fog, and despair over and over, until they finally come to the realization that when you tempt the devil, the devil usually wins. Think of unhealthy foodlike substances like the devil. You'll be more successful if you avoid them altogether.

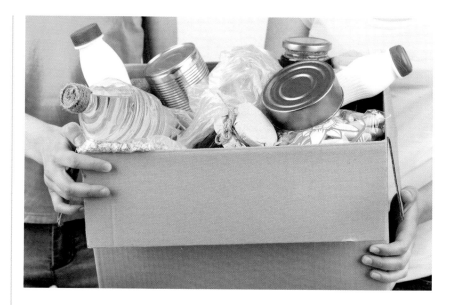

If the food you're getting rid of is simply not "optimal" for the highest level of performance, you may consider giving it to a homeless shelter. However, if it's truly toxic, please just get rid of it. Homeless people are the last ones we should be making sicker with toxic food. And please do not send your leftover candy to the troops we rely on to protect our country! The candy drives I see outside my daughter's school and the local grocery stores, collecting candy and baked goods for the troops, drive us crazy. These are our heroes. They deserve delicious, nutritious food that will help them focus at the highest level possible. It's not just you they are protecting. Their lives depend on it! Toxic "foodlike substances" lead to bad decision making.

Here's a list of what to toss:

- ► The majority of processed foods. Most contain lots of unhealthy fat, sugar, corn syrup, artificial sweeteners, and other ingredients that you'll be avoiding. Beware of any products containing more than five ingredients or ingredients you can't pronounce. Read the labels. It will be eye opening.
- ► All foods that contain high-fructose corn syrup, sugar, artificial sweeteners, soy, trans fat, or hydrogenated or partially hydrogenated fat.
- ► The following cooking oils: vegetable oils such as corn oil, safflower oil, canola oil, and soy-based oils.
- ► Cereal and other grain-based foods.
- ► Bread, pasta, and other foods that contain gluten.
- ► Fruit juice. Even if it's 100 percent fruit, juice causes unhealthy blood sugar spikes. Whenever fruit sugar is unwrapped from its fiber source, it can turn toxic in your liver.

- ▶ Foods that contain genetically modified ingredients.
- ▶ Foods that contain milk or other dairy products. The exception is a bit of goat or sheep milk yogurt and cheese if you're not sensitive or allergic to them, or organic ghee.
- ▶ Cookies, cakes, candy, and other sweets.
- ▶ Condiments such as ketchup, barbecue sauce, and mustard (unless it's natural), which are usually packed with sugar, salt, and artificial ingredients and food coloring. Soy sauce contains gluten (usually), soy, and excessive sodium. Mustard that is gluten free and sugar free can stay. On rare occasions that you need soy sauce, choose organic, low-sodium sauce, which is gluten free.
- ▶ Jams, jellies, and pancake syrup. They are pure sugar. Most "pancake" syrup contains no maple at all! It is high-fructose corn syrup and artificial flavoring.

Stock Up on Brain Warrior Basics

Now that you've purged your pantry of unhealthy processed foods, you have space for whole, nutritious foods that will fuel your brain and body with an abundance of vitamins, minerals, antioxidants, and anti-inflammatory compounds they need for excellent health and peak performance. It's time for a trip to the grocery store, health food store, or farmers' market to start stocking up on the Brain Warrior Basics:

- ▶ Vegetables and more vegetables. Purchase fresh, organic produce when possible and skip the white potatoes.
- ▶ Small amounts of fruit. The best choices are blueberries, raspberries, strawberries, and blackberries, as they don't affect blood sugar as much as starchy fruits like bananas. They are also super packed with brain-boosting antioxidants. However, berries should always be organic, as they absorb more pesticides than nearly any other fruit.
- ▶ Meat, fish, and poultry, including wild salmon, tuna, herring, chicken and turkey, lamb, and lean beef. Buy meats and poultry that are grass-fed, free-range, hormone free, and antibiotic free.
- ▶ Eggs. When possible, choose organic, DHA-enriched eggs from pasture-raised chickens
- ▶ Coconut wraps, zucchini wraps, and other bread replacements. See brand list on pages 338–39.
- ▶ Raw, unsalted seeds and nuts. Be sure to choose raw nuts and seeds, because when nuts and seeds are roasted, their oils oxidize and they are robbed of their health benefits.

- ▶ Fresh and dried herbs and spices. They supercharge your health benefits and contain fantastic flavor.
- ▶ Healthy oils such as coconut oil, almond oil, macadamia nut oil, and olive oil.
- ▶ Hummus, salsa, and guacamole. For dipping raw vegetables.
- ▶ Shirataki noodles. These are a gluten-free, high-fiber alternative to pasta. Our favorite brand is Miracle Noodle because they don't contain soy.
- ▶ Unbleached sea salt. To be used in *small* amounts instead of bleached table salt.
- ▶ Salt substitute (potassium chloride). It's a great substitute for many people on a low-sodium diet.
- ▶ Unsweetened almond milk or hemp milk. Drink these instead of cow's milk.
- ▶ Nut and seed butter. Almond butter and macadamia nut butter are perfect replacements for peanut butter.
- ▶ Goji berries.
- ▶ Raw, shredded coconut, unsweetened.
- ▶ Vegan protein powder, sugar free.
- ▶ Flax, hemp, and chia seeds.
- ▶ Freeze-dried greens.
- ▶ Ghee. If you prefer a buttery taste and are not vegan, use this for cooking at high temperatures.
- ▶ Organic, low-sodium tamari sauce or any gluten-free soy sauce.
- ▶ Coconut milk creamer (plain flavor) or coconut milk.
- ▶ Stevia sweetener. Use this in place of sugar. Liquid stevia is less bitter.
- ▶ Erythritol sweetener. Use this in place of sugar for baking.
- ▶ Raw, unsweetened cocoa. Not commercial cocoa.
- ▶ Raw cacao nibs.
- ▶ Dark chocolate, sugar free and dairy free. Find chocolate sweetened with stevia or erythritol.
- ▶ Dried beans and lentils. Consume only in limited amounts.
- ▶ Lots of travel-sized storage containers, ice packs, and coolers for packing leftovers and on-the-go lunches and snacks.

The Environmental Working Group (EWG) is a wonderful resource for budget-conscious Brain Warriors who are passionate about consuming clean food. The EWG has a regularly updated list of nonorganic produce that contains the most pesticides, the "Dirty Dozen." The EWG also lists nonorganic produce with the least amount of pesticides and harmful chemicals called the "Clean Fifteen." Try to avoid purchasing nonorganic produce from the "Dirty Dozen," as pesticides have been linked to increased risk of many brain disorders like ADHD and Alzheimer's disease, cancer, diabetes and hormonal disturbances.

Reading Sugar on Labels: How Much and What Kind of Sugar Is Okay?

Let's face it: it's simply not realistic to get rid of ALL sugar from your diet, at least not if you ever want to eat another salad or bowl of mixed berries. All vegetables and fruit contain sugar, along with the myriad of disease-fighting plant compounds and antioxidants that help keep your brain young. We don't advocate that you eliminate these powerful foods from your diet, but we do want you to pay attention to how much sugar you are consuming overall. It's a matter of consuming low-glycemic foods (explained in detail in the book *The Brain Warrior's Way*) that give you the most positive nutritional impact.

One of the main reasons we've listed the nutritional information on these recipes is so you know how much sugar you're consuming in a day. Healthy, wholesome fat and clean protein aren't the major health stealers in most recipes. It's the high sugar content and simple carbohydrates.

Here are some simple tips to help you understand food labels, especially sugar.

1. When reading food labels, the first thing you want to notice is the quality of the ingredients. Make sure you can pronounce them and that your grandmother would recognize them as food. There are a few exceptions, like stevia and erythritol, which are actually naturally occurring ingredients that may not have been popular items fifty years ago. Generally, food is not the best place for chemicals with scientific-sounding names.

2. Check out the amount of carbohydrates compared to fat and protein. Make sure your diet isn't heavy with simple carbohydrates. One quick way to determine if it's a simple carbohydrate is to see how much fiber it contains. Fiber is a special carbohydrate that is vital to gut health and doesn't elevate blood sugar. You can deduct the fiber content from the overall carb count.

3. Look at the sugar content. If it has more than five grams of sugar, it's a red flag. Be cautious. Less sugar is always better. This doesn't mean you can never have foods with five grams of sugar, but avoid processed foods and baked goods with high-fructose corn syrup and especially high sugar content. A green juice without any fruit can contain up to six or seven grams of sugar, but it is extremely detoxifying and loaded with nutrition. We'd rather have you choose the green drink than the giant cookie. If you know something contains high

amounts of sugar, have a smaller amount so you don't get a large sugar jolt.

4. You will notice that the recipes in this book that contain the highest amounts of sugar are the salads and smoothies and recipes with lots of vegetables, especially tomatoes. The desserts are actually very low in sugar. Fruit is one of the fastest ways to increase your overall sugar consumption. We still want you to eat some fruit, but the sugar content is why we tell you to limit fruit to one or two pieces each day. Consider these facts as you put your menu together.

5. The higher the sugar is on the ingredient list, the more sugar the product contains.

6. Beware of sneaky trans fats. The idea that all trans fats have been removed from our food supply is false. If the label lists partially hydrogenated oil, it contains trans fat. As long as there is not more than 0.5 gram of trans fat per serving, manufacturers do not have to list it. To get around this, food companies have decreased the portions that they consider a serving size. Packaged snack foods that consumers consider one serving are often listed as up to four servings or more on the label. That means there could be 2 grams of trans fat in that one snack.

Why All the Fuss over Something as Natural as Fruit?

Up until the early 1800s there was no efficient way to store and can fruit and vegetables, which meant people usually ate them seasonally. People would often eat more of these delicious foods when they were available, knowing they would not have them for many months. What they were *not* able to do was eat five or six pieces of fruit every day out of convenience, or add fruit jams, jellies, and spreads filled with sugar all day long as we do now. Add to that processed snack foods, trans fat, and lots of chemicals, and we now have a perfect storm for chronic illness. It's not a coincidence that with the revolution in industrialization, farming, and food storage came chronic illness the likes of which mankind had never seen in history. Be conscious of the food you consume. We recommend one piece of fruit each day to people who are diabetic or insulin resistant. If you are healthy, active and have stable blood sugar, you may be able to tolerate two pieces of fruit without problems.

The Importance of Oil and Fat

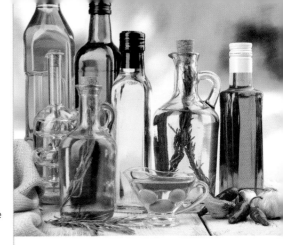

Although olive oil and other unsaturated fats (usually liquid at room temperature) are nutritious when consumed in raw form, they oxidize and become harmful when heated to high temperatures. When oils reach their smoke point during cooking, they break down, lose nutritional value, and become toxic.

For cooking I usually use coconut oil, ghee, or macadamia nut oil. Grape seed oil has a high smoke point and is a less expensive option. However, it has been shown to be more inflammatory than some of the previous oils mentioned. All of these oils have a higher smoke point than olive oil, so they can get hotter without breaking down. Often you don't even need oil for cooking! Most of the recipes in this book suggest using vegetable broth for sautéing instead of oil. In most cases, it works just as well. Save the calories for your salad dressing.

Organic, unrefined, expeller-pressed, and cold-pressed oils are the healthiest. Processing strips oils of all nutritional value, leaving them as nothing more than liquid fat, and not the healthy kind. You can find unrefined oils in most health food stores. As a rule, oils should be colored somewhat the shade of the source they came from. For example, if olive oil has a light, clear color, it has been processed and stripped of its natural character. Olive oil should have a slight green tint. Oils are best stored in dark-colored glass bottles and should be kept in the refrigerator for extended storage time.

Stay away from cooking with flax oil. There is an ongoing debate as to whether flax oil is a good source of omega-3 fatty acids but, in truth, it can also cause inflammation. Flaxseeds are very healthy because they contain lignans, a type of antioxidant, but when the oil is removed from the seed, it can become pro-inflammatory. Also, while flax oil contains some omega-3 fatty acids, it is higher in the pro-inflammatory omega-6 fatty acids, which negates the omega-3s. Flaxseeds are great for you, but flax oil? Not so much.

One of the few dairy products I like to cook with is organic ghee, also called clarified butter. The milk proteins have been removed and the remaining product is safe for cooking and it's not processed like other butter substitutes.

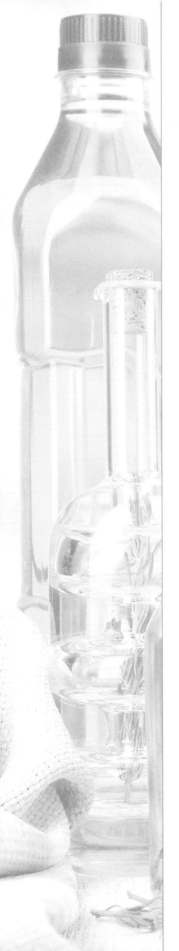

COOKING OIL GUIDE

Best Oils for Cooking at High Temperatures

When frying, braising, broiling, or any other cooking method at high temperatures, it's best to use oils and fats that can be heated to high temperatures before they begin to smoke. When marinating meats in the refrigerator prior to cooking, you'll want to choose an oil that remains liquid at cool temperatures, unlike ghee or coconut oil.

SFA=Saturated MFA=Monounsaturated PUFA=Polyunsaturated

TYPE OF OIL	TYPE OF FAT	SMOKE POINT
Unrefined Coconut Oil	86% SFA	450° F
Ghee	63% SFA	480° F
Avocado Oil	70% MUFA	500° F
Macadamia Nut Oil	80% MUFA	420° F
Rice Bran Oil	38% MUFA to 37% PUFA	415° F
Palm Oil	54% SFA	455° F

Oils That Are All Right for Cooking at Lower Temperatures

For heating or sautéing at low temperatures, the following oils are safe options. With the exception of cacao butter, these oils are usually liquid at room temperature.

TYPE OF OIL	TYPE OF FAT	SMOKE POINT
Olive Oil	73% MUFA	370° F
Grape Seed Oil	71% PUFA	420° F
Cacao Butter	60% SFA	370° F

Avoid Cooking with These Oils

While some of these oils appear to have a high smoke point, they are not stable fats and they oxidize quickly with heat, which is why you should never cook with them.

TYPE OF OIL	TYPE OF FAT	SMOKE POINT
Canola Oil	64% MUFA	400° F (most GMO)
Safflower Oil	76% PUFA	250 to 510° F
Sesame Seed Oil	43% MUFA to 43% PUFA	450° F
Sunflower Oil	19% MUFA to 63% PUFA	225 to 400° F
Vegetable Shortening	34% SFA to 52% PUFA	330 to 440° F
Corn Oil	59% PUFA	440° F (most GMO)
Soybean Oil	23% MUFA	495° F (most GMO)

Preparing Poultry, Meat, and Seafood

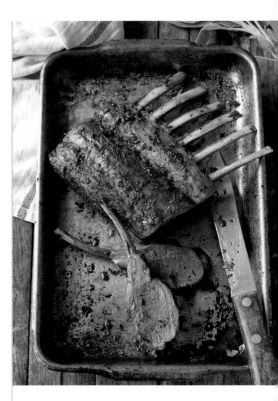

Generally speaking, cooking methods that require lower heat or less cooking time are healthier because they prevent a process that creates high levels of advanced glycation end products (AGEs). Dietary advanced glycation end products (AGEs) are created by cooking meat, poultry, and seafood at high heat due to the chemical reactions that take place between carbohydrates, protein, and fat. AGEs can lead to inflammation, diabetes, and increased risk of cancer and Alzheimer's disease. As the protein that is necessary for healthy cells becomes damaged, vital organs also become damaged. Skin being the largest organ of the human body, damage to protein in skin caused by AGEs may be seen in the form of wrinkles!

This doesn't mean you have to toss your favorite grill. But understanding a few simple concepts can dramatically boost your mental health, energy, and vitality. If you love grilling, try turning it down and cooking over lower heat for a longer period, or try a stove-top grill, which doesn't expose meat to the open flame and gives you more control over the temperature. You'll get that grilled effect without the associated risks.

Healthy Cooking Guide

Healthiest Methods

- ▶ **Baking:** A dry-heat method of cooking, usually in an oven, at moderate temperatures. Poultry and seafood are sometimes covered during the baking process to prevent browning and preserve moistness.

- ▶ **Poaching:** Usually cooked in water or broth below boiling point of 160 to 180 degrees F, poaching can be done in a pan over the cooktop or in the oven. While poaching is a popular way to prepare fish, it's also a great way to prepare poultry. The intense flavor you may lose from charring or frying, you will make up in spades with moisture. Be sure to check poultry with a thermometer. An internal temperature of 160 to 170 degrees F indicates that poultry is finished cooking.

- ▶ **Boiling:** Usually done in boiling water or broth. The advantage is that poultry and certain types of seafood or meat cook quickly and remain moist and tender. Be sure to check poultry with a thermometer.

Next Best Methods

▶ **Stir-fry:** Traditionally, stir-fry recipes call for oil and very hot cooking temperatures. However, oil is optional. One of the most flavorful and healthy ways to stir-fry is with low-sodium vegetable broth or a little water. This method requires less cooking time due to smaller chunks of meat.

▶ **Braising:** When braising, you brown meat or poultry in a hot pan for a short time, then allow it to simmer in a covered pan or Crock-Pot for a long period of time. To improve on the health aspect of traditional methods (browning in fat or heavy oil), try removing as much fat as possible and use a small amount of oil or broth instead. Slow-cooking in broth is a great way to impress guests because the result is fabulously tender meat or poultry.

▶ **Broiling:** Cooking quickly on high, intense heat under the broiler in an oven seals the outside of many dishes, while leaving the inside juicy and tender. However, be careful about the amount of charring that broiling produces. Try to broil on the lowest setting possible. One way to decrease the amount of time under the broiler is to start with broiling, then finish off by poaching.

GRILLING GUIDE

Grilling	How Long	How Hot
Meat	3 to 5 minutes per inch of thickness	145° at center
Poultry	3 to 5 minutes per inch of thickness	160 to 170° at center
Fish	2 to 3 minutes per inch of thickness	135° at center

Least Healthy Methods

▶ **Roasting:** A dry-heat method of cooking, with a temperature of 300 degrees F or above, usually in an oven. Meat, poultry, or fish should be left uncovered so heat penetrates evenly. The difference between roasting and baking is the temperature. Roasting is achieved with more intense heat to produce a browned surface. Also, meat is often left uncovered during roasting to allow for caramelizing of sauces or browning of the surface. Avoid caramelizing food when possible for best health.

▶ **Grilling:** Rapid cooking on a rack over coals, electric coil, or open fire with intense heat. This traditional favorite is easy and produces incredible flavor. But like broiling, the intense heat and close proximity to fire (especially with open-fire grilling) can increase charring. To decrease charring, remove excess fat, start with grilling (and turn frequently), then finish off with poaching or baking. You can also try a stove-top grill, which doesn't expose meat to the open flame. Consider cooking high-quality cuts of meat (not poultry) medium or medium rare.

- **Microwave:** Quickly reheating in a microwave, or an occasional meal in a bind, isn't so bad. If it's a choice between a quick healthy snack heated in the microwave for thirty seconds or a trip to the donut shop, the microwave wins, hands down. However, try to avoid making the microwave your best friend. Microwave cooking is an extremely rapid cooking method using electromagnetic radiation. The water molecules in food vibrate violently in the microwaves, creating friction, which heats food. Microwaving food not only changes the molecular structure of what it heats; it destroys the nutritional value of food. Multiple studies from Russia found that nearly all food cooked in microwave ovens were changed in some way, and nearly all contained carcinogenic agents after being microwaved.

- **Frying:** Rapid cooking of food in some form of oil or fat, at very high temperatures. Frying can be done in a hot skillet or in a deep fryer by submerging the food completely in oil. Previously, most studies linked fried foods to heart disease, diabetes, and many other illnesses. However, more recent studies from Spain have shown that the actual frying process may not be the culprit, as much as the type of oil and the frying method. Don't fry food in canola oil, corn oil or soybean oil. In addition to being highly inflammatory, the majority of these oils come from GMO crops. Use oils that don't break down at high temperatures such as coconut oil or macadamia nut oil, or ghee. Grape seed oil is an affordable alternative. While grape seed oil is affordable, it's not as optimal for health as the other choices. Also, minimize the frying time by cooking food with another method of cooking (such as baking), then finish off by lightly frying in a hot pan for a few seconds. Fry food in a pan instead of a deep fryer, and minimize the amount of oil. This will still give you the result you are looking for without the excess oil.

- **Caramelizing:** A method of browning carbohydrates like sugar on the surface of certain foods, usually at temperatures above 300 degrees F. When carbohydrates are broken down in the heating process they become simple sugars, like fructose. Fructose is toxic to your liver. When protein is heated together with sugar at high temperatures in a cooking process, advanced glycation end products (AGEs) form, which, as discussed earlier, cause rapid aging, damage to vital organs, and even wrinkles!

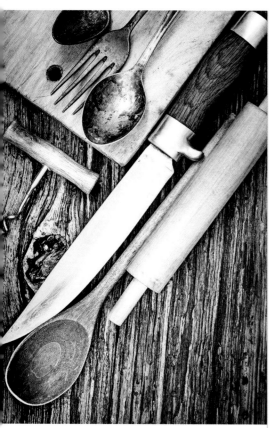

Equipment and Tools

A Brain Warrior's kitchen is a place of healing. Think of your kitchen like a "farmacy." If food is medicine, you will need proper tools to prepare it.

Having the basic kitchen utensils is critical to cooking success. Here's a list of regularly used utensils in our kitchen, and throughout the recipes in this book:

- ▶ Airtight storage containers, various sizes
- ▶ Box grater
- ▶ Citrus zester
- ▶ Colander
- ▶ Cooking spatulas—for high heat
- ▶ Cutting boards, meat safe
- ▶ Knives:
  - Boning knife for trimming fat
  - Chef's knife, 5-inch blade and 12-inch blade
  - Meat cleaver
  - Paring knife
  - Serrated knife for slicing tomatoes and bread
- ▶ Knife sharpener
- ▶ Lemon and orange juicer
- ▶ Mandoline slicer for thinly slicing vegetables and fruit
- ▶ Measuring cups and spoons, all sizes
- ▶ Meat tenderizer for pounding
- ▶ Meat thermometer
- ▶ Microplane grater
- ▶ Mixing bowls, various sizes
- ▶ Parchment paper
- ▶ Pizza cutter
- ▶ Pot holders
- ▶ Pyrex measuring cups, small and large
- ▶ Rubber spatulas
- ▶ Slotted cooking spoons
- ▶ Solid cooking spoons
- ▶ Soup ladle
- ▶ Strainer for vegetables and pasta
- ▶ Tongs, various sizes
- ▶ Vegetable peeler
- ▶ Whisks, various sizes
- ▶ Wooden spoons
- ▶ Zoodle Slicer (vegetable pasta maker)

- Food processor
- Handheld electric mixer
- High-powered blender
- Immersion blender
- KitchenAid stand mixer is helpful
- Toaster or toaster oven

Pots and pans are best with sturdy bottoms. Nonstick pans can be convenient, but avoid Teflon. Ceramic is best as a nonstick option. Over time, try to collect the following:

- Baking dishes, 8 x 8, 9 x 11, 9 x 13 inches, and 8-inch round
- Baking sheets, multiple sizes
- Muffin tins, regular and mini
- Pots for sauces and soups, several sizes
- Roasting pan, 14 x 10 inches
- Skillets, multiple sizes
- Soufflé dishes
- Stockpot (large pot for making soups)
- Stove-top grill

ADDITIONAL SUPPLIES:

- Candy papers
- Kebab skewers
- Muffin papers
- Parchment paper
- Self-sealing bags
- Tinfoil
- Wooden ice pop sticks

A Note About Nutritional Information and Recipes

Optional ingredients are not counted in the nutritional information listed at the bottom of each recipe. All ingredients marked "optional" or "add to taste" are excluded for lack of objective information.

Any recipe including salt in the ingredient list may be altered for low-sodium diets. Simply reduce the amount of salt according to your nutritional and health needs or eliminate altogether. Salt or salt substitute may be added as desired after the meal preparation is complete.

"Watering your brain is the quickest way to perk up your energy and strength."

WATER YOUR BRAIN
EACH MORNING!

Being hydrated increases your physical power by 19 percent. Being dehydrated by only 2 percent has a dramatically negative impact on cognitive function. A cup of warm lemon water infused with ginger is a stimulating, detoxifying way to wake up. Not only will you be more focused; you'll be stronger in the gym and you'll have greater aerobic capacity. What happens when you drink the juice of one lemon and ½ teaspoon of grated fresh ginger added to 16 ounces of warm water each morning?

1. The powerful flavonoids and antioxidants along with hydration are the best gift you can give your brain in the morning.
2. Citric acid in lemon helps aid digestion.
3. Increases vitamin C intake, which is good for your skin and immunity.
4. Flavonoids in lemon help balance pH to aid in detoxification.
5. Lemon and ginger have powerful anti-inflammatory properties.
6. Lemon and ginger contain powerful antioxidants to help fight free radicals.
7. The pectin fiber in lemons aids in craving control.
8. Ginger is soothing to the intestinal tract and may reduce symptoms of upset stomach, nausea and heartburn.
9. Ginger is neuroprotective, which means that it helps to prevent or slow the aging process of brain cells.
10. Ginger has been used as a natural pain reliever for centuries due to its anti-inflammatory properties.

Follow with a hydrating, power-packed smoothie containing another 16 ounces of water. By the time you hit the gym, boardroom, or classroom, you'll be hydrated, nourished, and brainpowered up!

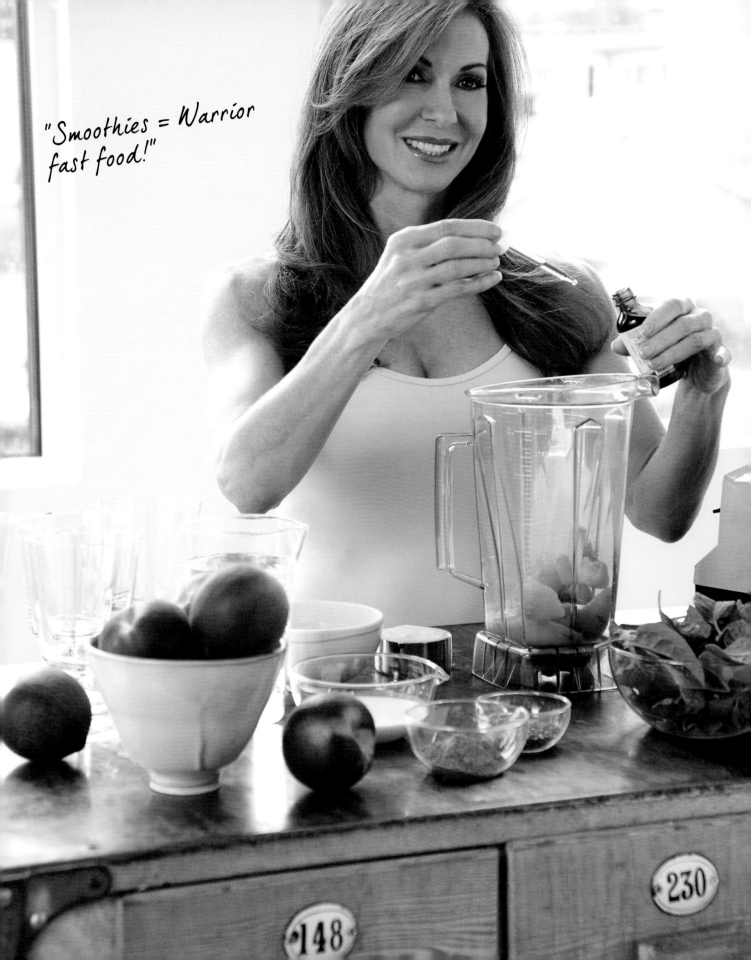

"Smoothies = Warrior fast food!"

Smoothies and Breakfast Drinks

■

The warrior has only one true friend. Only one man he can rely on. Himself. So he feeds his body well; he trains it; works on it. Where he lacks knowledge he studies. But above all he must believe. He must believe in his strength of will, of purpose, of heart and soul.

—DAVID GEMMELL, *QUEST FOR LOST HEROES*

Smoothies are a Brain Warrior's "fast food." They are quick, easy, nourishing, and hydrating. Your brain is 80 percent water, and hydrating first thing in the morning is one of the best things you can do for your brain. But I'm not talking about commercial sugar bombs loaded with fruit juice. These smoothies are very loaded with micronutrients, healthy fat, and protein to increase your focus and energy, to jump-start your brain. It's the perfect send-off for a victorious day!

Brain Warrior
Smoothie Strategies

1. Never add more than ½ to ¾ cup fruit per serving.

2. Add at least 16 to 20 ounces water to boost hydration.

3. Add a small amount of healthy fat such as coconut butter or nut butter.

4. Use sugar-free, plant-based protein powder.

5. Boost your antioxidant level by adding at least one cup of green leafy veggies.

6. Increase fiber and omega-3 fatty acids with flaxseed, hemp, or chia seeds.

Note: The carb load in most smoothies is not as high as it may seem because the fiber content is so high. Fiber is a nondigestible carbohydrate that is essential for bowel health. To determine the net carb load, subtract the fiber from the total carbs. Also, even though the fruit content in these recipes is kept to a minimum, notice that natural sugar adds up quickly with fruit and vegetables. That's why I'd like you to avoid commercial smoothies that contain excessive fruit.

■

Detoxifying Green Juice

People often ask us if fresh juice is healthy. There is one test: look to see if it's green, and make sure it doesn't contain fruit juice. Eating fruit is healthy; juicing fruit is pure sugar.

PREPARATION:

1. Place a large bowl or jar under the spout of the juicer.

2. Process all produce through a juicer and catch in the jar or bowl.

3. Drink fresh or freeze for future desserts.

> **NOTE:** It's very difficult to calculate exact nutritional information for fresh juice. Information is based on the quality of the produce, variances in juicers, amount of pulp and fiber left in juice, how much juice is extracted from produce, etc. The nutritional information below is an estimation based on 8-ounce serving sizes.

SERVES 2

INGREDIENTS:
5 cups spinach

4 cups torn chard leaves or kale, thick stems removed

1 large cucumber (about 3 cups, sliced into rounds)

4 celery stalks (about 4 cups, roughly chopped)

2 cups cilantro

OPTIONAL INGREDIENTS:
1 ounce fresh ginger (for peppery taste)

4 tablespoons fresh squeezed lemon juice

NUTRITIONAL INFORMATION
PER SERVING: 80.0 calories, 6.1g protein, 13.0g carbohydrates, 4.2g fiber, 7.0g sugar, 0.0g fat, 0.0g saturated fat, 0.0mg cholesterol, 105.0mg sodium

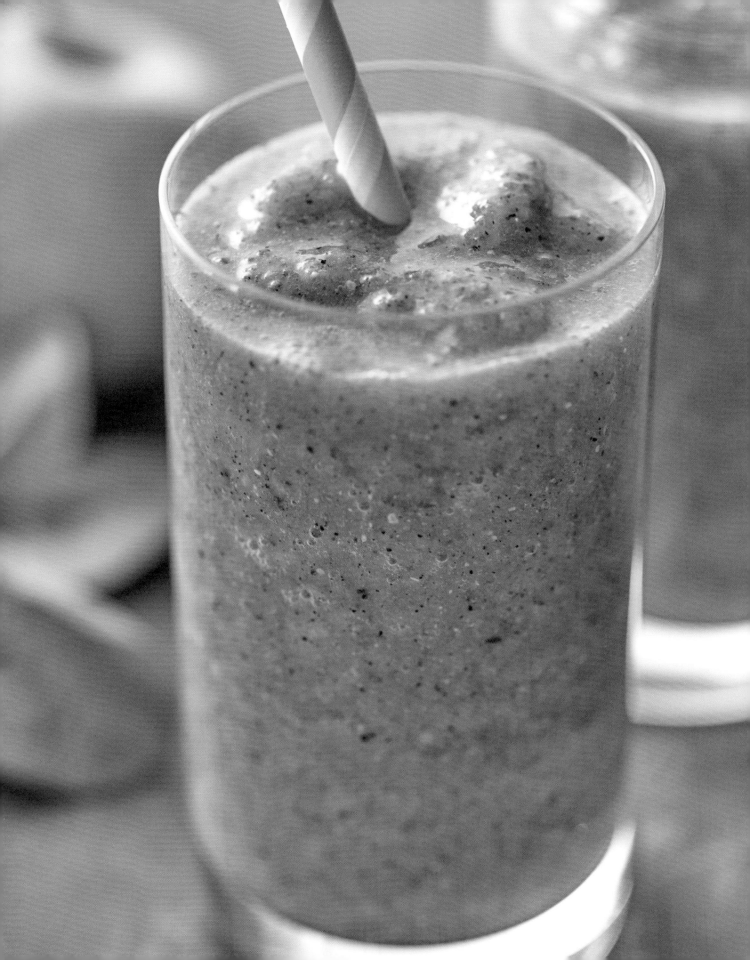

Super-Focus Smoothie

It's a good idea to keep some green tea brewed and refrigerated if you like iced tea or green tea smoothies like this one. It's easy to make, good for you, and a delicious brain-focusing beverage to replace coffee. And the cayenne pepper in this recipe really revs up the metabolism!

PREPARATION:

Blend all ingredients in a high-powered blender until smooth. Divide evenly between two glasses. Serve cold.

> **NOTE:** Chia seeds or hemp seeds can be substituted for flaxseed meal if you prefer them or if they are more readily available.

SERVES 2

INGREDIENTS:
24 ounces iced green tea

1 large green apple, cored and quartered

2 scoops vanilla protein powder (plant based, sugar free)

2 cups spinach

1 teaspoon cinnamon

½ teaspoon nutmeg

2 tablespoons flaxseed meal

1 cup ice, approximately

OPTIONAL INGREDIENTS:
¼ teaspoon cayenne pepper

5 to 10 drops liquid stevia, vanilla flavored

1 teaspoon freeze-dried greens (or use scoop included with greens)

superfoods: 1 tablespoon acai or goji powder

NUTRITIONAL INFORMATION PER SERVING: 226 calories, 25.3g protein, 16.2g carbohydrates, 9.1g fiber, 7.4g sugar, 11.5g fat, 1.0g saturated fat, 0.0mg cholesterol, 208.4mg sodium

Cherry Mint Blast

I like my delicious Cherry Mint Blast smoothie extra minty, with the chocolate protein powder.

INGREDIENTS:

1 cup frozen cherries

1 to 2 tablespoons fresh mint, according to taste

2 cups spinach or kale, thick stems removed

2 tablespoons hemp seeds

2 scoops chocolate or vanilla protein powder (plant based, sugar free)

3 cups cold water, or to taste

OPTIONAL INGREDIENTS:

5 to 10 drops liquid stevia, chocolate, vanilla or berry flavored

1 teaspoon freeze-dried greens (or use scoop included with greens)

2 tablespoons coconut butter

superfood: 1 tablespoon pomegranate powder

PREPARATION:

Blend all ingredients in a high-powered blender until smooth. Divide evenly between two glasses. Serve cold.

> **NOTE:** Chia seeds or flaxseed meal can be substituted for hemp seeds if you prefer them or if they are more readily available.

NUTRITIONAL INFORMATION PER SERVING: 231.0 calories, 25.7g protein, 21.1g carbohydrates, 4.2g fiber, 7.2g sugar, 7.0g fat, 0.3g saturated fat, 0.0mg cholesterol, 23.7mg sodium

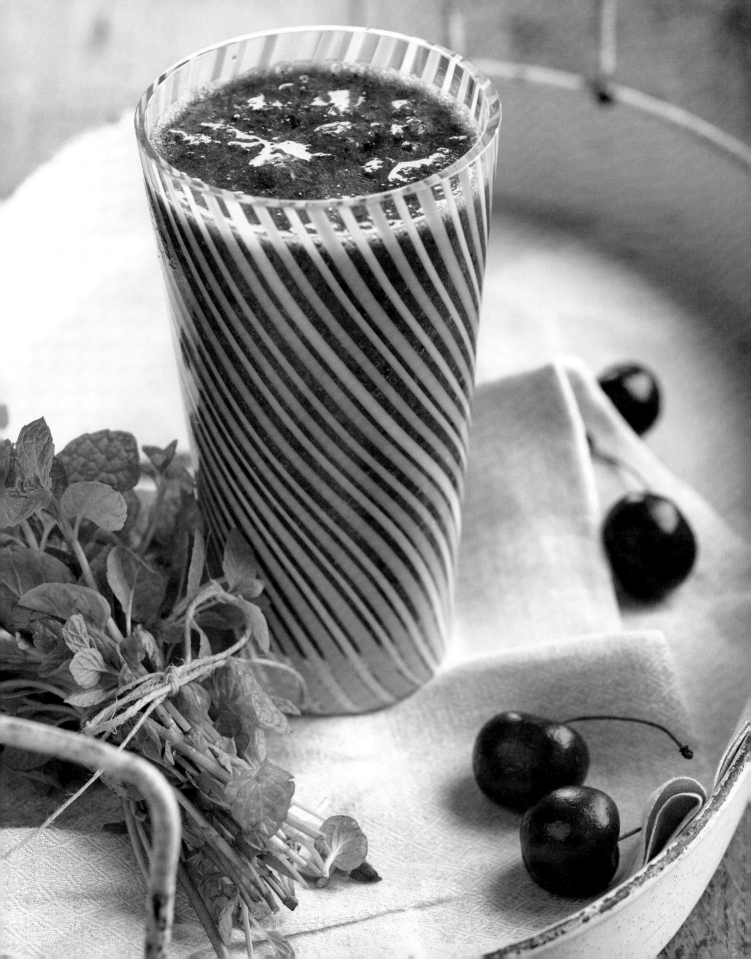

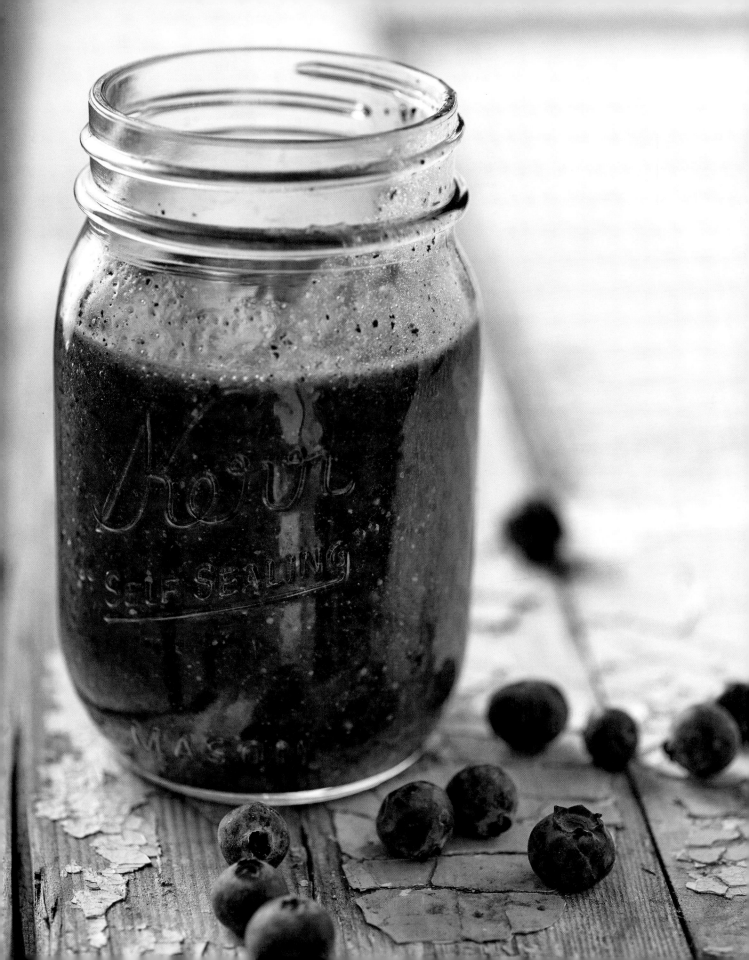

Coconut Berry Cooler

PREPARATION:

Blend all ingredients in a high-powered blender until smooth. Divide evenly between two glasses. Serve cold.

> **NOTE:** Chia seeds or hemp seeds can be substituted for flaxseed meal if you prefer them or if they are more readily available.

SERVES 2

INGREDIENTS:

1 cup frozen blueberries or blackberries

2 cups spinach or kale with thick stems removed

2 scoops chocolate or vanilla protein powder (plant based, sugar free)

2 tablespoons coconut butter

2 tablespoons flaxseed meal

24 to 30 ounces cold water

OPTIONAL INGREDIENTS:

1 cup ice, approximately

5 to 10 drops liquid stevia, chocolate, vanilla, or berry flavored

1 teaspoon freeze-dried greens (or use scoop included with greens)

superfoods: 1 tablespoon acai or goji powder

NUTRITIONAL INFORMATION PER SERVING: 305.5 calories, 25.7g protein, 25.4g carbohydrates, 12.0g fiber, 7.6g sugar, 15.6g fat, 8.4g saturated fat, 0.0mg cholesterol, 42.1mg sodium

Peachy Keen Chia Chiller

SERVES 2

INGREDIENTS:

1 fresh pitted peach or 1 cup frozen peach slices

2 tablespoons chia seeds

½ cup light coconut milk

2 cups spinach or chard leaves

2 scoops vanilla protein powder (plant based, sugar free)

1 cup ice, approximately

24 to 30 ounces cold water (or replace half with unsweetened almond milk)

OPTIONAL INGREDIENTS:

½ cup plain coconut milk yogurt or goat milk yogurt

5–10 drops liquid stevia, vanilla flavored

1 teaspoon freeze-dried greens (or use scoop included with greens)

superfoods: 1 tablespoon maca powder

PREPARATION:

Blend all ingredients in a high-powered blender until smooth. Divide evenly between two glasses. Serve cold.

> **NOTE:** Hemp seeds or flaxseed meal can be substituted for chia seeds if you prefer them or if they are more readily available.

NUTRITIONAL INFORMATION PER SERVING: 223.0 calories, 23.7g protein, 18.0g carbohydrates, 7.6g fiber, 5.7g sugar, 8.5g fat, 3.5g saturated fat, 0.0mg cholesterol, 23.7mg sodium

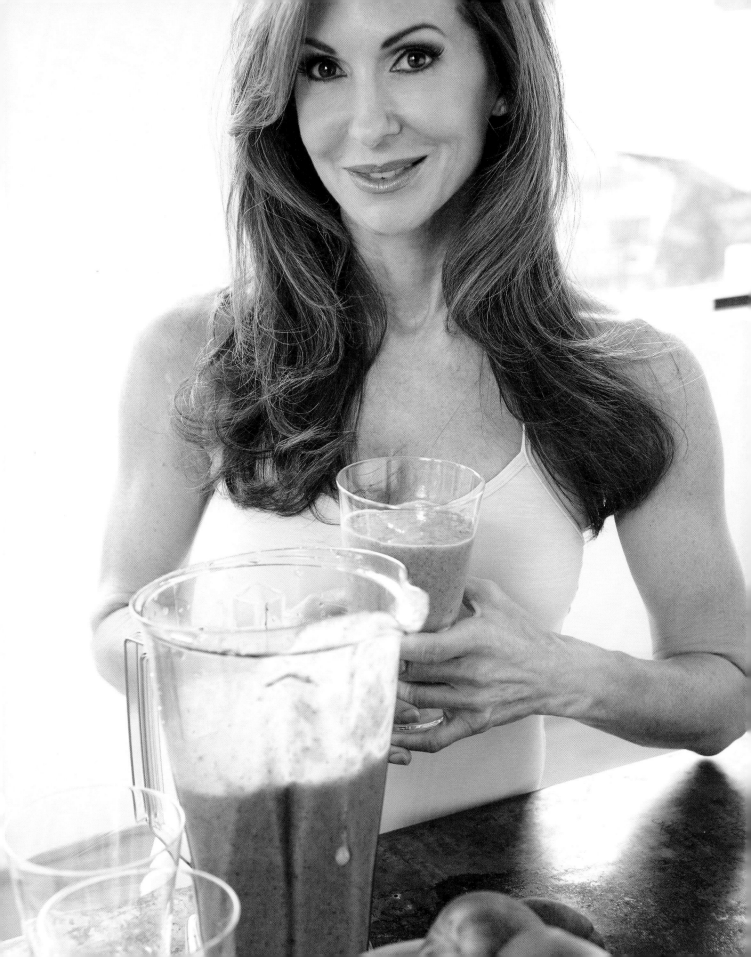

Tropical Hurricane Shake-Up

INGREDIENTS:

1 cup frozen pineapple

2 cups kale, thick stems removed

1 teaspoon spirulina

2 scoops vanilla protein powder (plant based, sugar free)

2 tablespoons flaxseed meal

1 cup ice, approximately

24 to 30 ounces cold water or half plain water, half coconut water

OPTIONAL INGREDIENTS:

5 to 10 drops liquid stevia, chocolate, vanilla, or berry flavored

1 teaspoon freeze-dried greens (or use scoop included with greens)

2 tablespoons coconut butter

Superfoods: 1 tablespoon lucuma powder

PREPARATION:

Blend all ingredients in a high-powered blender until smooth. Divide evenly between two glasses. Serve cold.

> **NOTE:** Chia seeds or hemp seeds can be substituted for flaxseed meal if you prefer them or if they are more readily available.

> **NOTE:** Lucuma powder comes from the lucuma fruit and is considered a superfood because it packs a nutrient-dense punch. Lucuma contains beta-carotene, iron, zinc, vitamin B_3, calcium and protein. It also has a wonderful maplelike flavor and is lower glycemic than most sweeteners.

NUTRITIONAL INFORMATION PER SERVING: 228.0 calories, 26.g protein, 27.1g carbohydrates, 9.6g fiber, 2.1g sugar, 7.3g fat, 0.5g saturated fat, 0.0mg cholesterol, 36.2mg sodium

Daybreak Green Tea Latte

This is another of Daniel's favorite drinks when he has a craving for something sweet and warm. It is totally satisfying and filling without the fat, sugar, and calories of a traditional chai tea latte . . . and with all the benefits of green tea at the same time.

PREPARATION:

1. Heat almond milk in medium saucepan over medium heat until milk begins to boil. Turn off heat immediately or milk will boil over.

2. Pour milk into a teapot to keep warm while steeping, or divide evenly between two cups.

3. Add a tea bag to each cup and let steep for five minutes.

4. Add 5 drops stevia to each cup (or to taste). Serve hot.

SERVES 2

INGREDIENTS:

20 to 24 ounces plain almond milk (unsweetened)

2 green chai tea bags

5–10 drops liquid stevia, vanilla or cinnamon flavored

NUTRITIONAL INFORMATION PER SERVING: 60.0 calories, 2.0g protein, 3.0g carbohydrates, 2.0g fiber, 0.0g sugar, 5.0g fat, 0.0g saturated fat, 0.0mg cholesterol, 270.0mg sodium

"Some days you just want to wake up and enjoy the morning without starting with a heavy meal. These simple, satisfying breakfast drinks will stimulate your brain, while soothing your senses. Daniel and I love sipping them on cozy weekend mornings while focusing on all we are grateful for."

Wake-Up Call Cappuccino

Here's to guilt-free morning comfort! By brewing half-caffeinated coffee and mixing it with almond milk, it becomes "quarter caf." You get the morning comfort and boost without the unnecessary caffeine. By adding coconut oil and ghee, it becomes a meal replacement: coconut oil has medium-chain triglycerides that are great for your brain, and ghee has short-chain fatty acids that are gut healing.

PREPARATION:

1. Using a coffeemaker of your choice, brew a pot of half-caffeinated coffee, using equal parts caffeinated and decaffeinated coffee. If you prefer, you may use only decaffeinated coffee.

2. While coffee is brewing, heat 2 cups almond milk on stove top or in microwave. If heating on stove top, watch closely; almond milk boils over quickly. If heating in the microwave, place in microwave-safe cup and heat for 2½ to 3 minutes.

3. Pour 2 cups coffee, the warm almond milk, and stevia, coconut oil, and ghee, if desired, in a blender. Blend for 10 to 15 seconds, until froth begins to form. Divide between two large mugs and dust each mug with cinnamon as desired.

SERVES 2

INGREDIENTS:
organic caffeinated coffee

organic decaffeinated coffee

2 cups plain almond milk (unsweetened)

OPTIONAL INGREDIENTS:
liquid stevia to taste: chocolate, hazelnut, or English toffee

1 to 2 teaspoons coconut oil

1 to 2 teaspoons ghee

cinnamon

NUTRITIONAL INFORMATION
PER SERVING: 40.0 calories, 1.0g protein, 2.0g carbohydrates, 1.0g fiber, 0.5g sugar, 3.0g fat, 0.0g saturated fat, 0.0mg cholesterol, 180.0mg sodium

Pumpkin Spice-Up Cappuccino

SERVES 2

INGREDIENTS:

organic caffeinated coffee

organic decaffeinated coffee

2 cups plain almond milk, unsweetened

pumpkin spice–flavored liquid stevia to taste

1 teaspoon pumpkin pie spice

1 tablespoon coconut oil

OPTIONAL INGREDIENTS:

1 to 2 teaspoons ghee

cinnamon

This is Daniel's favorite way to start the morning. Adding coconut oil and ghee provides short- and medium-chain fatty acids to support gut health. It also makes the cappuccino creamy and creates some amazing foam. However, if you're calorie conscious, simply eliminate the oils and you'll reduce the calories by more than half.

PREPARATION:

1. Using a coffeemaker of your choice, brew a pot of half-caffeinated coffee, using equal parts caffeinated and decaffeinated coffee. If you prefer, you may use only decaffeinated coffee.

2. While coffee is brewing, heat 2 cups almond milk on stove top or in microwave. If heating on stove top, watch closely; almond milk boils over quickly. If heating in the microwave, place in microwave-safe cup and heat for 2½ to 3 minutes.

3. Pour 2 cups coffee, warm milk, and all other ingredients into a blender and cover. Blend for 10 to 15 seconds, until froth begins to form. Divide between two large mugs and dust each mug with cinnamon as desired.

NUTRITIONAL INFORMATION PER SERVING: 81.1 calories, 0.8g protein, 1.5g carbohydrates, 0.8g fiber, 0.0g sugar, 8.7g fat, 5.9g saturated fat, 0.0mg cholesterol, 135.0mg sodium

Focus and Energy Mochaccino

Warriors need high-powered fuel for a high-powered life! This Focus and Energy Mochaccino is one of my favorite morning comfort drinks because it serves a dual purpose. Besides being delicious and nutritious, it can quickly become a meal on the run by adding a scoop of protein powder and a tablespoon of coconut oil. Mornings in our house are extraordinarily busy, and there are days that these two-in-one recipes come in handy. By brewing "half-caf" coffee and adding a cup of almond milk, you've created a nice comfort drink with less than the caffeine of a small cup of coffee. It also tastes just as great made with decaffeinated coffee.

PREPARATION:

1. Using a coffeemaker of your choice, brew a pot of half-caffeinated coffee, using equal parts caffeinated and decaffeinated coffee. If you prefer, you may use only decaffeinated coffee.

2. While coffee is brewing, heat 2 cups almond milk on stove top or in microwave. If heating on stove top, watch closely; almond milk boils over quickly. If heating in the microwave, place in microwave-safe cup and heat for 2½ to 3 minutes. When milk is warm, pour about 12 ounces of coffee and milk into blender.

3. Add stevia and cacao.

4. If desired, add protein powder and coconut oil.

5. Blend for about 15 seconds. Start on low and increase speed to medium high. Blending creates a nice froth. If you prefer not to have a frothy drink, blend on low setting for about 5 seconds, until ingredients are thoroughly mixed.

6. Divide between two mugs and dust each mug with cinnamon as desired.

> **NOTE:** Try the equally amazing vanilla version of this drink by simply swapping the stevia and the protein powder with vanilla-flavored versions and omitting the cacao powder.

SERVES 2

INGREDIENTS:
organic caffeinated coffee

organic decaffeinated coffee

2 cups almond milk, unsweetened

5–10 drops chocolate-flavored liquid stevia, or to taste

1 tablespoon raw cocoa, increase as desired

OPTIONAL INGREDIENTS:
2 servings chocolate protein powder (plant based, sugar free)

1 tablespoon coconut oil

cinnamon

NUTRITIONAL INFORMATION PER SERVING FOR MOCHA: 40.0 calories, 1.0g protein, 3.0g carbohydrates, 3.0g fiber, 0.0g sugar, 1.5g fat, 0.0g saturated fat, 0.0mg cholesterol, 180.0mg sodium

NUTRITIONAL INFORMATION PER SERVING FOR 1 SCOOP PROTEIN POWDER AND COCONUT OIL: 162.0 calories, 19.5g protein, 8.5g carbohydrates, 4.5g fiber, 0.0g sugar, 5.5g fat, 6.0g saturated fat, 0.0mg cholesterol, 0.0mg sodium

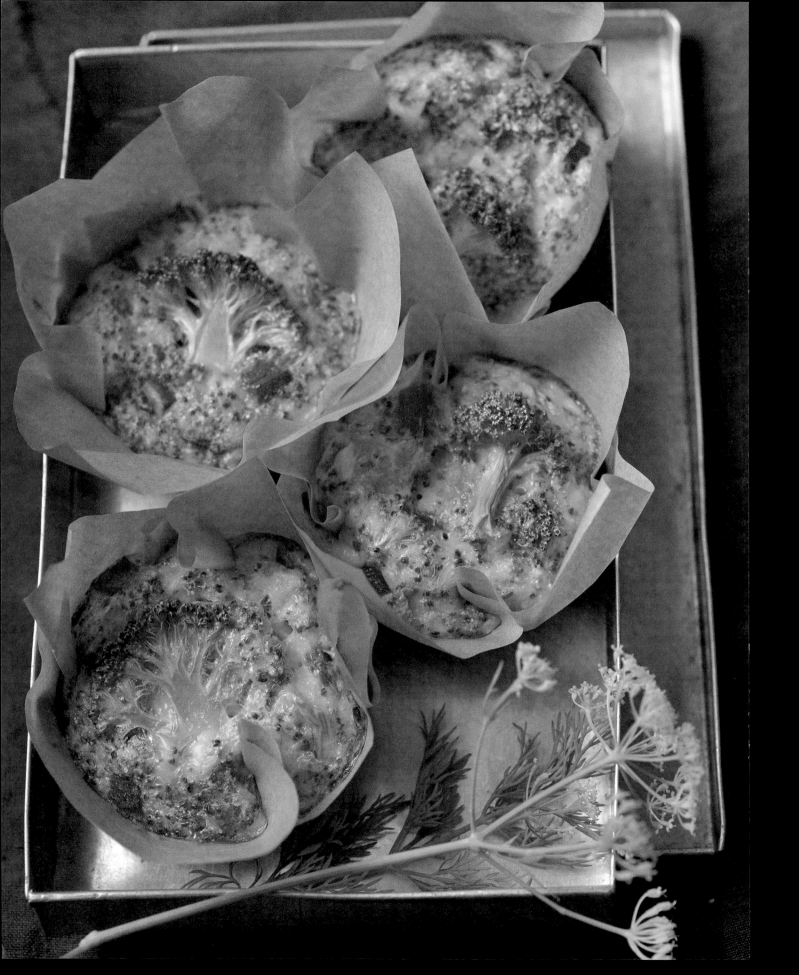

Breakfast

■

Success is nothing more than a few simple disciplines
practiced every day!

—JIM ROHN

Food fuels success or failure, and it starts with breakfast. What you eat first thing in the morning will determine how you feel all day. Starting your day with simple carbohydrates will quickly elevate blood sugar and insulin, trigger inflammation, create brain fog, and lead to cravings that you will fight for the rest of the day.

Having a thoughtful breakfast of protein, healthy fat, and *smart* carbohydrates will increase focus and energy. Also, it balances the hormones of metabolism that send the signal to your brain that you're full and satisfied. You'll be less likely to crave unhealthy snacks when you eat a Brain Warrior breakfast. Eat simple carbs and you will crave simple carbs and sugar. Don't eat them, don't crave them. It's that simple.

Adjust your nutrition based on your demands. For example, if you're an athlete, you need more high-quality fuel, especially carbs. But if you're a keyboard warrior, focus more on protein for brain focus. Carbs will slow you down and make you thick around the middle.

Purchasing the highest-quality ingredients that are practical for your budget is important for your brain and body. For example, organic DHA-enriched eggs from pasture-raised chickens are higher in omega-3 fatty acids and don't contain hormones and antibiotics that may be harmful. Also, berries and apples are best purchased organic when possible because they hold more pesticides than any other fruit. But if you are on a tight budget, buying nonorganic bananas and oranges might not be the end of the world because of the thick skin.

Brain Warrior Breakfast Strategies

If you're like most of the people we work with, time is the greatest obstacle to getting a great breakfast in the morning. These simple strategies are how we manage to keep our hectic mornings healthy. Most of the people we coach have told us that this helps them stay away from the donut shop on the way to work.

1. Make a list of five super-simple breakfast recipes you love, and keep it where you can see it. Be sure to automatically add the ingredients to your weekly shopping list so they're always on hand. Our favorites are One-Minute Avocado Egg Basket, Cherry Mint Blast smoothie, Brainberry Muffins, Omega Egg Burrito to Go, and Focus and Energy Mochaccino.

2. Get prepared for the week. For example, measure smoothie ingredients into wet and dry containers. Dry ingredients go in the cabinet, and wet ingredients (fruit, greens, and stevia) go in the freezer. Then just put everything in a blender and add water and nut butter.

3. Bake a dozen muffins and freeze half. The rest will keep in the refrigerator for a week. Just heat and go.

4. Organize cabinets for quickest accessibility. For example, have everything you need for smoothies in one cabinet, in the same place you store the blender.

5. Keep coconut wraps handy for turning a quick morning scramble into a breakfast burrito on the run.

■

Island-Style Egg Burrito

This recipe is a great way to get picky little eaters interested in something other than donuts and waffles. The coconut adds a sweet taste to the eggs, giving them a fun twist.

PREPARATION:

1. Whisk eggs in a bowl.

2. Add shredded coconut, coconut cream and salt if desired and whisk together until well blended.

3. Scramble egg mixture in a medium nonstick pan over medium heat until fluffy, mixing and turning continuously until thoroughly cooked.

4. Remove from heat and set aside until just warm.

5. Divide evenly between two coconut or lettuce wraps. Top each with bananas or drizzle each with about ½ teaspoon maple syrup if desired.

6. Roll wrap like a burrito and roll in parchment paper.

7. Serve warm.

NOTE: Refrigerate a can of coconut milk and skim the thicker cream off the top to get the coconut cream for this recipe.

SERVES 2

INGREDIENTS:
4 large eggs
¼ cup shredded coconut, unsweetened
2 tablespoons coconut cream
sea salt to taste
2 coconut wraps or lettuce wraps

OPTIONAL INGREDIENTS:
1 teaspoon maple syrup
½ banana, sliced

NUTRITIONAL INFORMATION PER SERVING WITH COCONUT WRAP:
305.5 calories, 14.0g protein, 7.1g carbohydrates, 2.1g fiber, 1.4g sugar, 20.9g fat, 10.3g saturated fat, 372.0mg cholesterol, 405.5mg sodium

Tanana Pancakes

SERVES 2
(8 TO 10 SMALL PANCAKES)

INGREDIENTS:

½ cup fresh strawberries, stems removed

3 eggs

1 banana

1 teaspoon almond butter

½ teaspoon baking powder

1 teaspoon arrowroot

OPTIONAL INGREDIENTS:

1 teaspoon coconut oil

2 tablespoons flaxseed meal

Our grandson Liam calls me "Tanana," which just melts me. Liam loves these delicious pancakes, so they are dedicated to him.

We recommend skipping the maple syrup for this recipe. The banana and strawberry make it sweet enough.

PREPARATION:

1. In advance, blend strawberries in a high-powered blender until mixture is a saucelike consistency. Place sauce in a small serving bowl and set aside.

2. Place all other ingredients in a blender and blend on medium speed for 30 seconds or until mixture is thoroughly blended. Instead of using a blender, you may place ingredients in a bowl and use an immersion blender.

3. Heat a ceramic nonstick pan or griddle or spray with a light coat of coconut oil cooking spray.

4. Ladle small circles of batter onto the heated pan, about 3 inches in diameter (about the size of an average can top). If you make them too large, they will burn and be difficult to turn. Watch closely, as they cook quickly—usually about 30 to 45 seconds per side.

5. Plate pancakes, and spoon a small amount of strawberry sauce over the top.

NOTE: Swap strawberries with your favorite berry or seasonal fruit.

NUTRITIONAL INFORMATION PER SERVING: 185.2 calories, 11.0g protein, 15.4g carbohydrates, 3.4g fiber, 7.7g sugar, 9.6g fat, 2.6g saturated fat, 279.0mg cholesterol, 229.7mg sodium

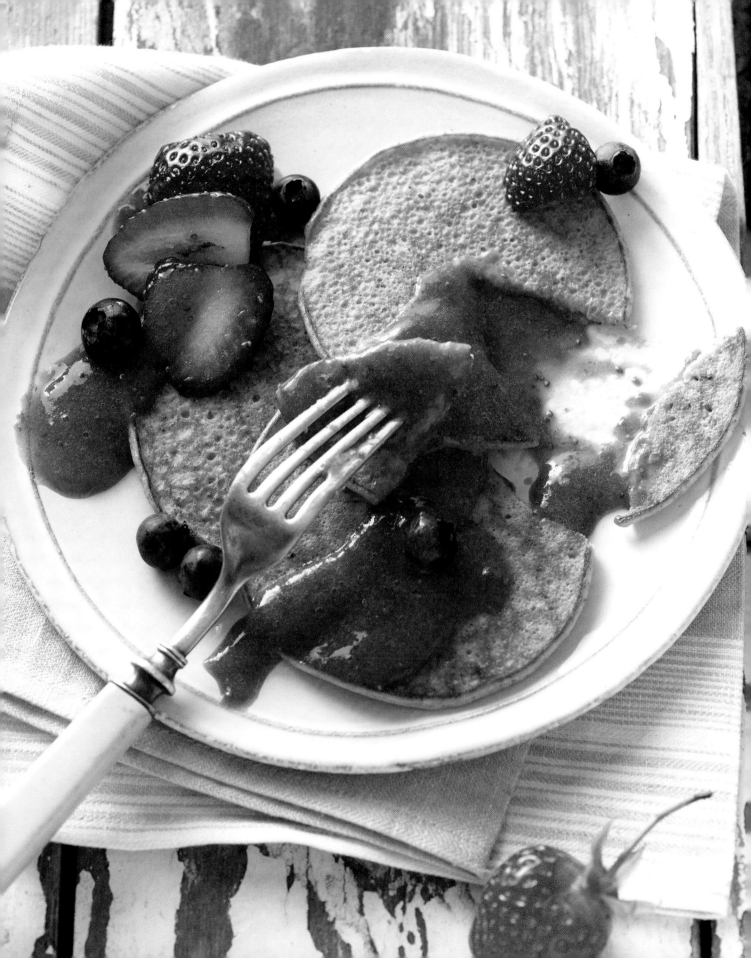

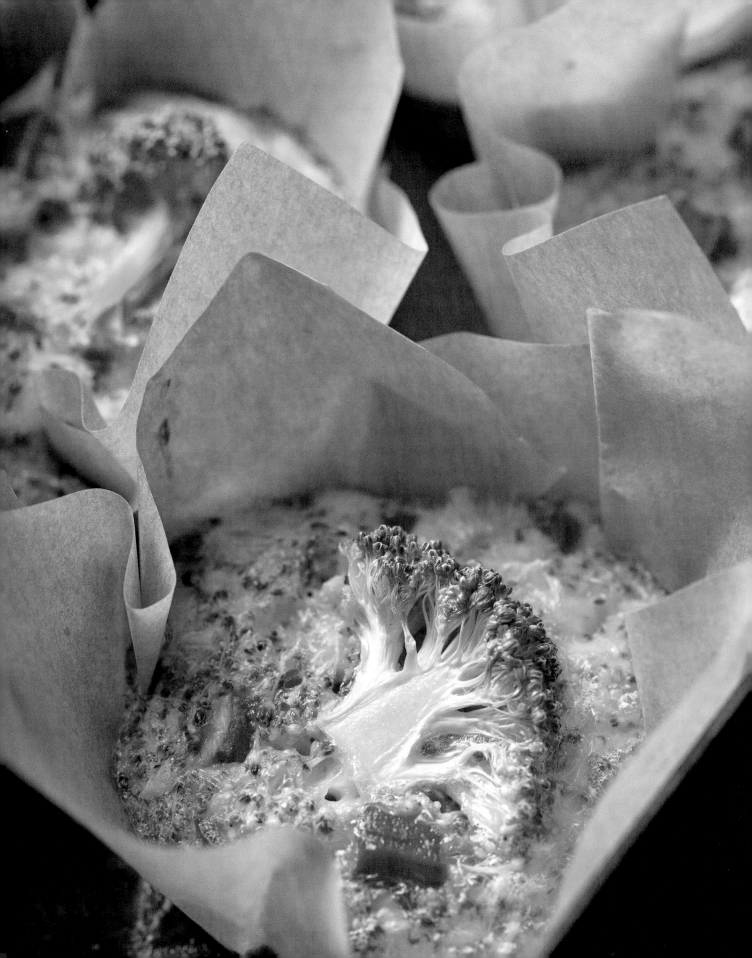

Muffin Tin Egg Frittatas

PREPARATION:

1. Heat oven to 350 degrees F, and coat a twelve-muffin tin with coconut oil cooking spray. Silicone muffin pans also work really well in this recipe and need no cooking spray.

2. Whisk together the eggs, salt, and pepper.

3. Stir in the broccoli slaw, bell pepper, and walnuts.

4. Divide mixture evenly in the prepared muffin tin.

5. Bake for 20 minutes or until eggs are set.

NOTE: This recipe can be halved and cooked in the microwave in a pinch. Use individual microwave-safe soufflé bowls or small microwave-safe cups. Microwave for about 1 minute each or until the egg is set.

NOTE: Using muffin papers as shown is an option for making these simple frittatas look elegant while ensuring they don't stick to the pan.

SERVES 6

INGREDIENTS:
coconut oil nonstick cooking spray

8 eggs

½ teaspoon salt

pinch of pepper

2 cups broccoli slaw (shredded broccoli, usually sold preshredded)

½ cup chopped red bell pepper

½ cup walnuts, finely chopped

NUTRITIONAL INFORMATION PER SERVING: 92.3 calories, 5.9g protein, 3.3g carbohydrates, 1.7g fiber, 1.7g sugar, 6.5g fat, 1.4g saturated fat, 124.0mg cholesterol, 155.5mg sodium

Brainberry Muffins

INGREDIENTS:

⅔ cup coconut flour

½ teaspoon salt

1 teaspoon baking powder

¼ teaspoon cinnamon

8 eggs

1 teaspoon pure vanilla extract

3 tablespoons maple syrup

½ cup erythritol

½ cup coconut milk

½ cup coconut butter, softened

1 cup blueberries

OPTIONAL CRUMBLE TOPPING:

¼ cup almond meal

½ cup slivered almonds

1 tablespoon maple syrup

1 tablespoon erythritol

2 tablespoons coconut butter, softened

We used to play a game with Chloe when she was a toddler to teach her which foods were good for her brain and which were bad for her brain. By the time she was three she called blueberries "brain berries—God's candy." She would also ask if they were organic because nonorganic blueberries hold more pesticides than any other fruit, which is really bad for the brain!

PREPARATION:

1. Heat oven to 350 degrees F. Prepare a twelve-muffin tin pan, lining each muffin cup with muffin papers, or spray with coconut oil nonstick cooking spray.

2. In a large bowl whisk together coconut flour, salt, baking powder, and cinnamon. Create a well in the center of the dry ingredients and add the eggs, vanilla extract, maple syrup, erythritol, coconut milk, and coconut butter.

3. Whisk together the liquid ingredients in the center and then whisk in the dry ingredients. Keep whisking for 1 to 2 minutes or use a handheld electric mixer.

4. Fold in the blueberries and let the mixture sit for 5 minutes. The batter will thicken as the coconut flour absorbs the liquid.

5. Combine all ingredients for the topping, if desired, and set aside.

6. Using a spoon, evenly distribute muffin batter between twelve muffin cups in the tin. Then sprinkle the topping evenly on each of the muffins.

7. Bake for 35 minutes and serve warm.

> NOTE: Swap blueberries for cranberries for a delicious holiday treat!

> NOTE: Baking often requires a small amount of either maple syrup or raw honey for consistency. Replacing it completely with stevia or erythritol is possible, but won't usually yield the same moisture content and flavor. That's why I've learned to combine ingredients. While each tablespoon of maple syrup yields about 1.1 gram of sugar per muffin in this recipe, compare that to the average blueberry muffin, which contains a whopping 30 grams of sugar. Most of the sugar in these muffins comes from the blueberries.

NUTRITIONAL INFORMATION PER SERVING: 168.9 calories, 5.8g protein, 23.0g carbohydrates, 12.9g fiber, 7.2g sugar, 10.0g fat, 6.9g saturated fat, 124.0mg cholesterol, 114.5mg sodium

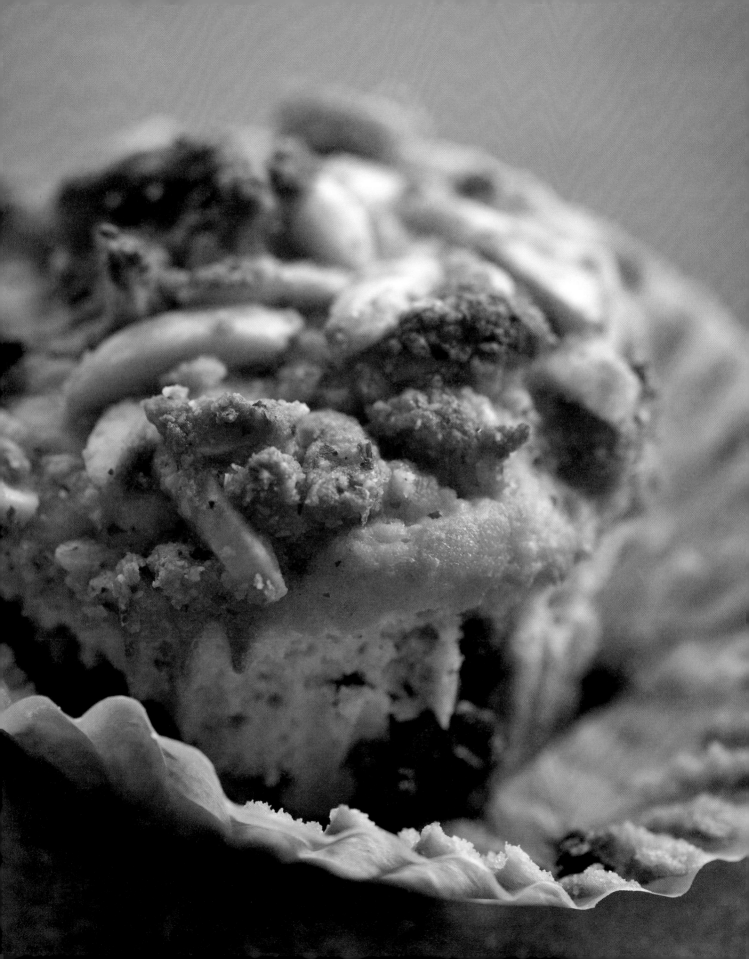

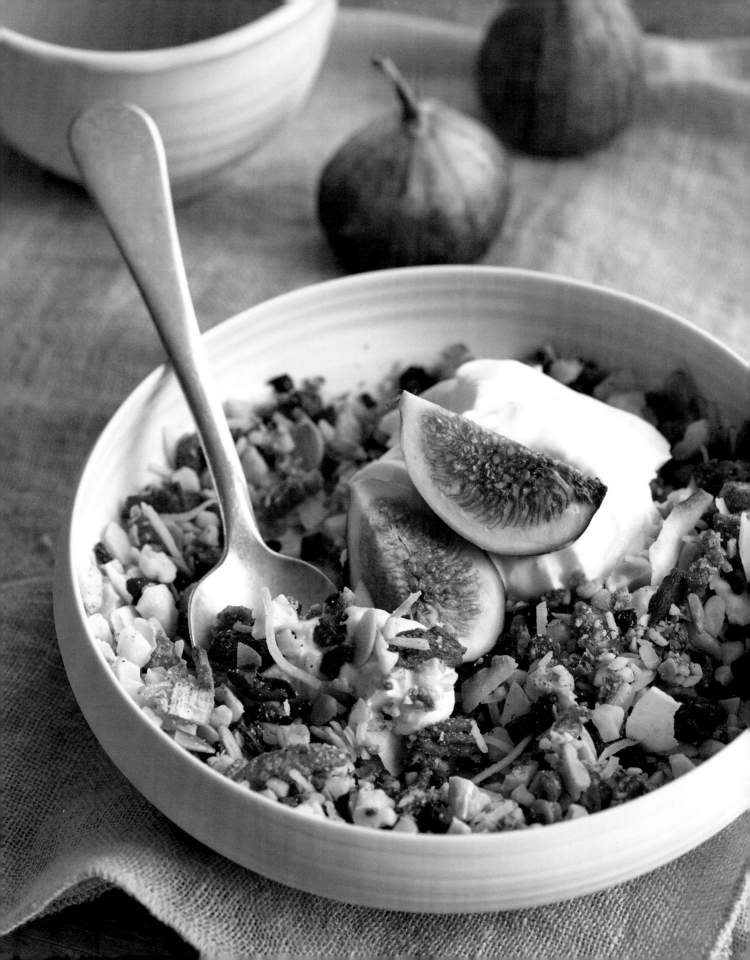

Sunrise Grainless Granola

Making granola takes an investment of time, but it's a very versatile food for breakfast, snacks and dessert. When making granola I usually double or triple the recipe and freeze leftovers. When I'm in a hurry I simply combine the raw nuts and seeds with almond milk and skip the baking process.

If you really want the most nutritional value from nuts, try soaking them prior to preparing granola. This will increase the preparation time significantly, so plan in advance. Soaking nuts and seeds initiates sprouting. In addition to making them easier to digest, sprouting improves the absorption of protein and vitamins in nuts and seeds. To soak the nuts and seeds, place them in a large bowl and add cold water to cover. Place in the refrigerator for 7–24 hours. Remove from water without rinsing in order to preserve nutritional value. Place soaked nuts and seeds in a dehydrator set at 140 degrees F for 12 hours, or place in conventional oven set at 170 degrees F for 5–6 hours. Adjust time as necessary until nuts and seeds are dry and crisp but not burnt. Once the nuts and seeds are dehydrated, continue with the preparation steps below.

PREPARATION:

1. Preheat oven to 200 degrees F and spray a large baking sheet with coconut oil nonstick cooking spray.

2. Add nuts, seeds, coconut, and goji berries or dates to a food processor and pulse a few times until coarsely chopped to the consistency of granola (be careful not to overprocess). Depending on the size of your processor, you may have to do this in two steps. Remove the mixture from processor and put in a large bowl.

3. In a small bowl, whisk egg white, water and maple syrup. Add in vanilla and spices as desired. Mix well. Slowly drizzle egg mixture over nut and seed blend. Blend well with clean hands, covering granola mixture with a light coat of the liquid.

4. Spread mixture evenly over a large baking sheet and bake for 45–60 minutes or until mixture is dry and forms small clusters. Remove from heat and allow to cool prior to serving.

5. Place ¼ cup of the granola in each bowl. Add ½ cup almond, coconut or hemp milk into each bowl of granola.

6. Top each bowl with ¼ cup yogurt of your choice if desired.

7. Place remaining granola in an airtight container. Be sure to freeze leftover granola within several days.

SERVES 12

INGREDIENTS:
coconut oil nonstick cooking spray

½ cup shaved almonds

½ cup chopped cashews

½ cup walnut halves

½ cup pecan halves

½ cup pumpkin seeds or sunflower seeds

½ cup shredded coconut, unsweetened

¼ cup chopped goji berries *or* ¼ cup dates

1 egg white

2 teaspoons water

1 tablespoon maple syrup

OPTIONAL INGREDIENTS:

½ teaspoon pure vanilla extract

1 teaspoon cinnamon or nutmeg

½ teaspoon salt

¼ cup almond, coconut *or* hemp milk per serving

¼ cup plain coconut milk yogurt *or* goat milk yogurt per serving

NUTRITIONAL INFORMATION PER SERVING: 199.0 calories, 4.6g protein, 10.0g carbohydrates, 3.1g fiber, 5.2g sugar, 16.9g fat, 4.3g saturated fat, 0.0mg cholesterol, 52.0mg sodium

Country-Style Biscuits

SERVES 8

INGREDIENTS:

2 cups almond flour

1 teaspoon baking powder

¼ cup coconut oil, ghee, or butter (grass-fed dairy)

¼ cup full-fat coconut milk, cream skimmed from top (reserve remaining coconut milk for future use)

2 eggs

OPTIONAL INGREDIENTS:

¼ teaspoon salt

favorite herbs: rosemary, thyme, sage, etc.

Enjoy the comforts of a homemade country breakfast without the health problems associated with heavy country-style cooking.

PREPARATION:

1. Preheat oven to 400 degrees F.

2. Line a baking sheet with parchment paper or lightly spray with coconut oil cooking spray to prevent sticking.

3. In a large bowl blend almond flour, baking powder, salt if desired, and your favorite herbs.

4. Add coconut oil, ghee, or butter and coconut milk to flour mixture. Mix all ingredients thoroughly with a handheld electric mixer, or by hand using a spoon or spatula.

5. In a separate bowl, using a handheld electric mixer, mix eggs until frothy but not stiff. You can also use your blender on lowest setting. Mix eggs for about 2 minutes.

6. Add eggs to flour mixture and gently fold in with mixing spatula or handheld electric mixer on low setting until thoroughly combined.

7. Scoop with large spoon or ice cream scooper onto baking sheet. Gently flatten top to form rounded biscuits instead of balls. Mixture should make about 8 biscuits.

8. Bake for 18 to 20 minutes or until golden brown on top.

9. Serve with Guiltless Gravy (page 244).

NUTRITIONAL INFORMATION PER SERVING: 230.0 calories, 6.6g protein, 5.9g carbohydrates, 3.1g fiber, 1.3g sugar, 21.6g fat, 8.7g saturated fat, 41.0mg cholesterol, 17.0mg sodium

Pleasing Pumpkin Pancakes

PREPARATION:

1. Combine all pancake ingredients, along with optional ingredients as desired, in a blender. Mix on low-medium speed until thoroughly blended.

2. Spray a nonstick skillet, griddle, or crepe pan with coconut oil spray, and heat to medium low. Allow griddle or pan to get hot before adding batter.

3. Add batter in small circles, about the size of sand dollars. Pour batter directly from blender. I don't waste the time pouring batter into a bowl; batter will cook very quickly. Flip pancakes after 30 to 45 seconds on each side or when pancakes start to bubble. Be sure to keep pancakes small, as they will cook more evenly and not burn.

4. Enjoy with a drizzle of maple syrup or Silky Coconut Whipped Cream (page 251).

> **NOTE:** Add 5 to 10 drops pumpkin spice–flavored stevia and a teaspoon of maple syrup to ¼ cup coconut whipped cream for a unique fall topping.

INGREDIENTS:
coconut oil nonstick cooking spray

2 eggs

¼ cup organic canned pumpkin

1 tablespoon almond butter

½ to 1 teaspoon pumpkin pie spice (depending on desired spiciness)

¼ teaspoon baking powder

OPTIONAL INGREDIENTS:
1 teaspoon pure vanilla extract

1 tablespoon flaxseed meal

2 teaspoons arrowroot (for thicker pancakes)

NUTRITIONAL INFORMATION PER SERVING: 136.9 calories, 7.8g protein, 5.4g carbohydrates, 1.9g fiber, 1.6g sugar, 9.4g fat, 2.0g saturated fat, 186.0mg cholesterol, 169.9mg sodium

Omega Egg Burrito to Go

SERVES 1

INGREDIENTS:

coconut oil nonstick cooking
spray

1 egg

¼ cup chopped veggies on hand
or ½ cup spinach

a dash of your favorite spices

1 coconut wrap, plain or curry
flavor

¼ avocado, sliced

2 ounces low-sodium smoked
salmon

salt and pepper, to taste

I like to keep nitrate-free "lox" on hand for when we are on the run. Traditional smoked salmon can be high in polyaromatic hydrocarbons (PAH), created from the smoke of wood or coal as it burns. They're also found in high concentrations in commercial liquid smoke, used to speed up the smoking process of seafood and meat. PAH is believed to cause cancer. While cold smoking without nitrates and liquid smoke eliminates this substance, it also decreases the shelf life. Make sure you consume the higher-quality salmon in a reasonable time frame. Also, if you're on a low-sodium diet, make sure you look for low-sodium smoked salmon. It can mean a difference of over 1,200 milligrams of sodium in one serving. I prefer low-sodium smoked salmon to avoid water retention.

PREPARATION:

1. Spray a small nonstick skillet with coconut oil spray. Over medium-low heat, scramble the egg. As egg is scrambling, add chopped veggies or spinach, stirring regularly. If preferred, you can heat the salmon for the last few seconds of cooking. I prefer not to heat the salmon and save this step. Add spices as desired. Curry or chili powder adds a tasty twist.

2. Remove egg mixture from heat when cooked (usually cooks within 2 to 3 minutes). Allow to cool for 1 minute. (If the egg is too hot, it will wilt the coconut wrap.)

3. While egg is cooling, place coconut wrap on a square of parchment paper. Place egg mixture on wrap lengthwise at one end, to accommodate rolling (like a burrito).

4. Top with avocado and smoked salmon. Sprinkle with salt and pepper as desired.

5. Make a small fold at the bottom of the wrap, so contents don't fall out. Roll tightly. Wrap parchment paper around burrito and fold the top down.

NUTRITIONAL INFORMATION PER SERVING: 317.3 calories, 18.4g protein, 6.9g carbohydrates, 6.0g fiber, 1.5g sugar, 20.5g fat, 6.1g saturated fat, 199.0mg cholesterol, 300mg sodium for low-sodium smoked lox

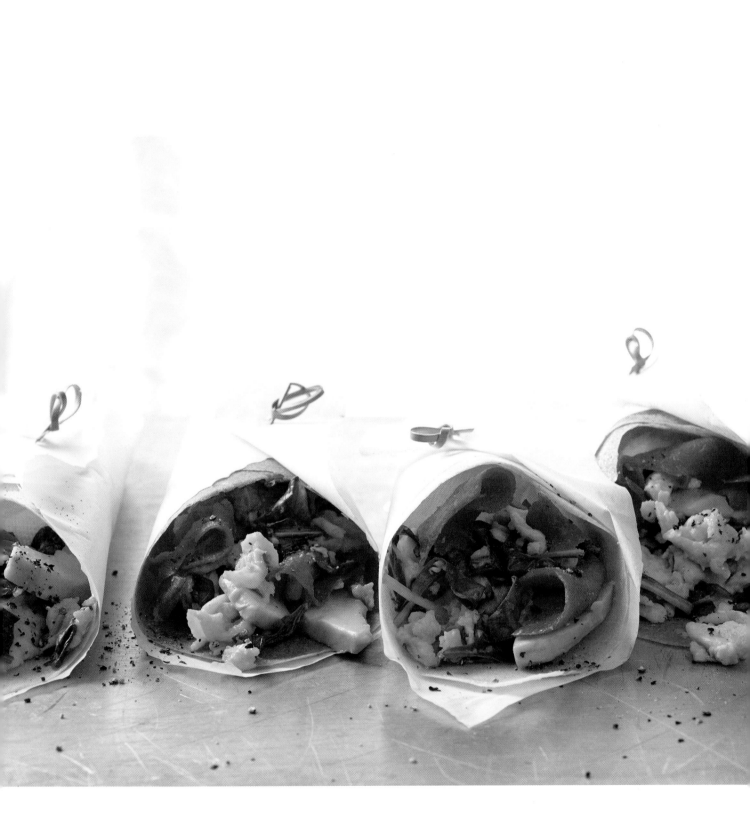

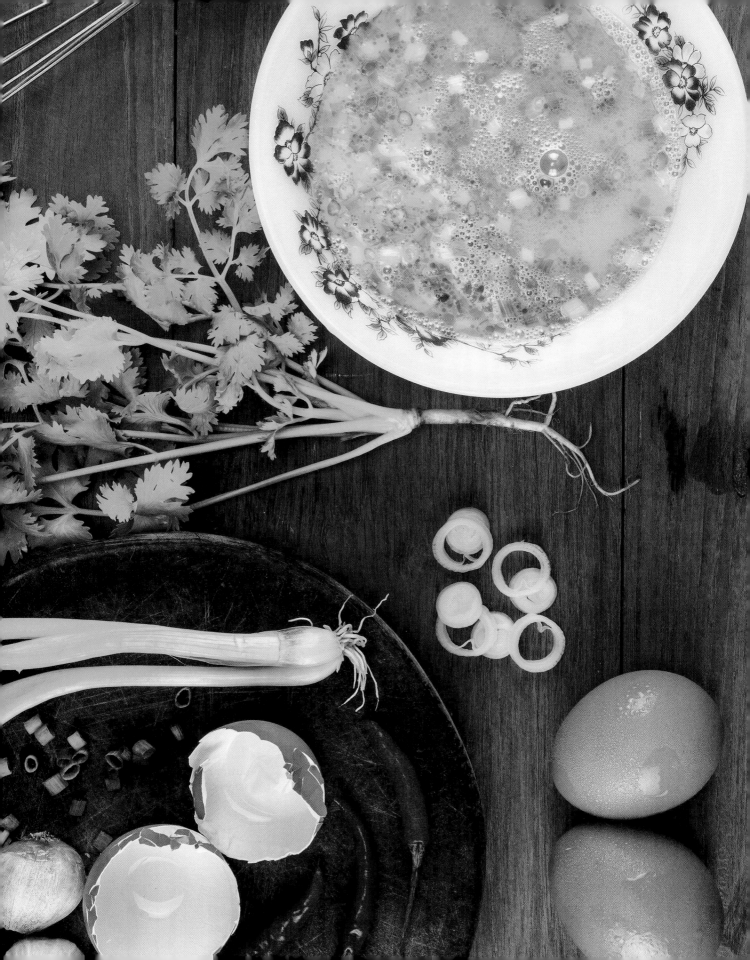

Spanish Scramble

This is one of our favorite recipes for making use of leftovers. It is super simple, satisfying, and delicious.

PREPARATION:

1. Place eggs in a mixing bowl and whisk until yolks are blended with whites.

2. If onion and garlic are desired, heat oil in medium pan over medium heat. Add onion and sauté for two minutes. Add garlic for another minute or two. If you're not adding onion and garlic, spray a medium pan with coconut cooking oil or use a nonstick pan and place over medium heat.

3. Add egg mixture to pan for a minute and begin to stir with a spatula or wooden spoon. As eggs begin to form, add chicken. Continue cooking for several minutes until eggs are no longer liquid or runny, 3 to 4 minutes. Add salt and pepper as desired.

4. Divide eggs evenly between two plates. Top with avocado slices and spoon two tablespoons salsa over the top. Serve hot.

SERVES 2

INGREDIENTS:
4 eggs
½ cup diced chicken, cooked
salt and pepper to taste
avocado, sliced
¼ cup Restaurant Style Salsa (page 235)

OPTIONAL INGREDIENTS:
1 tablespoon coconut, ghee or macadamia nut oil, only if sautéing onion and garlic
¼ cup diced onion
1 garlic clove, minced

NUTRITIONAL INFORMATION PER SERVING: 293.9 calories, 26.7g protein, 6.6g carbohydrates, 3.5g fiber, 0.5g sugar, 17.9g fat, 4.5g saturated fat, 407.1mg cholesterol, 316.8mg sodium

Speedy Seafood Omelet

SERVES 2

INGREDIENTS:

4 eggs

¼ teaspoon white pepper

2 teaspoons macadamia nut oil, coconut oil, or ghee

4 green onions, diced

6 shrimp, peeled, deveined, and cooked

salt to taste

OPTIONAL INGREDIENTS:

1 teaspoon minced fresh ginger (or ¼ teaspoon dried)

½ cup bean sprouts

¼ avocado, sliced

This is another favorite in our house because it gives us an opportunity to make use of leftover seafood. You can use any seafood you happen to have. Shrimp, salmon, halibut, scallops, and crab work great. Since we tend to have leftover shrimp quite often, I'm including that in the recipe.

PREPARATION:

1. Place eggs and pepper in a bowl and whisk until mixed thoroughly. Set aside.

2. Heat oil in a medium-sized omelet pan over medium heat. Add green onions and fresh ginger if desired. Sauté for 1 minute. If using dried ginger, add to egg mixture.

3. Add egg mixture to pan and allow it to spread evenly. Cover skillet for about 60 seconds to give eggs a chance to set. Remove cover and gently lift edges to check for doneness. When eggs are firm enough, but not overcooked, flip the omelet like a large pancake and allow it to cook for about another minute.

4. As soon as you flip the omelet, add shrimp. Don't add them too soon or they will become tough. You just want them to get warm. Add salt to taste.

5. Remove from heat. Gently fold omelet in half, and divide into two equal servings.

6. Place each half on a plate and top with avocado and bean sprouts if desired.

NUTRITIONAL INFORMATION PER SERVING: 189.2 calories, 13.1g protein, 4.3g carbohydrates, 0.7g fiber, 0.4g sugar, 13.2g fat, 3.7g saturated fat, 372.0mg cholesterol, 143.2mg sodium

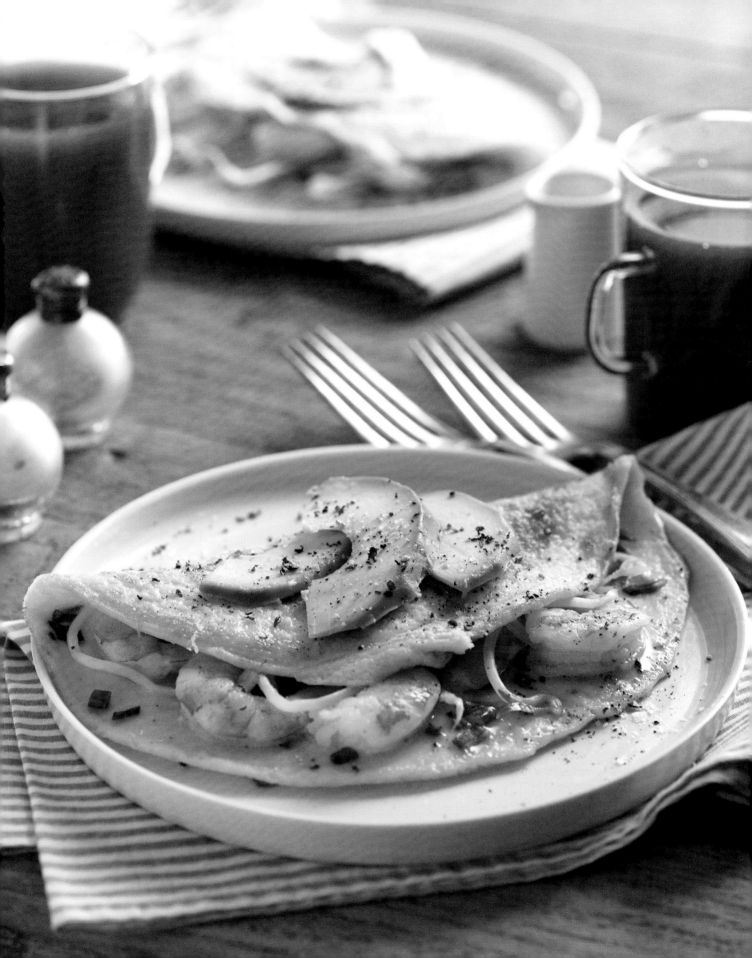

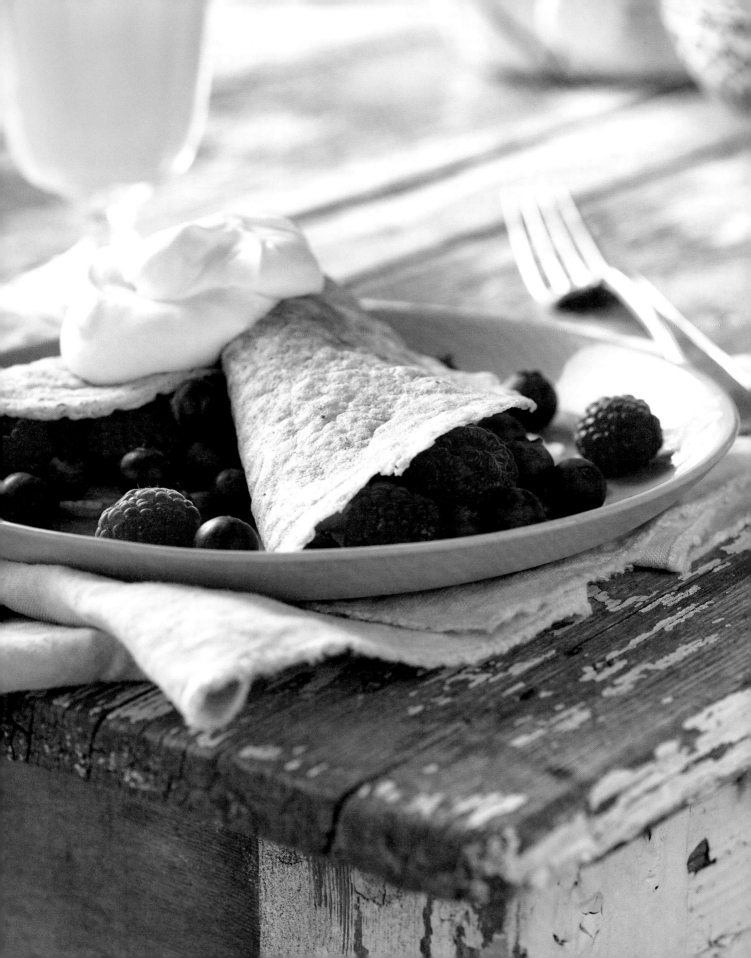

Super-Simple Crepes

PREPARATION:

1. In a large mixing bowl, combine the dry ingredients first: the flour, flaxseed meal, and baking powder.

2. Add the egg whites, almond milk, and vanilla if desired. Using a handheld electric mixer at medium speed or a whisk, beat until batter is smooth. Do not allow to rest for long, as the flaxseed tends to thicken the batter over time. For best results, the batter should be thin.

3. Spray a nonstick crepe pan with coconut oil and heat over medium heat. Pour a little less than ¼ cup of the batter into the pan (just enough to cover the pan with a thin layer), tilting the pan with a circular motion so that the batter coats the pan evenly. Cook the pancake for about 1 minute, until the bottom is golden brown. Loosen with a spatula, turn over, and cook the other side for about 30 seconds. It's all right to use your hand to help turn it. Remove the crepe and set aside on a plate, then repeat with the remaining batter.

4. Place two crepes on each plate and fill with fruit of your choice. Fold over or roll crepe.

5. Top with Silky Coconut Whipped Cream or drizzle with Mood-Boosting Chocolate Sauce.

> **NOTE:** Be sure you use flaxseed meal and not whole flaxseed. The crepes will not cook the same and will have an odd texture if you use flaxseed.

> **NOTE:** In a pinch, I just use the coconut fat from coconut milk instead of taking time to make coconut whipped cream, as it has a similar consistency. Put a can of coconut milk in the refrigerator for a couple of hours. When the fat floats to the top, scoop it off and place on the crepes.

SERVES 4

INGREDIENTS:

coconut oil nonstick cooking spray

CREPE
1 cup gluten-free all-purpose flour

2 tablespoons flaxseed meal

1 teaspoon baking powder

5 egg whites

1 cup plain unsweetened almond milk or rice milk

OPTIONAL INGREDIENT:
1 teaspoon pure vanilla extract

FILLING:
1 cup berries of your choice

TOPPING:
½ cup Silky Coconut Whipped Cream (page 251) or Mood-Boosting Chocolate Sauce (page 253)

NUTRITIONAL INFORMATION PER SERVING FOR CREPES: 156.9 calories, 10.3g protein, 23.8g carbohydrates, 4.3g fiber, 1.1g sugar, 2.9g fat, 0.1g saturated fat, 0.0mg cholesterol, 260.7mg sodium

NUTRITIONAL INFORMATION PER SERVING FOR STRAWBERRY FILLING: 12.2 calories, 0.9g protein, 2.8g carbohydrates, 0.7g fiber, 1.8g sugar, 0.1g fat, 0.0g saturated fat, 0.0mg cholesterol, 0.0mg sodium

NUTRITIONAL INFORMATION PER SERVING FOR 2 TABLESPOONS SILKY COCONUT WHIPPED CREAM: 69.0 calories, 0.7g protein, 1.7g carbohydrates, 0.0g fiber, 0.0g sugar, 7.2g fat, 6.3g saturated fat, 0.0mg cholesterol, 5.0mg sodium

NUTRITIONAL INFORMATION PER 1-TABLESPOON SERVING OF MOOD-BOOSTING CHOCOLATE SAUCE: 58.5 calories, 0.9g protein, 7.1g carbohydrates, 3.75g fiber, 0.0g sugar, 5.9g fat, 3.4g saturated fat, 0.0mg cholesterol, 0.9mg sodium

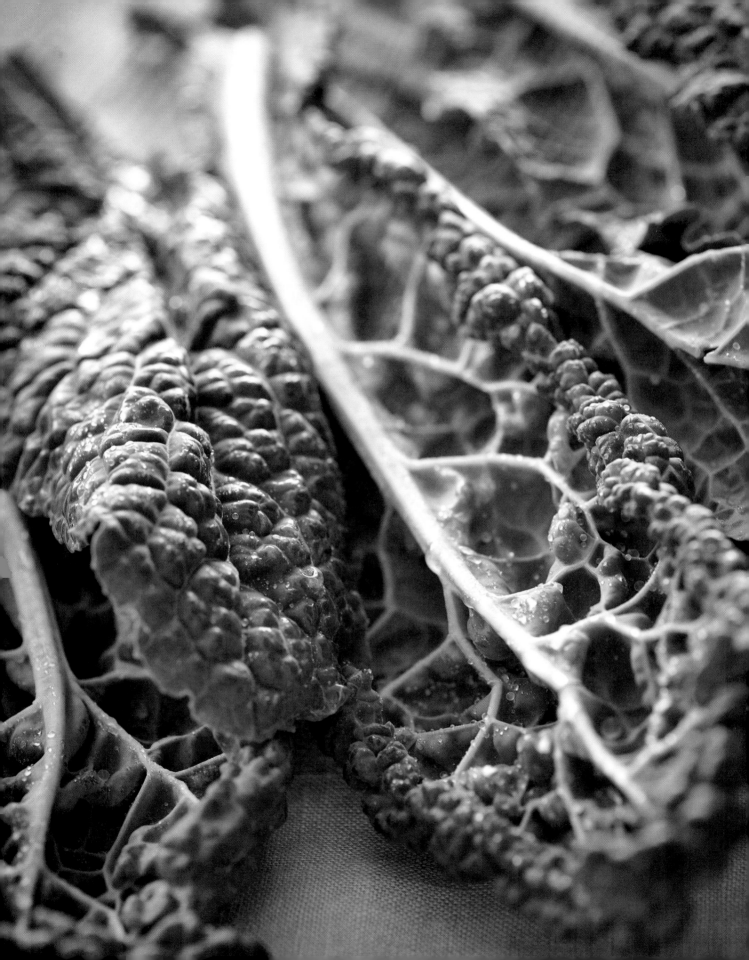

Salads

■

Today I will do what others won't, so tomorrow I can accomplish what others can't.

—JERRY RICE

Salads are a favorite in our home. We love eating foods of many colors: berries, veggies, pomegranate, grapefruit, and dark greens. We usually add a little avocado or a few nuts and top it off with a simple vinaigrette dressing. We're so full by the time we finish the salad that we consume much less of the "main course." In fact, in our home the "main course" is the salad and the veggies. The protein is the "side."

Brain Warrior
Salad-Saving Strategies

Now that you've committed to eating healthy, you might be happy to know a few simple tips that stretch your budget and your menu. Instead of throwing out leftover vegetables and salads, try:

1. Tossing leftover vegetables such as cabbage, kale, sweet potatoes, brussels sprouts, broccoli, or asparagus into a pot with some broth and spices to make a healthy soup.

2. Using lightly wilted spinach to make pesto.

3. Steaming leftover chard and serving it with a little garlic and olive oil as a side.

4. Pureeing cauliflower, bell peppers, and zucchini and adding it to chili for an antioxidant boost.

5. Using lettuce, bean sprouts, chopped veggies, and quinoa from any leftover salad to create a delicious stir-fry.

6. Adding leftover salad without the dressing to a morning smoothie for a power-packed breakfast.

■

Cruciferous Cold Slaw

PREPARATION:

1. Toss all the slaw ingredients in a large bowl.

2. Whisk together all the dressing ingredients.

3. Toss the slaw and dressing together and chill till serving.

INGREDIENTS:

SLAW:
1 cup shredded broccoli

2 cups shredded cabbage

1 cup shredded brussels sprouts

¼ cup raw pumpkin seeds

¼ cup goji berries

DRESSING:
2 tablespoons apple cider vinegar

2 tablespoons vegan mayonnaise or Nayonnaise (page 257)

1 tablespoon Dijon mustard

2 teaspoons raw honey

1 teaspoon fresh squeezed lemon juice

½ teaspoon salt

NUTRITIONAL INFORMATION PER SERVING FOR SALAD: 90.1 calories, 4.7g protein, 15.5g carbohydrates, 5.2g fiber, 6.4g sugar, 2.8g fat, 0.5g saturated fat, 0.0mg cholesterol, 92.8mg sodium

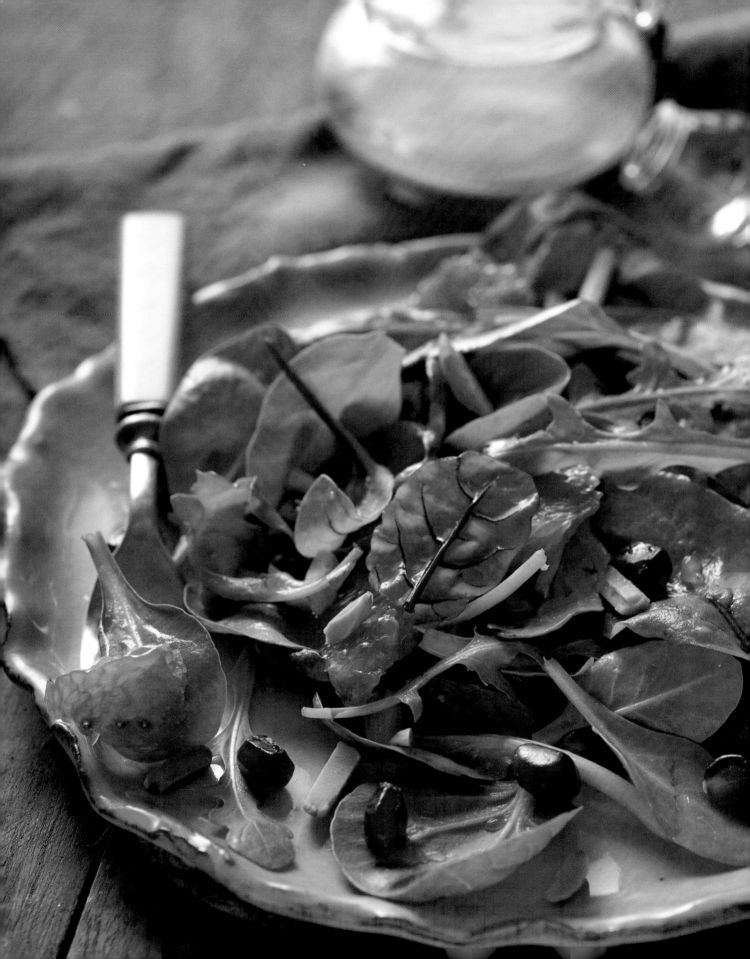

Savory Grapefruit Avocado Salad

PREPARATION:

1. In a blender, puree pink grapefruit juice, avocado, garlic, salt, and pepper to a creamy dressing consistency. If it is too thick, add a little cold water 1 teaspoon at a time or a little more juice.

2. If desired, lightly toast the pumpkin seeds or slivered almonds. (I prefer them raw.)

3. Toss the greens, grapefruit, and pomegranate seeds with the dressing, and top with pumpkin seeds or almonds.

4. Divide evenly among four salad plates and serve.

SERVES 4

INGREDIENTS:

DRESSING:
juice of 1 small pink grapefruit (about ¼ to ½ cup)

¼ avocado

¼ to ½ teaspoon minced garlic

OPTIONAL INGREDIENTS:
⅛ teaspoon salt and ground pepper combined

SALAD:
6 to 8 cups mixed greens

1 pink grapefruit, peeled and seeded with membrane removed-large dice

⅓ cup pumpkin seeds or slivered almonds

¼ cup pomegranate seeds

NUTRITIONAL INFORMATION PER SERVING FOR DRESSING:
17.5 calories, 0.3g protein, 4.3g carbohydrates, 1.3g fiber, 2.5g sugar, 0.1g fat, 0.0g saturated fat, 0.0mg cholesterol, 0.0mg sodium

NUTRITIONAL INFORMATION PER SERVING FOR SALAD: 139.6 calories, 5.7g protein, 21.4g carbohydrates, 2.4g fiber, 7.5g sugar, 4.5g fat, 0.8g saturated fat, 0.0mg cholesterol, 40.0mg sodium

Orange, Fennel, and Blueberry Salad

SERVES 4

INGREDIENTS:

SALAD:

6 cups mixed greens

1 fennel bulb, sliced very thin

2 oranges, peeled, with membranes removed, and cut into sections

½ cup blueberries

DRESSING (MAKES 8 SERVINGS):

juice of one orange

zest of one orange

1 tablespoon champagne vinegar

½ teaspoon salt

pinch of white pepper

½ cup extra-virgin olive oil

PREPARATION:

1. Place the greens in a large bowl or on individual salad plates, and arrange the fennel, oranges, and blueberries on top.

2. Mix all the ingredients for the dressing with a whisk until thoroughly combined, and drizzle on top.

NOTE: I always make extra dressing since we eat salads every day. Most of these dressings taste great on other salads or sides and can be preserved for over a week in the refrigerator. Extras and leftovers are the key to a healthy lifestyle for my family. Dressing lasts about ten days in the refrigerator. Since it's easier to make larger portions of dressing, I prefer to prepare enough for eight servings and refrigerate what's left over.

NUTRITIONAL INFORMATION PER SERVING FOR SALAD: 88.5 calories, 2.9g protein, 20.1g carbohydrates, 5.7g fiber, 5.4g sugar, 0.3g fat, 0.0g saturated fat, 0.0mg cholesterol, 69.0mg sodium

NUTRITIONAL INFORMATION PER SERVING FOR DRESSING: 122.5 calories, 0.2g protein, 2.2g carbohydrates, 0.0g fiber, 1.5g sugar, 16.0g fat, 2.0g saturated fat, 0.0mg cholesterol, 0.6mg sodium

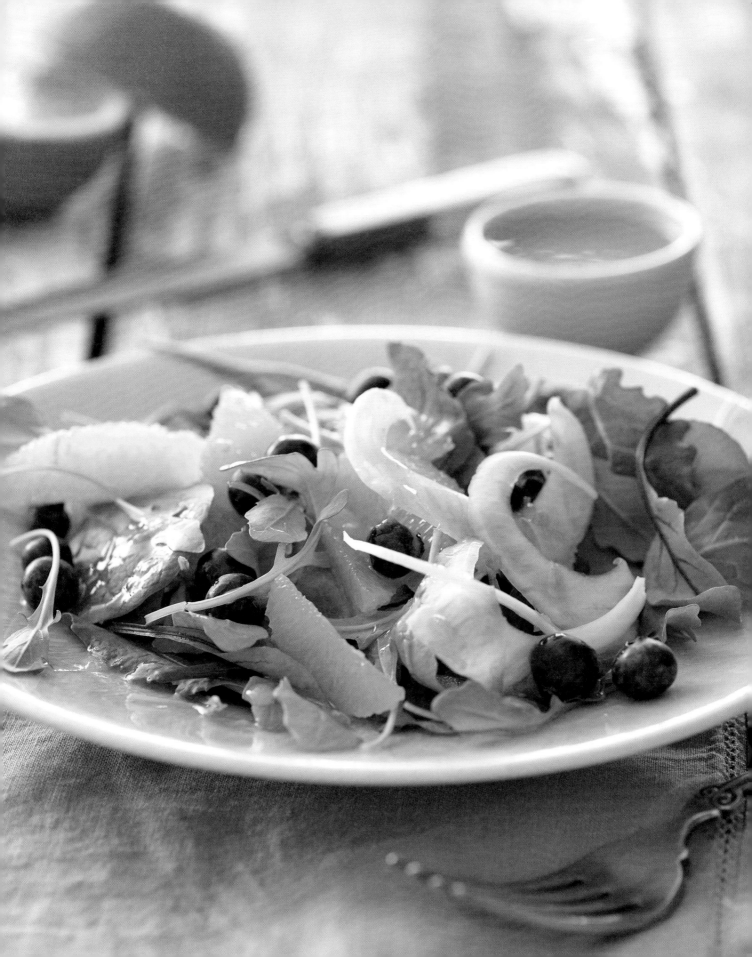

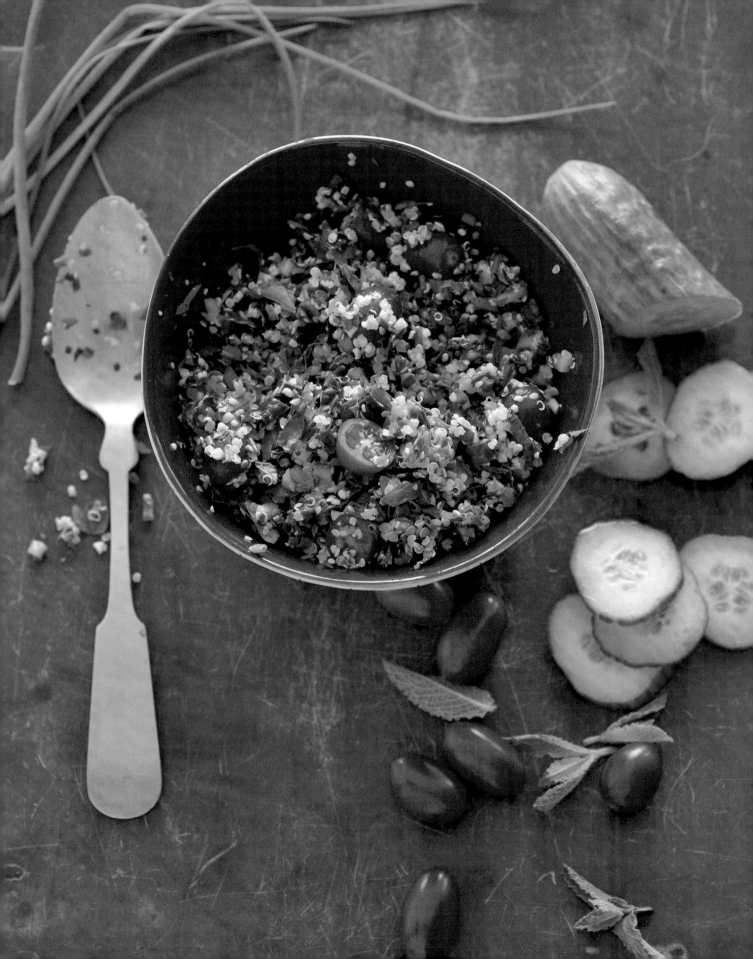

Kale and Quinoa Tabbouleh

PREPARATION:

1. Rinse quinoa. Add quinoa to a small pot. Cook according to the instructions on the package. You'll need one cup cooked. Reserve remaining quinoa for other uses.

2. Remove cover from pot after quinoa is finished cooking and place a clean towel over the pot. Let cool for at least 15 minutes. Remove towel, and fluff with a fork.

3. When quinoa is cool, combine quinoa with remaining salad ingredients in a large bowl.

4. In a medium-sized bowl, whisk dressing ingredients together, and add salt and pepper to taste.

5. Toss salad with dressing and serve.

SERVES 6

INGREDIENTS:

SALAD:
1 cup cooked quinoa
1 cup flat-leaf Italian parsley, finely chopped
¼ cup fresh mint, finely chopped
1 cup kale, finely chopped
1 cup fresh chives, finely chopped
1 cup Persian cucumber, or hothouse cucumber, seeded and diced small
½ cup hemp seeds
1 cup grape tomatoes, halved
zest of 1 lemon

DRESSING:
2 tablespoons extra-virgin olive oil
2 tablespoons fresh squeezed lemon juice, about 1 lemon
2 garlic cloves, minced
salt and pepper

NUTRITIONAL INFORMATION PER SERVING: 309.3 calories, 13.9g protein, 39.2g carbohydrates, 6.0g fiber, 2.5g sugar, 11.5g fat, 1.0g saturated fat, 0.0mg cholesterol, 25.1mg sodium

Wilted Kale and Strawberry Salad

SERVES 2

INGREDIENTS:

DRESSING:

2 tablespoons fresh squeezed lemon juice, about 1 lemon

2 tablespoons olive oil

1 teaspoon raw honey or real maple syrup

⅛ teaspoon salt

⅛ teaspoon pepper

SALAD:

1 bunch kale, thick stems removed and cut into bite-sized pieces

1 pound strawberries, stemmed and sliced

2 tablespoons fresh basil or mint, roughly chopped

½ cup chopped walnuts

OPTIONAL INGREDIENTS:

1 tablespoon macadamia nut oil

2 tablespoons crumbled or shredded goat cheese

To make this a complete meal, consider topping with leftover bison steak or chicken breast.

PREPARATION:

1. In a blender or food processor, combine all ingredients for the dressing. Mix on low speed for 1 to 2 minutes. Set aside until ready to use.

2. Rinse kale and shake off excess water.

3. Bring about an inch of water to a boil in the bottom of a medium pot. Place kale in a steamer basket and place in boiling water, making sure water doesn't touch the kale. Cover the pot and allow the kale to steam for 2 to 3 minutes. Remove kale from heat to prevent overcooking. You could also sauté the kale in a pan with a tablespoon of macadamia nut oil for about 2 minutes instead of steaming.

4. In a large bowl, toss kale, strawberries, fresh herbs, and walnuts with dressing. Top with goat cheese if desired.

5. Serve warm.

NUTRITIONAL INFORMATION PER SERVING: 300.0 calories, 6.5g protein, 18.4g carbohydrates, 7.0g fiber, 3.4g sugar, 26.5g fat, 2.7g saturated fat, 0.0mg cholesterol, 56.3mg sodium

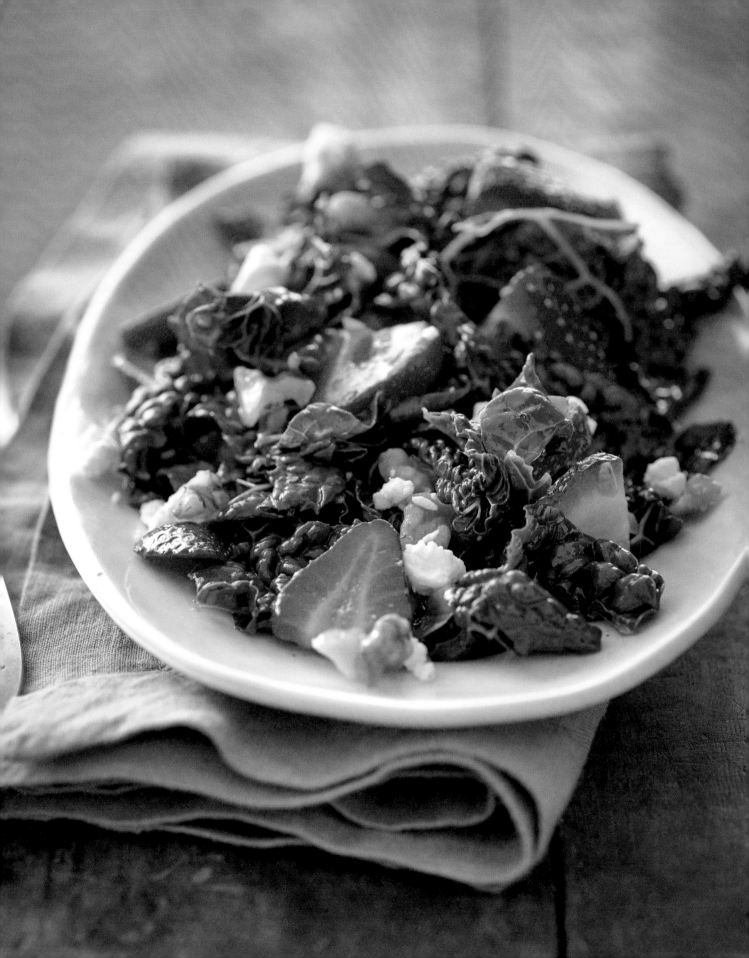

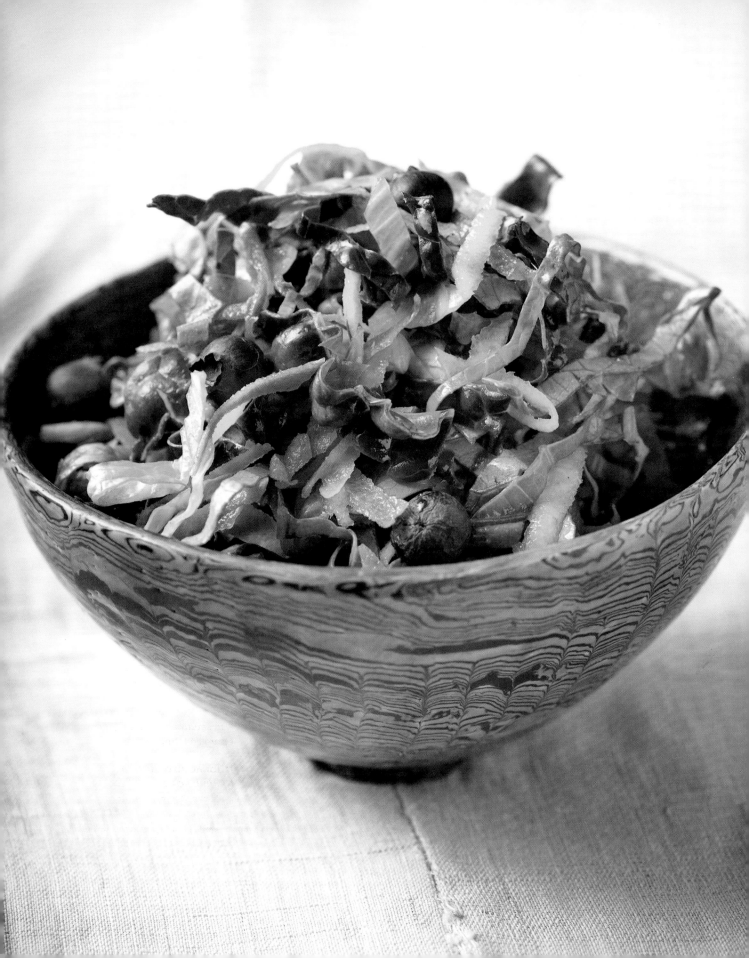

Shredded Rainbow Salad

PREPARATION:

1. Place the kale or chard in a large bowl and massage it with your hands for a minute to help break it down and make it tender.

2. Add the lettuce, beet, and carrots.

3. Whisk together the dressing ingredients in a separate bowl and toss with the salad.

4. Top with the golden berries or blueberries.

SERVES 4

INGREDIENTS:

SALAD:

1 small bunch kale or chard, thick stems removed and cut into very thin ribbons

1 small head romaine lettuce, cut into very thin ribbons

1 small golden beet, peeled, and shredded on a box grater

2 carrots, peeled, and shredded on a box grater

¼ cup golden berries or blueberries

DRESSING:

2 tablespoons apple cider vinegar

1 teaspoon raw honey or maple syrup

salt, to taste

pinch of white pepper

¼ cup extra-virgin olive oil

NUTRITIONAL INFORMATION PER SERVING FOR SALAD: 41.5 calories, 1.3g protein, 9.4g carbohydrates, 2.5g fiber, 5.3g sugar, 0.2g fat, 0.0g saturated fat, 0.0mg cholesterol, 44.0mg sodium

NUTRITIONAL INFORMATION PER SERVING FOR DRESSING: 115.0 calories, 0.1g protein, 1.5g carbohydrates, 0.0g fiber, 1.5g sugar, 12.6g fat, 1.8g saturated fat, 0.0mg cholesterol, 0.0mg sodium

Chicken Quinoa Chard Toss

SERVES 4

INGREDIENTS:

2 cups water

1 cup white quinoa, rinsed and drained

4 cups rainbow chard (or kale), thick stems removed and discarded, and chopped into bite-sized pieces

2 cups cooked chicken, diced

1 cup cherry tomatoes, halved or whole

salt and pepper as desired

dressing of your choice

¼ cup slivered almonds

OPTIONAL INGREDIENT:

½ cup green onions, thinly sliced

Adding leftover protein to salads is a great way to save time and create a hearty meal. I always make extra portions so I can have a healthy meal ready for my family within a few minutes. For a vegan version, leave out the chicken.

PREPARATION:

1. Bring water to a boil in a medium-sized pot. Stir in quinoa and reduce heat to medium low. Allow to simmer for about 15 minutes.

2. Stir in chard just before removing pot from heat.

3. Remove pot from heat. Cover the pot and allow to sit for 10 minutes.

4. Divide quinoa mixture evenly among 4 dishes, and top with diced chicken, tomatoes, and green onions if desired. Salt to taste.

5. Drizzle with Avocado Cilantro Dressing (page 241).

6. Sprinkle each plate with almonds.

NUTRITIONAL INFORMATION PER SERVING FOR SALAD: 178.1 calories, 16.1g protein, 13.9g carbohydrates, 7.1g fiber, 3.7g sugar, 5.5g fat, 0.3g saturated fat, 0.0mg cholesterol, 55.2mg sodium

Cashew Kale Salad with Chicken

PREPARATION:

1. Chop the chicken and set aside.

2. Finely slice the kale leaves, discarding the stems. (A shortcut is to roll the kale leaves and slice. Turn and slice in the opposite direction. Keep the pieces very small.)

3. Using a mandoline slicer set to the thinnest setting, shred the cabbage.

4. Finely chop the cilantro. Chop mint and slice scallions, if desired.

5. In a large salad bowl, combine the prepared salad greens.

6. In a blender, or a tall bowl if using an immersion blender, combine the dressing ingredients and proceed to blend on high for about 2 minutes. Once the dressing is smooth, toss it with the salad.

7. Top the salad with chicken and cashews.

> **NOTE:** You may want to consider purchasing cut-resistant gloves to go with your mandoline, as it is extremely sharp. I've seen even the most experienced chefs sustain terrible cuts if they aren't paying attention.

SERVES 4

INGREDIENTS:

SALAD:
1½ cups cooked chicken
1 bunch flat-leaf kale
1 cup shredded red cabbage
¼ bunch cilantro
½ cup unsalted cashews, chopped

OPTIONAL INGREDIENTS:
¼ cup fresh mint, finely chopped
2 scallions, sliced

DRESSING:
¼ cup olive oil or macadamia nut oil
1 tablespoon low-sodium tamari sauce
2 teaspoons sesame oil
2 teaspoons rice vinegar
1 tablespoon raw honey
salt and pepper, to taste

NUTRITIONAL INFORMATION PER SERVING FOR SALAD: 213.2 calories, 22.9g protein, 7.3g carbohydrates, 1.6g fiber, 2.1g sugar, 10.3g fat, 2.7g saturated fat, 52.7mg cholesterol, 61.0mg sodium

NUTRITIONAL INFORMATION PER SERVING FOR DRESSING: 148.0 calories, 0.3g protein, 4.6g carbohydrates, 0.0g fiber, 4.4g sugar, 14.9g fat, 2.2g saturated fat, 0.0mg cholesterol, 63.0mg sodium

Sesame Citrus Chicken Salad

SERVES 6

INGREDIENTS:

1 bunch (about 8 ounces) kale or chard, shredded, thick stems removed

¼ to ½ cup cilantro, chopped

2 navel oranges or 1 Ruby Red grapefruit, 1 juiced for dressing and 1 peeled and diced for salad

¼ teaspoon salt

½ teaspoon pepper

1 teaspoon raw honey

1 tablespoon toasted sesame oil

2 tablespoons toasted sesame seeds

2 tablespoons chopped raw pecans

3 cups grilled or baked chicken, diced

I like to use half kale and half chard when I make this recipe!

PREPARATION:

1. Place kale or chard and cilantro in large bowl.

2. In small bowl, whisk together the citrus juice, salt, pepper, honey, and sesame oil until blended.

3. Remove membranes and seeds from remaining orange or grapefruit, and dice.

4. Toss diced orange or grapefruit, sesame seeds, pecans, and dressing with the kale and cilantro. Refrigerate for 30 minutes prior to serving.

5. Serve salad on plates and top with diced chicken.

NUTRITIONAL INFORMATION PER SERVING: 145.8 calories, 10.1g protein, 8.5g carbohydrates, 2.9g fiber, 2.0g sugar, 8.8g fat, 1.2g saturated fat, 19.8mg cholesterol, 32.9mg sodium

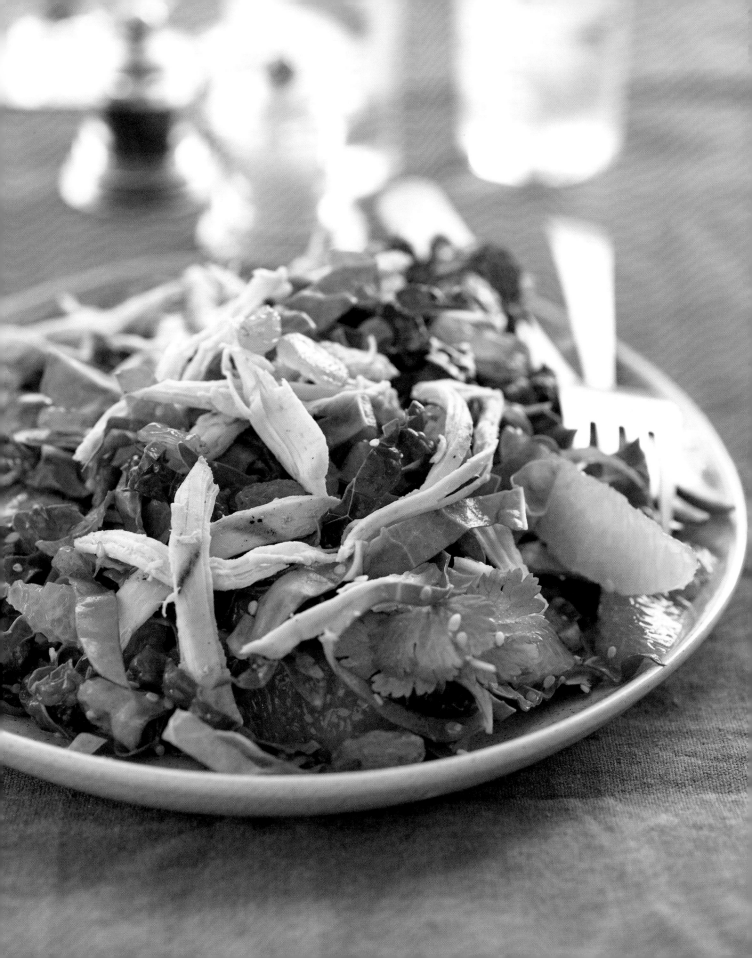

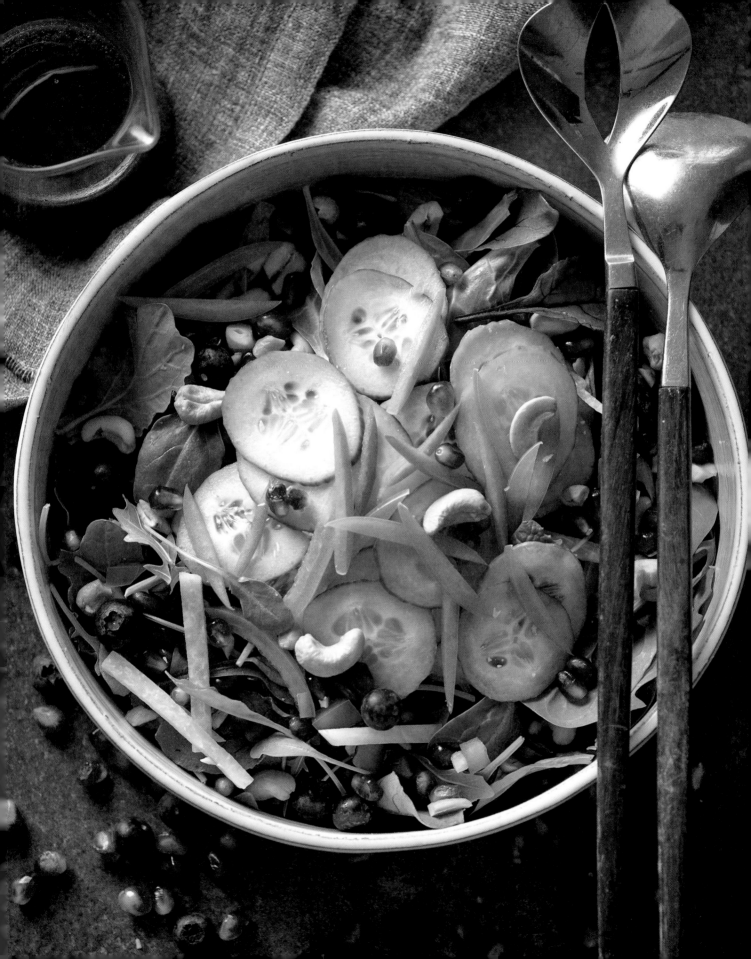

Festive Blueberry Pomegranate Salad

This is my go-to salad for nearly every holiday party. The festive colors are as beautiful for Independence Day celebrations as they are for winter holiday parties.

PREPARATION:

1. In a small bowl, mix balsamic vinegar and honey.

2. Slowly whisk in olive oil. Season with salt. Refrigerate until ready to serve.

3. Either place all salad ingredients together in a large salad bowl and toss with dressing, or assemble salad on a platter and drizzle with dressing.

4. For platter presentation: Lay salad greens evenly across a large platter. Place cucumber slices around the outer edge of the platter. Put the cashews in a narrow line down the center of the salad. Do the same with the blueberries, placing a line next to the line of cashews. Place a line of pomegranate seeds on the other side of the cashews. Sprinkle the jicama and bell peppers around the outer edges, just inside the cucumber.

> **NOTE:** Tossing the ingredients creates a pretty winter holiday feel, while laying the ingredients out in lines on a platter with red, white, and blue stripes creates a fun Independence Day presentation.

SERVES 4

INGREDIENTS:

DRESSING:
2 tablespoons balsamic vinegar
1 teaspoon raw honey
¼ cup olive oil
salt, to taste

SALAD:
8 cups mixed greens
1 Persian cucumber, sliced
½ cup chopped cashews
½ cup blueberries
½ cup pomegranate seeds
¼ cup jicama, diced
½ bell pepper, diced

NUTRITIONAL INFORMATION PER SERVING: 122.0 calories, 0.7g protein, 4.5g carbohydrates, 1.0g fiber, 3.1g sugar, 9.5g fat, 1.5g saturated fat, 0.0mg cholesterol, 8.5mg sodium

Sweet Potato Salad

SERVES 6

INGREDIENTS:

1 teaspoon salt

3 small sweet potatoes or yams (about 2 pounds)

½ cup red bell pepper, diced

½ cup celery, chopped

½ cup finely chopped kale, thick stems removed

¼ cup fresh chives, chopped

¼ cup fresh dill, chopped

DRESSING:

½ cup vegan mayonnaise or Nayonnaise (page 257)

2 tablespoons fresh squeezed lemon juice, about 1 lemon

1 teaspoon cumin

salt and pepper, to taste

We love this sweet and tangy replacement for potato salad on a hot summer day. It's loaded with nutrition and bursting with flavor!

PREPARATION:

1. Bring a large pot of water to boil and add salt.

2. Peel and cut sweet potato into ½-inch pieces.

3. Add the sweet potatoes to the boiling water, reduce to a simmer, and cook until they are fork tender, 5 to 10 minutes. Drain and let cool.

4. Make the dressing by whisking together the vegan mayonnaise or Nayonnaise with the lemon juice, cumin, and salt and pepper to taste.

5. Toss the dressing with the bell pepper, celery, kale, chives, and dill. Then carefully fold in the sweet potatoes so they don't fall apart and mash.

6. Serve cold or at room temperature.

NUTRITIONAL INFORMATION
PER SERVING: 201.1 calories, 1.7g protein, 19.9g carbohydrates, 3.5g fiber, 0.8g sugar, 12.2g fat, 0.7g saturated fat, 0.0mg cholesterol, 148.0mg sodium

"Don't underestimate the power of ordinary moments to create extraordinary habits."

—Daniel and Tana

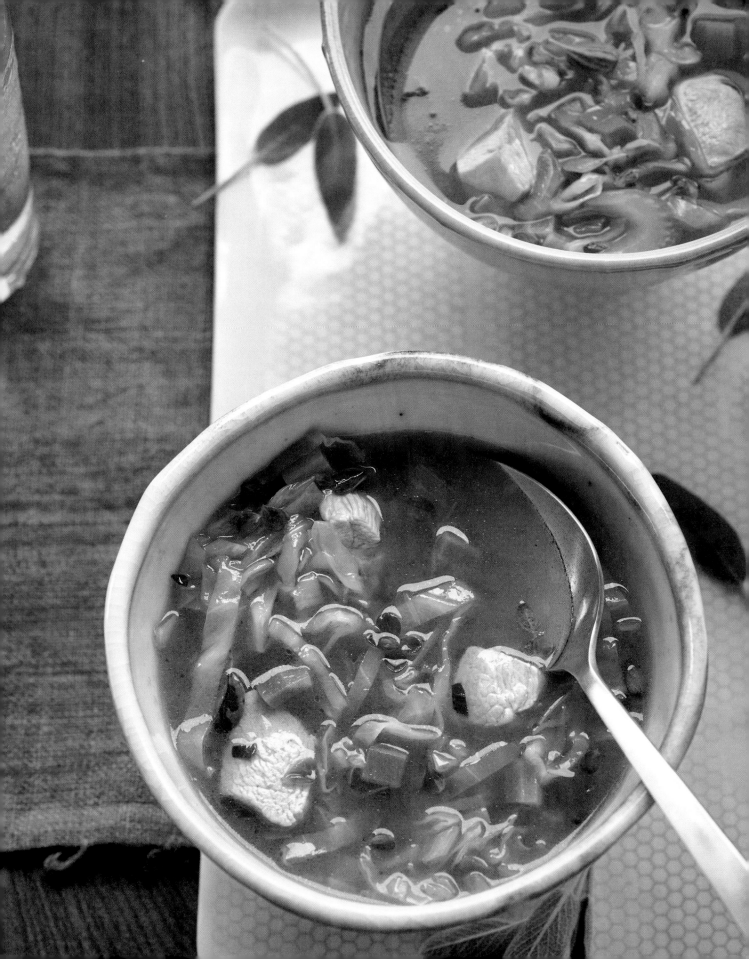

Soups and Stews

■

Your calm mind is your ultimate weapon against your
challenges. So relax.

—BRYANT MCGILL

Rest and relaxation are a crucial key to the success of a Brain
Warrior's journey, and there's nothing quite as relaxing and healing
for the body and mind as a warm bowl of soup or a hearty stew on a
cold winter night. These complete dishes can be a small starter, or robust
enough to be the main course. Be creative and add a little leftover protein
from the night before for a complete meal. Vegetarians can swap some
tofu or other protein quite easily in many of the recipes.

Like salads, soups are incredibly versatile. Use these recipes as a
template, and add your own touch. Make use of whatever vegetables
and herbs are available. The only rules are to create high-quality fuel that
serves your brain and body, and of course, to have fun.

Brain Warrior Savvy
Soup Strategies

1. Utilize leftover veggies before making a trip to the store.

2. Use substitutions. Don't be afraid to adjust the ingredients in a recipe to include fresh herbs you may have.

3. If you're a busy person, double the recipe and freeze leftover portions.

4. Buy seasonal and on sale. Because of long simmering times and slow cooking, soups are the perfect way to soften tougher cuts of meat that may be less expensive. Also, anything seasonal can be used.

5. Save time and make delicious soup by setting a Crock-Pot on a low setting so your soup is simmering while you're busy with other tasks.

■

USE THE BONES

Making bone broth is one of the easiest and healthiest things to do once you get into the habit of saving the bones from your meals, or asking the butcher for extra bones during your weekly shopping trip. Commercial broth is very high in sodium, so making bone broth is a great way to cut down on sodium if you're on a heart-healthy diet. I understand that many of you need recipes to be as convenient as possible, and packaged broth may be your preference, but take a look at the recipe below and you might be surprised at how easy this is. You just drop the bones in a Crock-Pot and let it go, just like Mom used to do.

There's a good reason that Mom's old-fashioned chicken soup was considered medicine for the body and soul. In the good ol' days, broth didn't contain a bunch of chemicals and it was made from real bones, which have a lot of healing power. Technically, most commercial broth doesn't contain much chicken or beef at all; hence it holds very little nutritional value. However, real bone broth, when made from the bones of organic, pasture-raised chickens and free-range animals, especially wild game, is chock-full of nutrients, minerals, and amino acids including:

- Glycine, which helps aid in wound healing, supports detoxification, and aids in the release of growth hormone.
- Proline, which aids in building and strengthening cells. This helps improve the strength of veins and skin, giving skin a healthier appearance.

Making bone broth is also a great way to make good use of leftover bones. After a meal, scrape excess meat from bones and refrigerate or freeze until ready for use.

Ingredients

2 to 3 pounds of bones from a healthy, grass-fed, hormone-free, antibiotic-free source
2 tablespoons apple cider vinegar

Optional Ingredients

herbs and spices of your choice
2 garlic cloves, minced

Preparation

1. Set a Crock-Pot on low. Add bones and just enough water to cover the bones.
2. Add apple cider vinegar.

3. For chicken broth, simmer for 4 hours. Other meats should simmer for a minimum of 6 hours, up to 24. The longer you simmer the bones, the more minerals and nutrients will be drawn out. However, you will need to replace evaporated water.

4. Twenty minutes before the broth is finished, add herbs and spices of your choice if desired.

5. For clear broth, skim froth and fat from top. This is not necessary, simply a preference.

6. When broth is ready, cool quickly to prevent bacterial accumulation. Fill a sink with cold water and place the pot directly in the water until cool enough to refrigerate.

7. If you plan to use the broth quickly, store in the refrigerator. Freeze any portions that will not be used within a week. Be sure to reboil any remaining broth before using to kill bacteria.

Note: I like to add garlic to my broth, but I don't add salt. You will add salt later when using broth to make other soups, so adding salt at this early stage will increase the sodium too much.

Note: While there isn't a set amount of bones to add when making broth, the more bones you add, the heartier the flavor will be.

Creamy Coconut Curry Soup

1. In a large pot, heat the coconut oil over medium-high heat, add the onion, and cook till soft.

2. Add the curry powder, stirring to coat the onions.

3. Add the cauliflower, the coconut milk, and enough water to just cover the cauliflower with liquid. Bring to a boil, then reduce to a simmer and cook until the cauliflower is soft, 15 to 20 minutes.

4. Ladle the cauliflower into a blender, filling the blender no more than halfway, then pulse till smooth. Repeat with remaining cauliflower, adding enough liquid to get a smooth soup.

5. Return the soup to the pan, and bring to simmer. Season with salt and pepper. Divide evenly in soup tureens and garnish each dish with a few cashew halves and a couple of mint or cilantro leaves.

NOTE: White pepper is great for white soups or sauces because it doesn't leave any black spots. It is stronger than pepper, so use carefully.

SERVES 4

INGREDIENTS:
1 tablespoon coconut oil

1 cup chopped onion

2 teaspoons curry powder

1 large head cauliflower, leaves removed, stems and florets chopped

1 (13½-ounce) can coconut milk

salt and white pepper, to taste

OPTIONAL INGREDIENTS:
halved cashews

mint leaves or cilantro to garnish

NUTRITIONAL INFORMATION PER SERVING: 115.6 calories, 5.0g protein, 15.7g carbohydrates, 6.3g fiber, 0.3g sugar, 5.3g fat, 4.1g saturated fat, 0.0mg cholesterol, 69.7mg sodium

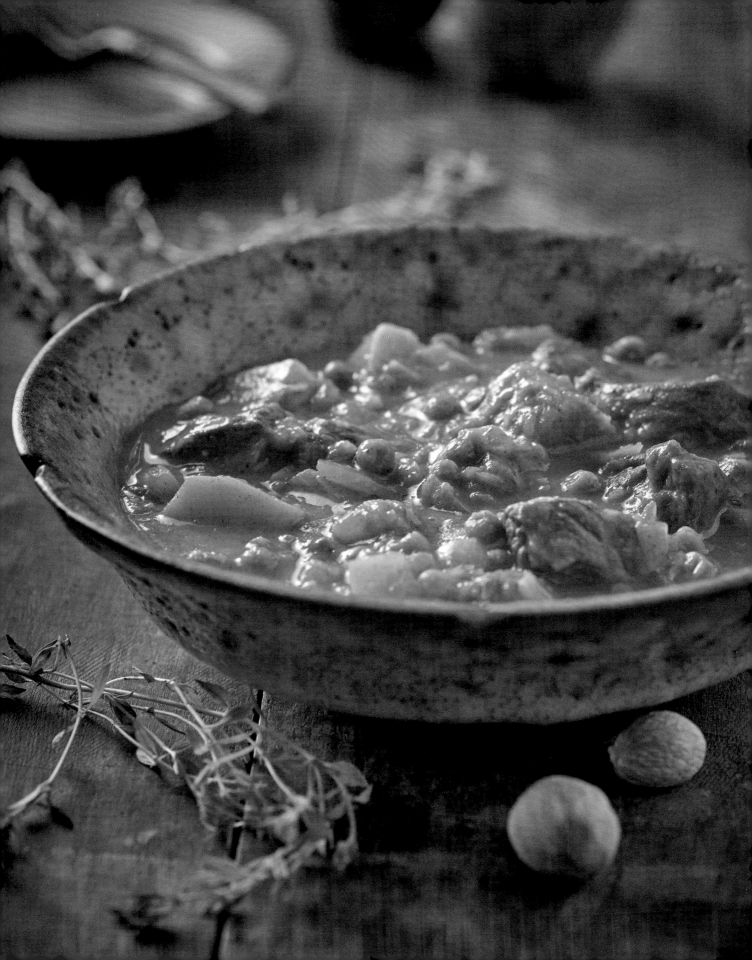

Moroccan Spiced Lamb Stew

PREPARATION:

1. Dice lamb into 1-inch cubes (or have the lamb cubed by the butcher in advance).

2. In a large pot or Dutch oven, heat the coconut oil over medium-high heat. Season the meat with salt and pepper, then add to pan and brown on all sides. Remove the meat from the pan and set aside.

3. Add the onion and yellow pepper to the pot and cook till tender.

4. Add the squash, cinnamon, and nutmeg. Stir gently.

5. Add the meat and tomatoes with juices. Add coconut milk. Bring to a boil, then turn heat down to a simmer and cook for 1½ hours, till the meat is tender.

6. Add peas and season with salt and pepper to taste.

NOTE: This stew can also be slow-cooked in a Crock-Pot. Put all ingredients except the peas in the Crock-Pot and cook on high for 4 hours or on low for 6 to 8 hours. Program the Crock-Pot to warm until ready to serve. Add the peas and season with salt and pepper right before serving.

SERVES 6

INGREDIENTS:

2 pounds lamb

2 tablespoons coconut oil

salt and pepper, to taste

1 onion, diced

1 yellow bell pepper, diced

1 small butternut squash, peeled, seeded, and cut into 1-inch cubes (about 3 cups)

1 teaspoon cinnamon

¼ teaspoon nutmeg

1 (28-ounce) can diced tomatoes with the juices

1 (13½-ounce) can coconut milk

1 cup frozen peas

NUTRITIONAL INFORMATION PER SERVING: 301.3 calories, 18.4g protein, 21.7g carbohydrates, 5.8g fiber, 4.5g sugar, 15.9g fat, 10.0g saturated fat, 50.0mg cholesterol, 305.8mg sodium

Smooth Sweet Potato Soup

SERVES 8

INGREDIENTS:

6 cups vegetable broth or bone broth (page 89), divided

½ cup diced onion

1 cup diced celery

3 tablespoons diced leeks

2 garlic cloves, minced

1½ pounds sweet potatoes, peeled and diced

½ teaspoon cinnamon

¼ teaspoon nutmeg

½ cup almond milk

1 teaspoon salt

1 teaspoon white pepper

OPTIONAL INGREDIENTS:

¼ cup sunflower seeds

2 tablespoons finely chopped fresh sage

¼ cup dried cranberries

cinnamon

PREPARATION:

1. Heat ¼ cup vegetable broth in large soup pot over medium heat. Sauté onion, celery, and leeks for 2 minutes. Then add garlic and sauté for another minute.

2. Add 4 cups vegetable broth, sweet potatoes, cinnamon, and nutmeg.

3. Bring to a boil, then reduce heat to medium low and simmer until potatoes are tender, about 10 minutes.

4. Use immersion blender or pour contents into a blender in batches. Blend until smooth.

5. Pour soup back into pot (if using a blender). Add almond milk. Then slowly add remaining broth according to preferred consistency. Add salt and pepper, to taste.

6. Ladle soup into bowls and garnish with sunflower seeds, sage, cranberries, and a sprinkle of cinnamon if desired.

> **NOTE:** For thinner soup, add a little more broth after blending, while soup is in the pot.

NUTRITIONAL INFORMATION PER SERVING: 81 calories, 2g protein, 17g carbohydrates, 2g fiber, 4.5g sugar, 0.0g fat, 0.0g saturated fat, 0.0mg cholesterol, 234.0mg sodium

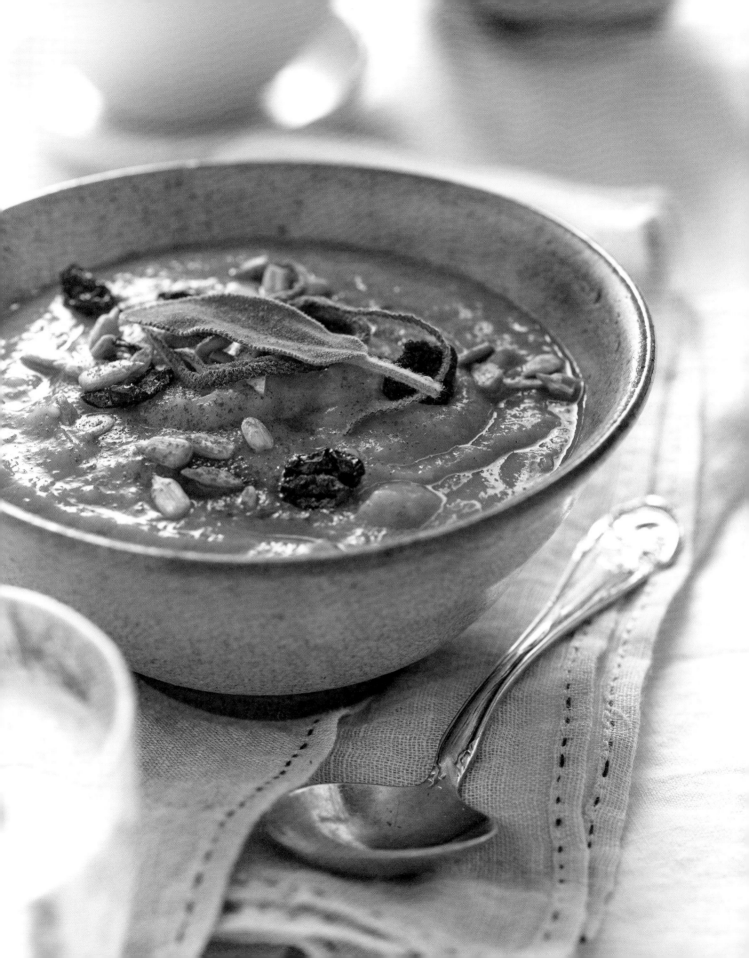

Crock-Pot Chicken Shawarma with Cilantro Garlic Oil

SERVES 4

INGREDIENTS:

CROCK-POT CHICKEN SHAWARMA

2 pounds boneless, skinless chicken thighs

1 red onion, sliced

5 garlic cloves, crushed

1 cup chicken broth or bone broth (page 89)

2 tablespoons fresh squeezed lemon juice, about 1 lemon

zest of 1 lemon

1 teaspoon pepper

1 teaspoon salt

1 teaspoon turmeric

2 teaspoons ground cumin

2 teaspoons sweet paprika

¼ teaspoon cinnamon

1 head butter lettuce and leaves separated for wraps

OPTIONAL INGREDIENTS:

pinch of red pepper flakes

1 cup sliced cucumber

1 cup chopped tomato

¼ cup chopped parsley

1 lemon, cut into wedges

CILANTRO GARLIC OIL

SERVES 8

¼ cup extra-virgin olive oil

¼ cup chopped cilantro

1 garlic clove

1 tablespoon fresh squeezed lemon juice, about ½ lemon

salt and pepper, to taste

PREPARATION:

1. Place chicken in Crock-Pot with onions and garlic.

2. Whisk chicken broth, lemon juice, zest, pepper, salt, turmeric, cumin, paprika, and cinnamon.

3. Pour liquids and spices over the chicken and cook on low for 6 hours. Can be left to warm after cooking.

4. Blend all ingredients for Cilantro Garlic Oil together until smooth.

5. Serve in lettuce cups or bowls like a stew. Drizzle each bowl or cup with 1 tablespoon Cilantro Garlic Oil and sprinkle with optional desired toppings.

NUTRITIONAL INFORMATION PER SERVING FOR SHAWARMA: 191.7 calories, 28.1g protein, 5.1g carbohydrates, 1.6g fiber, 0.3g sugar, 6.2g fat, 1.7g saturated fat, 115.8mg cholesterol, 407.1mg sodium

NUTRITIONAL INFORMATION PER SERVING FOR CILANTRO GARLIC OIL: 122.5 calories, 14g protein, 2.6g carbohydrates, 0.8g fiber, 0.2g sugar, 3.1g fat, 0.9g saturated fat, 57.9mg cholesterol, 203.0mg sodium

Zesty Crock-Pot Bison

PREPARATION:

1. Combine all in Crock-Pot and cook on low for 6 to 8 hours.

2. Shred beef. Adjust cinnamon, salt, and pepper to taste.

   NOTE: This recipe is delicious served with Cauliflower Rice Pilaf (page 187) or Zoodles (page 203).

(page 187) or Zoodles (page 203)

SERVES 6

INGREDIENTS:

1 pound beef or bison, free range, all natural

1 sweet onion, peeled and cut in quarters

4 carrots, peeled and quartered

2 sweet potatoes, quarterd

2 rutabaga, peeled and quartered

1 celery root, peeled and cut in quarters

5 garlic cloves, peeled and smashed

8 sage leaves, roughly chopped

1 tablespoon fresh or 1 teaspoon dried thyme leaves

1 teaspoon dried rosemary, crushed

1 cup beef broth

1 to 2 teaspoons salt as desired

1 teaspoon pepper

NUTRITIONAL INFORMATION PER SERVING: 282.5 calories, 37.3g protein, 10.1g carbohydrates, 1.4g fiber, 3.6g sugar, 9.4g fat, 3.7g saturated fat, 100.9mg cholesterol, 86.0mg sodium

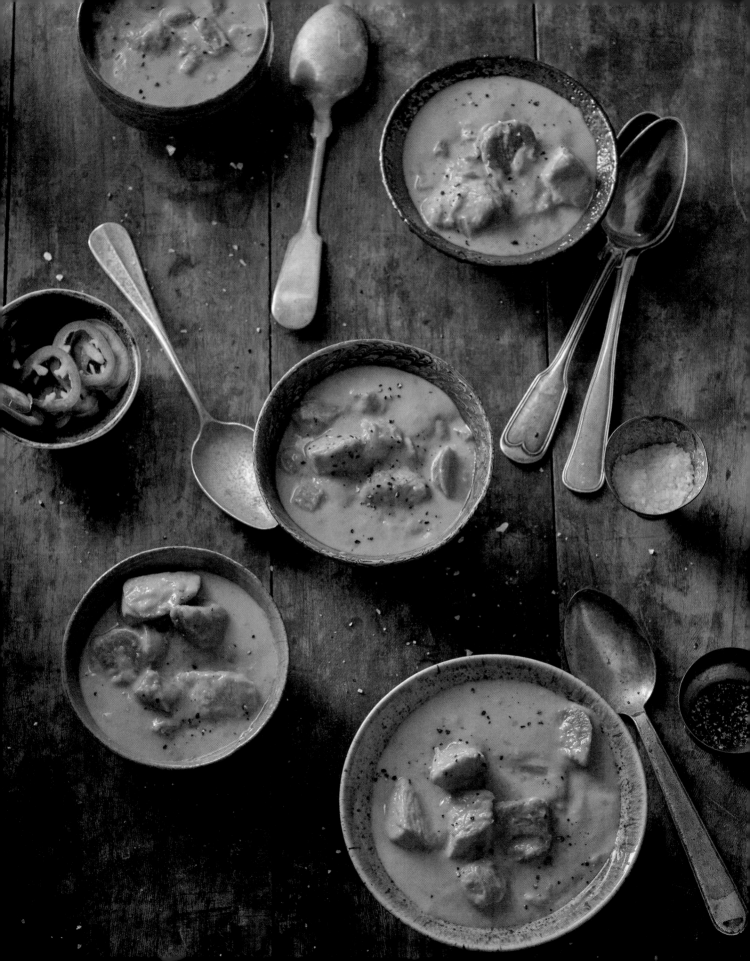

Chicken Yam Chowder

PREPARATION:

1. In a large pot, heat oil over medium heat and cook chicken until white on all sides and cooked through. Remove from pan and set aside.

2. Add onions, carrots, and celery over medium-high heat until they are soft.

3. Add the yams and chicken broth. Bring to a boil and simmer until they are tender, 15 to 20 minutes.

4. Remove half the broth and vegetables and put in a blender. Puree till smooth, and return to the pot.

5. Add the chicken and the coconut milk, and bring to a simmer. If the soup is too thick, add more broth or water to get your desired consistency.

6. Season with salt and pepper.

7. Ladle into tureens and top with jalapeño if desired.

SERVES 6

INGREDIENTS:

1 tablespoon coconut oil

1 pound boneless, skinless chicken breasts, cut into 1-inch strips

1 cup chopped onions

1 cup chopped carrots

1 cup chopped celery stalks

3 cups yams or sweet potatoes, chopped into 1-inch pieces

3 cups low-sodium chicken broth or bone broth (page 89)

1 (13½-ounce) can coconut milk

salt and pepper

OPTIONAL INGREDIENT:

1 jalapeño, seeds removed, chopped

NUTRITIONAL INFORMATION PER SERVING: 241.0 calories, 19.1g protein, 24.6g carbohydrates, 4.0g fiber, 2.0g sugar, 7.8g fat, 8.1g saturated fat, 46.0mg cholesterol, 91.0mg sodium

Mushroom Cashew Cream Soup

SERVES 6

INGREDIENTS:

2 tablespoons avocado oil or macadamia nut oil

1 cup chopped onion

1 cup chopped carrots

1 cup chopped celery

4 garlic cloves, chopped

1 pound cremini or white mushrooms, roughly chopped

5 cups low-sodium vegetable broth or bone broth (page 89)

½ teaspoon dried thyme

¾ cup raw cashews

salt and pepper, to taste

PREPARATION:

1. In a large pot, heat oil and sauté the onions, carrots, and celery till soft.

2. Add the garlic and half the mushrooms, and sauté for 3 to 4 minutes.

3. Add the broth, thyme, and cashews, and simmer for 20 to 30 minutes.

4. Puree the soup in a high-powered blender until smooth. Add more broth if you need to thin it.

5. Return the soup to the pot and add the remaining mushrooms. Bring to a boil, then simmer till mushrooms are cooked. Season with salt and pepper to taste.

NUTRITIONAL INFORMATION PER SERVING: 259.0 calories, 2.4g protein, 17.4g carbohydrates, 3.1g fiber, 3.9g sugar, 18.0g fat, 0.5g saturated fat, 124.0mg cholesterol, 124.0mg sodium

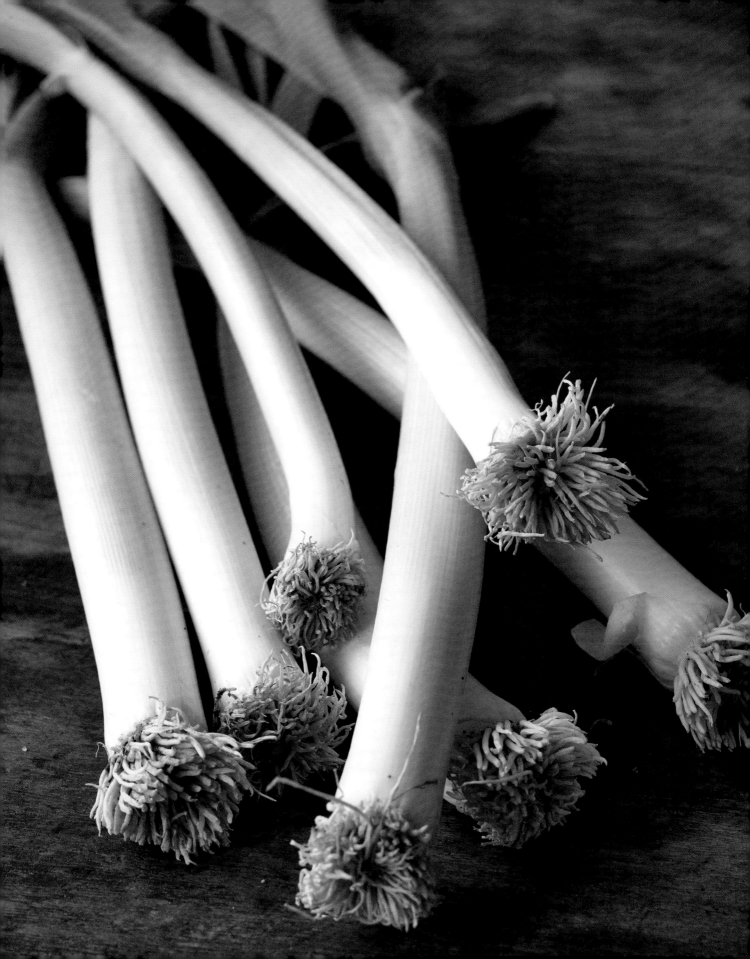

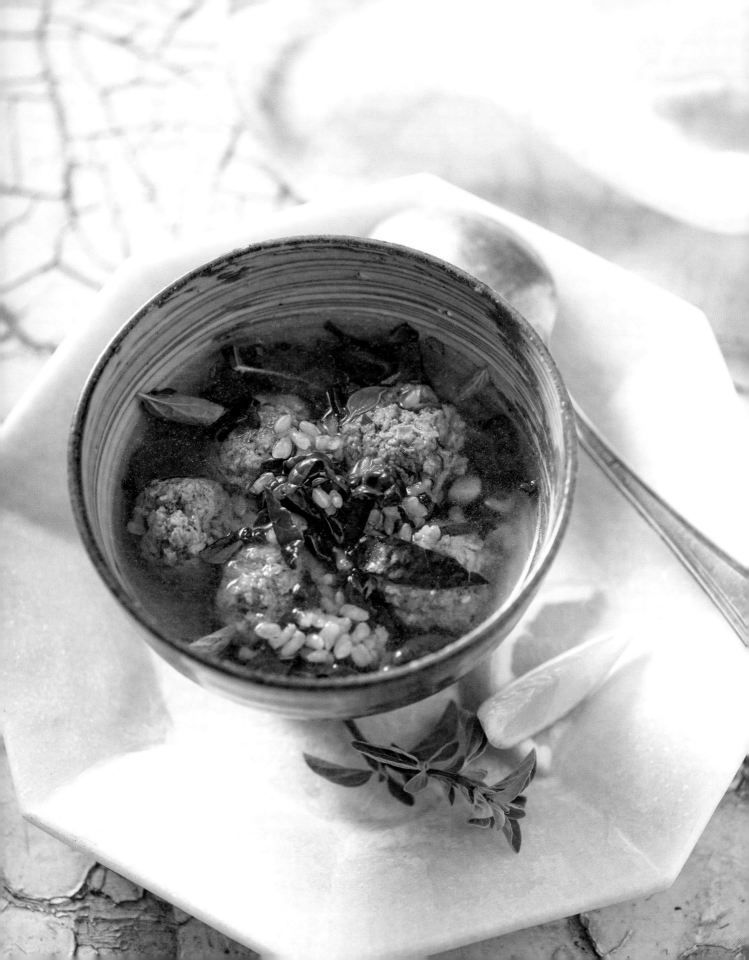

Peppy Meatball Soup

PREPARATION:

1. In a large pot, bring the broth to a boil and reduce to a simmer.

2. Mix meatball ingredients together and form into small bite-sized meatballs.

3. Place the meatballs in the pot with broth and simmer until cooked through, 6 to 7 minutes.

4. Add the kale, lemon juice, oregano, and rice if desired, and simmer until the kale is wilted, a couple of minutes.

5. Season to taste with salt and pepper.

6. Ladle into soup tureens and serve hot.

SERVES 8

INGREDIENTS:

MEATBALLS:
1 pound ground turkey

1 teaspoon fresh oregano, finely chopped, or ½ teaspoon dried

½ onion, grated

zest of one lemon

2 garlic cloves, minced

2 tablespoons parsley, chopped

SOUP:
8 cups low-sodium chicken broth or bone broth (page 89)

2 cups finely chopped kale, thick stems removed (about 1 bunch)

4 tablespoons fresh squeezed lemon juice, about 2 lemons

2 teaspoons fresh oregano, chopped, or ½ teaspoon dried

½ teaspoon salt

pepper, to taste

OPTIONAL INGREDIENT:
1 cup cooked brown rice

NUTRITIONAL INFORMATION PER SERVING: 108.0 calories, 12.9g protein, 5.0g carbohydrates, 1.1g fiber, 1.6g sugar, 4.7g fat, 2.1g saturated fat, 45.0mg cholesterol, 187.0mg sodium

Cream of Asparagus Soup

SERVES 6

INGREDIENTS:

1 pound asparagus

1 to 2 tablespoons ghee or coconut oil

½ onion, peeled and diced

¼ cup chopped celery

1 tablespoon arrowroot, rice flour, or any gluten-free flour dissolved in water

3 cups low-sodium vegetable or chicken broth

salt and pepper, to taste

1 teaspoon dried or 1 tablespoon fresh chopped tarragon

OPTIONAL INGREDIENTS:

1 leek, chopped, white and light green parts only

2 tablespoons full-fat coconut milk

PREPARATION:

1. Cut off asparagus tips and reserve. Discard tough ends (the last two inches) and chop remaining stems into 2-inch segments.

2. In medium-sized soup pot, heat ghee or oil. Sauté onions, celery, leeks, and asparagus stems over medium heat for about 5 minutes.

3. Add arrowroot and stir until well blended. Stir continuously for about 1 minute more.

4. Transfer vegetable mixture to a blender. Add about 1 cup stock (enough to help mixture blend easily). Blend well and transfer back to pot.

5. Add remaining stock to pot gradually, stirring out any lumps. Bring soup to a boil, then reduce heat and simmer until the soup is smooth and thickened, 30 to 40 minutes. Stir frequently.

6. Add coconut milk, if desired, for a creamy consistency. Add salt and pepper to taste.

7. Add asparagus tips to soup and simmer 5 to 10 minutes. Add tarragon for flavor and garnish with a sprig of fresh tarragon if desired.

8. Serve warm.

NUTRITIONAL INFORMATION PER SERVING: 80.0 calories, 3.0g protein, 10.0g carbohydrates, 2.0g fiber, 0.0g sugar, 4.0g fat, 1.0g saturated fat, 0.0mg cholesterol, 84.0mg sodium

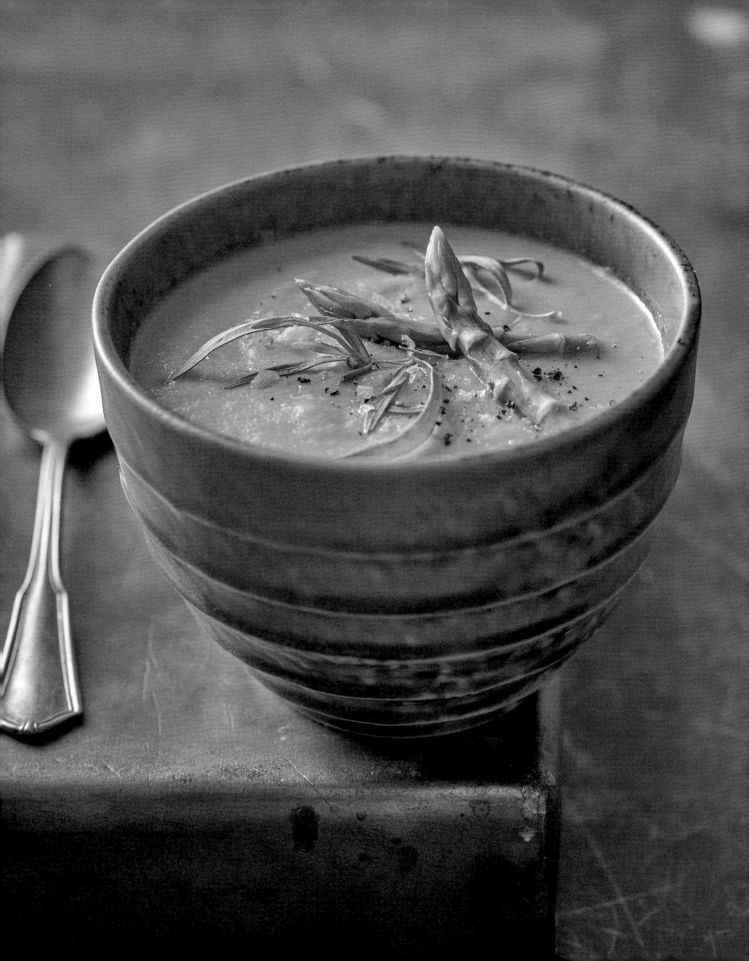

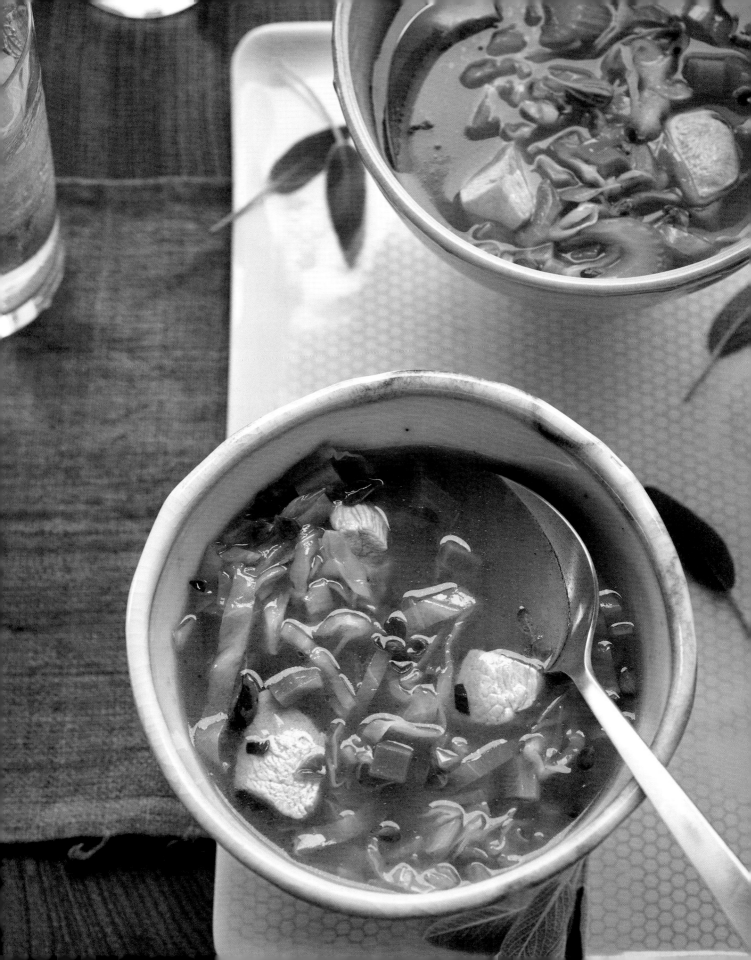

Healing Chicken Herb Soup

PREPARATION:

1. Dice chicken.

2. In large pot, heat oil over medium-high heat. Add garlic, celery, onion, and carrot and sauté for 2 to 3 minutes, stirring frequently.

3. Add chicken and cook for 4 more minutes.

4. Stir in water, vegetable broth, onion powder, marjoram, and sage. Bring to a boil, reduce heat, and simmer for 15 to 20 minutes.

5. Add cabbage and simmer for 5 minutes. Season with salt and pepper as desired.

6. Ladle into soup bowls and top with parsley. Serve hot.

SERVES 6

INGREDIENTS:

8 ounces chicken breast

2 tablespoons coconut oil or macadamia nut oil

2 garlic cloves, minced

2 celery stalks, sliced

½ sweet onion, diced

1 carrot, peeled and diced

1 cup water

5 cups low-sodium vegetable broth or bone broth (page 89)

1 teaspoon onion powder

½ teaspoon dried marjoram or 1 tablespoon fresh

½ teaspoon dried sage or 1 tablespoon fresh

1½ cups shredded green cabbage

salt and pepper, to taste

OPTIONAL INGREDIENT:

2 tablespoons fresh chopped parsley or 2 teaspoons dried parsley

NUTRITIONAL INFORMATION PER SERVING: 158.9 calories, 11.2g protein, 16.0g carbohydrates, 4.9g fiber, 3.7g sugar, 6.4g fat, 4.5g saturated fat, 21.7mg cholesterol, 135.0mg sodium

Lentil Vegetable Soup

INGREDIENTS:

¼ cup low-sodium vegetable broth or 1 tablespoon coconut oil for sautéing

4 celery stalks, cut into ½-inch pieces

1 carrot, cut into ½-inch pieces

1 red bell pepper, chopped

2 onions, chopped

2 garlic cloves, minced

6 cups water

6 cups no-salt-added vegetable broth or bone broth (page 89)

2 cups red lentils

¼ cup brown rice

½ teaspoon curry powder

½ teaspoon ground cumin

1 tablespoon lemon pepper

1 teaspoon pepper

1 tablespoon fresh lemon juice

OPTIONAL INGREDIENTS:

1 tablespoon fresh marjoram, finely chopped

1 tablespoon fresh sage, finely chopped

1 teaspoon garlic salt or to taste

This is an Amen household favorite on cool winter nights. It's simple and filling.

PREPARATION:

1. In a large soup pot, heat vegetable broth or coconut oil. Sauté celery, carrot, bell pepper, onion, and garlic for about 5 minutes.

2. Add water and vegetable broth or bone broth to pot. Stir in lentils and rice. Cover and bring to a boil. Reduce heat and simmer, stirring occasionally, for about 25 minutes.

3. Stir in curry, cumin, lemon pepper, pepper, and herbs and garlic salt if desired. Simmer uncovered for about 20 minutes, or until lentils fall apart and mixture thickens.

4. Stir in lemon juice.

5. Ladle soup into bowls and serve hot.

   NOTE: To make this a complete meal, consider adding some diced chicken or turkey. Vegetarians can add a bit of organic tofu.

NUTRITIONAL INFORMATION PER SERVING: 245.0 calories, 14.4g protein, 41.4g carbohydrates, 8.9g fiber, 5.5g sugar, 3.1g fat, 1.6g saturated fat, 0.0mg cholesterol, 787.0mg sodium

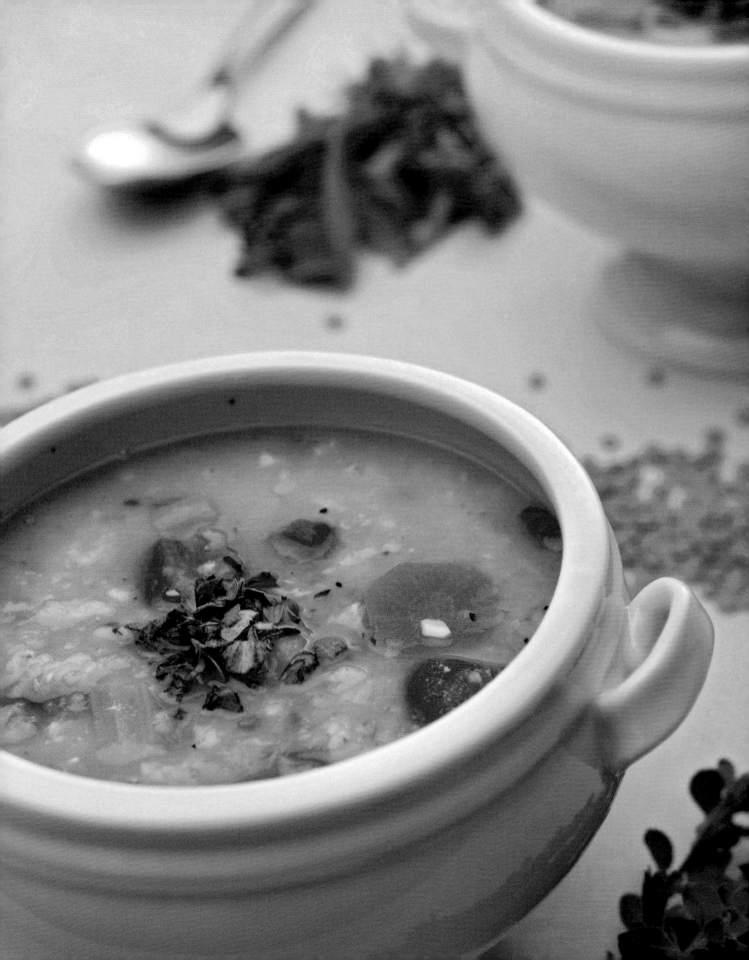

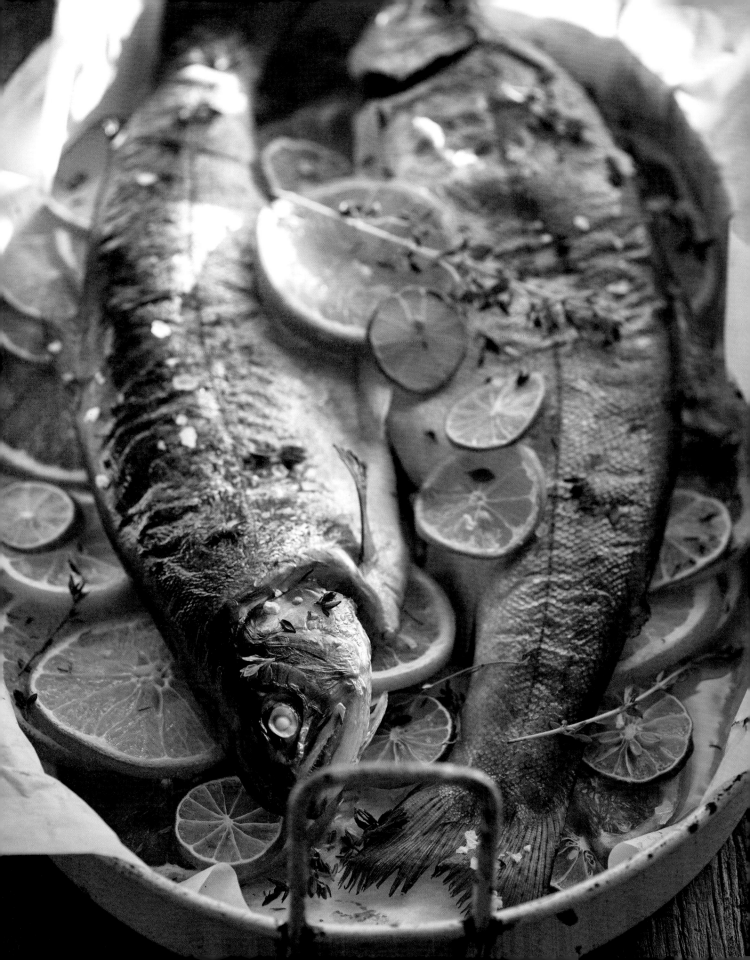

From the Sea

∎

It all begins and ends in your mind. What you give power
to has power over you if you allow it.

—LEON BROWN

People who eat fish at least once a week have larger brains and more activity in the frontal lobes, according to a study by Cyrus Raji from UCLA. When it comes to the brain, size matters! With a healthy brain come better decisions and a better life, as well as less risk of Alzheimer's disease. But knowing which seafood is healthiest to eat can be tricky these days, as it changes with current events from radiation levels to environmental contamination. Seafoodwatch.org is a wonderful website that is kept up-to-date with the healthiest fish for you as well as what is best for the environment. The recipes in this book are based on the best current seafood choices.

It's important to choose line-caught seafood when possible. However, many sustainable, responsible farms are following new protocols that actually make their fish safer than those caught in the wild in some cases, as a result of environmental pollution. Also, some of these farms work responsibly to protect the environment and natural resources. For a complete list go to seafoodwatch.org.

Brain Warrior
Fresh Fish Strategies

1. Purchase fresh fish from a reputable source.

2. Make sure flesh is moist and bright, not dull and dry when purchasing, and doesn't smell overly fishy.

3. Cook as soon as possible. Freeze uncooked portions. Store cooked seafood in airtight containers, but do not freeze cooked seafood.

4. Make use of leftovers within two days of cooking.

5. Leftovers: Flake salmon for salmon salad. Shellfish is great in omelets. Whitefish is perfect for fish tacos.

■

Fresh and Tangy Trout

PREPARATION:

1. Preheat oven to 400 degrees F and line a baking sheet with parchment paper. Use enough paper to wrap around the fish and make a fold. Place fish fillets on parchment paper.

2. Cut grapefruit or one orange in half. Lightly squeeze juice from half grapefruit or one orange onto both sides of fish. Spread garlic evenly over fillets, add salt and pepper as desired and top with whole thyme sprigs.

3. Thinly slice the remaining grapefruit or orange and spread evenly over fish fillets, covering the thyme.

4. Fold parchment paper over fish and wrap the edges over itself a couple of times. If you prefer your fish crisper on the surface, skip covering with parchment paper. The paper keeps it moist and from drying out.

5. Bake for 10 to 12 minutes depending on desired doneness.

6. Remove from paper and serve with a large salad or sweet potatoes.

SERVES 4

INGREDIENTS:
4 (6-ounce) trout fillets
1 sweet Ruby Red grapefruit (use 1½ oranges if grapefruit isn't in season)
salt and pepper to taste
12 stems fresh thyme

OPTIONAL INGREDIENT:
2 garlic cloves, minced

NUTRITIONAL INFORMATION PER SERVING: 277.9 calories, 39.2g protein, 5.6g carbohydrates, 0.1g fiber, 5.0g sugar, 9.9g fat, 2.8g saturated fat, 117.3mg cholesterol, 95.2mg sodium

Creamy Pesto Halibut

SERVES 4

FOR CREAMY PESTO:
¼ cup walnuts

1 teaspoon minced garlic

1 cup fresh or ⅓ cup dried basil leaves

½ cup spinach leaves

1 tablespoon olive oil

¼ to ⅓ cup almond milk or ½ cup coconut milk

zest of 1 lemon

FOR FISH:
1 teaspoon ghee, macadamia nut oil, or coconut oil

4 (4-ounce) wild halibut fillets

2 tablespoons fresh squeezed lemon juice, about 1 lemon

OPTIONAL INGREDIENTS:
¼ teaspoon salt

pepper, to taste

PREPARATION FOR CREAMY PESTO :

1. In a food processor or blender, place walnuts, garlic, basil, and spinach and blend for 30 seconds.

2. Add olive oil, milk, and lemon zest and blend. Set aside.

PREPARATION FOR FISH:

1. Heat ghee or oil in large sauté pan over medium heat and sear halibut fillets on one side until a golden crust forms and the fish is done on the bottom, 1 to 2 minutes. Gently turn the fish and cover to finish cooking through, about 2 minutes. The fish is ready when it starts to flake.

2. While fish is cooking, in separate small saucepan, warm Creamy Pesto on medium-low heat and reserve until fish is cooked.

3. Place a fillet on each plate, drizzle with lemon and spread the pesto on top (about 2 tablespoons per dish).

NUTRITIONAL INFORMATION PER SERVING: 269.2 calories, 25.6g protein, 2.7g carbohydrates, 1.5g fiber, 0.4g sugar, 17.3g fat, 2.6g saturated fat, 47.8mg cholesterol, 74.9mg sodium

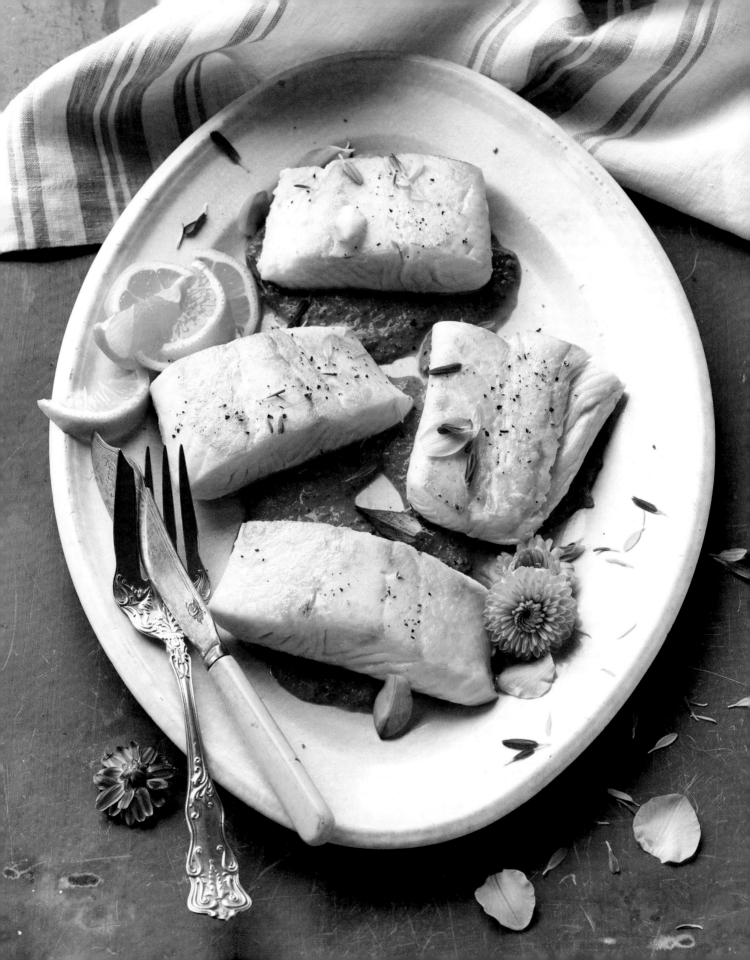

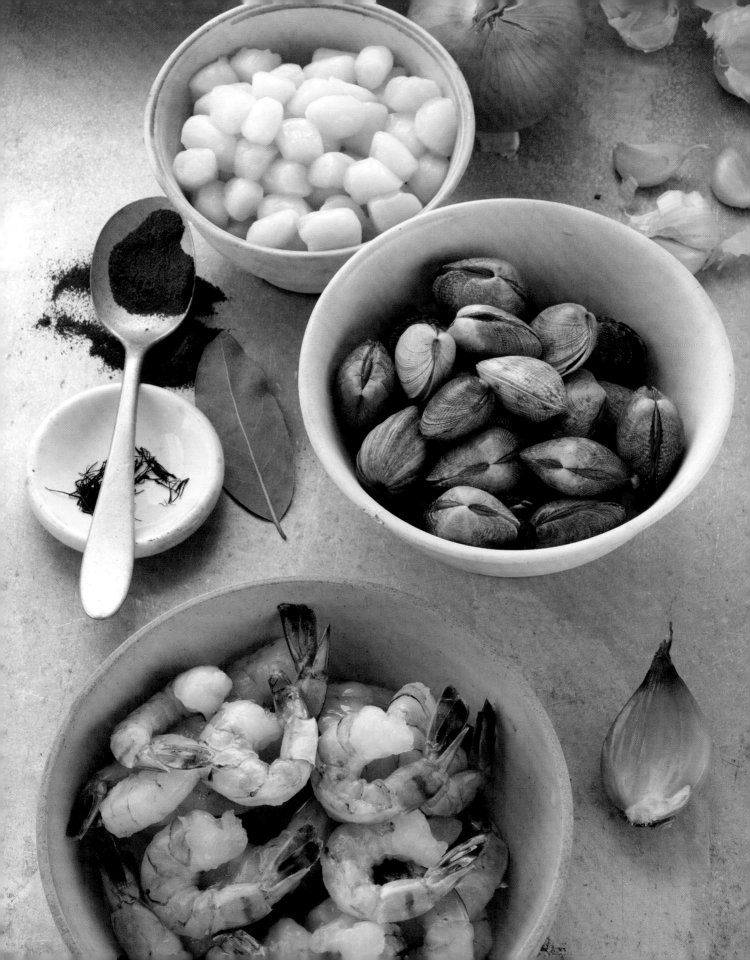

Curried Saffron Bouillabaisse

PREPARATION:

1. Heat ghee or oil in a large, deep pan over medium heat. Sauté onions and garlic for 3 to 5 minutes, until soft.

2. Add the curry paste and stir for another minute.

3. Stir in tomatoes and vegetable broth and bring to a light boil. Add saffron, ginger, and chili powder, if desired.

4. Reduce heat to simmer and add fish. Gently stir and turn fish after a couple of minutes. Cook fish for 5 to 7 minutes, until fish is no longer opaque and flakes easily.

5. Ladle into bowls and serve hot.

> **NOTE:** Get creative and add shrimp, scallops, or fresh fish of your choosing.

SERVES 4

INGREDIENTS:

1 tablespoon ghee or macadamia nut oil

1 large onion, chopped

2 garlic cloves, chopped

1 to 2 tablespoons red curry paste, gluten free (Thai Kitchen brand is decent)

2 ripe tomatoes or 1 (15-ounce) can tomatoes, diced

1 cup low-sodium vegetable broth or bone broth (page 89)

1 pound halibut or other whitefish fillet, skinned and cut into chunks

OPTIONAL INGREDIENTS:

pinch of saffron threads (use a bit less curry paste if adding saffron)

1 teaspoon grated fresh ginger

1 teaspoon chili powder

NUTRITIONAL INFORMATION PER SERVING: 227.0 calories, 30.9g protein, 7.7g carbohydrates, 0.9g fiber, 0.3g sugar, 7.2g fat, 4.2g saturated fat, 54.7mg cholesterol, 328mg sodium

Prosciutto Maple Salmon

SERVES 2

INGREDIENTS:

2 (4- to 6-ounce) salmon fillets

salt and pepper, to taste

2 slices of uncured prosciutto or ham

1 tablespoon ghee, macadamia nut oil, or coconut oil

1 tablespoon maple syrup

"Uncured" meat simply means it doesn't contain sodium nitrate. Unfortunately it's a bit misleading, as many forms of meat still require some form of "curing" in spite of eliminating the sodium nitrate. Ham, bacon, and lunch meat are examples of meat that still requires "curing" in some form. That form is typically through the use of salt—lots of salt—and spices. Be cautious if you're on a low-sodium diet, and read labels.

PREPARATION:

1. You may use the oven or cook in a pan. For oven-baked option, preheat oven to 375 degrees F.

2. Rinse salmon and pat dry with paper towels. Season with salt and pepper.

3. Wrap salmon in prosciutto or ham.

4. Heat oil in medium pan on medium-high heat. Place fillets in oven-safe pan and cook for about 2 minutes on each side until ham is light golden brown.

5. Brush both sides with maple syrup before transferring to the oven. Transfer the entire pan to the oven with the fish. Bake for 5 to 10 minutes depending on preferred doneness.

6. If you prefer to panfry, simply turn heat down to medium and turn the fish every minute or two for 5 to 7 minutes depending on preferred doneness.

7. Remove from oven or pan. Add salt and pepper to taste. Serve hot.

> **NOTE:** *Pan roasting* refers to a cooking technique in which meat, poultry, or fish is seared at higher temperatures in a pan prior to being transferred to the oven. Not only does it seal in juices, but this technique also reduces cooking time.

NUTRITIONAL INFORMATION PER SERVING: 171.8 calories, 11.3g protein, 4.4g carbohydrates, 0.0g fiber, 3.0g sugar, 12.3g fat, 6.8g saturated fat, 43.3mg cholesterol, 744.2mg sodium

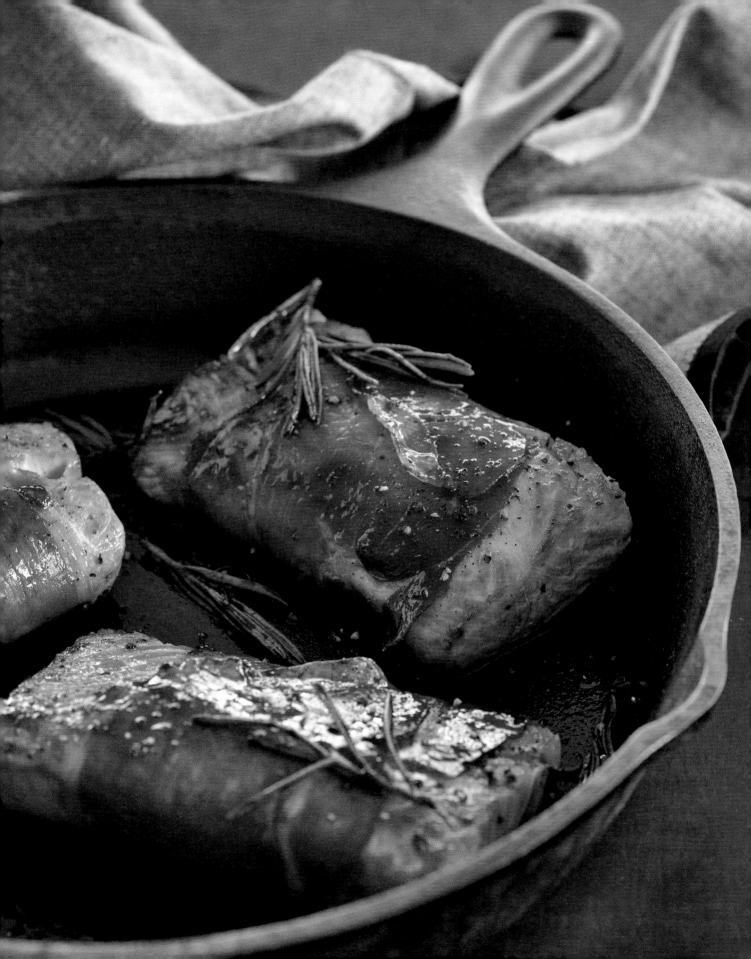

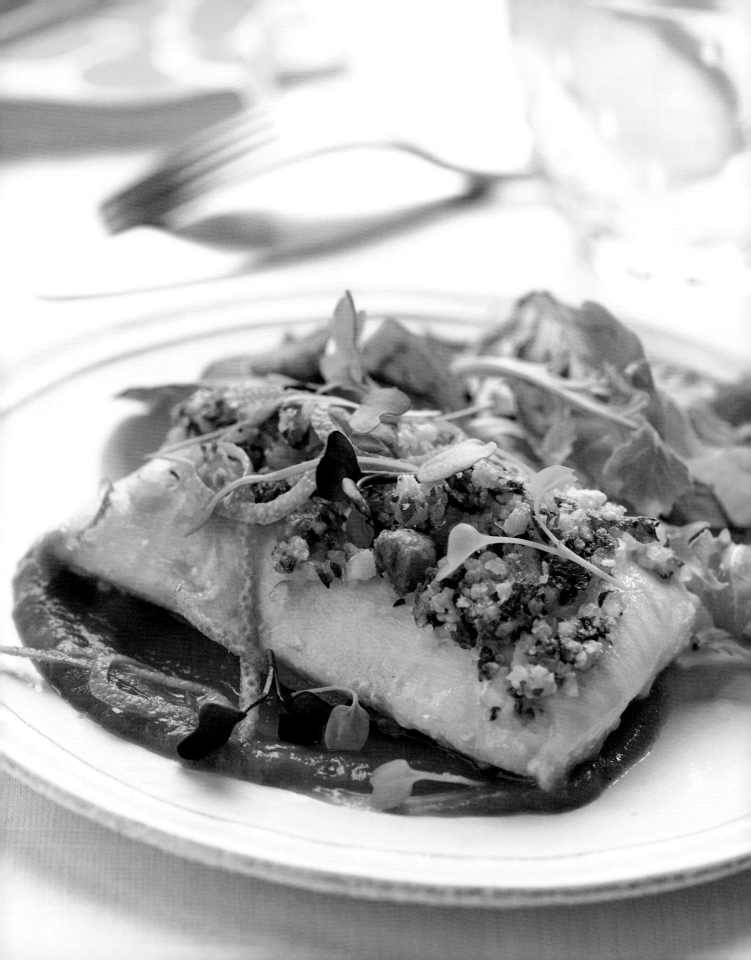

Macadamia-Crusted Mahimahi

The herb-infused crust make this dish heavenly. Have some fun and try using different blends of herbs. Marjoram, cilantro, and even mint add extraordinary flavor. For summer parties, I use edible flowers to garnish the plates. They're beautiful and delicious!

PREPARATION:

1. Heat oven to 375 degrees F.

2. In a food processor, pulse macadamia nuts, garlic, herbs, and orange zest to create a crumble topping. You want a fine crumbly consistency, but not mushy.

3. Place the fish on a baking sheet lined with parchment paper. Top the fillets equally with the macadamia and herb crumble. Refrigerate until ready to bake.

4. Optional (not necessary, but delicious): Put broth in a medium saucepan and bring to a boil. Reduce heat to medium. Reduce vegetable broth until it is similar in consistency to light gravy. It will actually become glazelike. This may take 20 to 30 minutes. Keep warm.

5. Bake for 8 to 12 minutes depending on desired doneness, or until it flakes easily.

> **NOTE:** This recipe is great served over Butternut Squash Puree (page 183).

SERVES 4

INGREDIENTS:
2 tablespoons chopped macadamia nuts

1 tablespoon minced garlic

1 tablespoon fresh oregano,

1 tablespoon fresh basil

1 tablespoon orange zest

4 (4-ounce) wild mahimahi fillets

salt and pepper, to taste

OPTIONAL INGREDIENTS:
4 cups vegetable broth for glaze drizzle

1 tablespoon fresh cilantro or other favorite herb

NUTRITIONAL INFORMATION PER SERVING: 149.3 calories, 20.8g protein, 2.8g carbohydrates, 1.6g fiber, 0.4g sugar, 6.6g fat, 0.9g saturated fat, 80.0mg cholesterol, 95.7mg sodium

Kickin' Popcorn Shrimp

SERVES 6

INGREDIENTS:

POPCORN SHRIMP:
½ cup coconut oil for frying

4 eggs

6 to 6½ tablespoons Kickin' Chili Spice Blend (see below)

¾ cup almond flour

1 pound small shrimp, peeled and deveined

KICKIN' CHILI SPICE BLEND:
3 tablespoons garlic powder

1 tablespoon paprika

4 teaspoons onion powder

1 teaspoon cayenne pepper

1 teaspoon chili powder

2 teaspoons salt

OPTIONAL INGREDIENTS FOR KICKIN' CHILI SPICE BLEND:
1 teaspoon your favorite dried herbs, such as oregano, basil, etc.

NUTRITIONAL INFORMATION PER SERVING: 348.2 calories, 19.3g protein, 2.8g carbohydrates, 1.5g fiber, 0.7g sugar, 29.0g fat, 17.3g saturated fat, 195.3mg cholesterol, 592.0mg sodium

The kids in our family love helping in the kitchen when they hear we're having popcorn shrimp! There's something fun about it. I'm not sure if it's the name, the preparation or the taste, but it's always a great time. However, one word of caution: The oil gets very hot and can splatter. Avoid having little faces near the hot pan while the shrimp is cooking.

PREPARATION:

1. Prepare work space. Line a large plate or baking sheet with several layers of paper towels and set aside. Put coconut oil in a large pan and have it ready to go, but don't turn on heat yet.

2. Place eggs in a large bowl and whisk thoroughly.

3. In another large bowl, mix Kickin' Chili Spice Blend and flour thoroughly.

4. When you have egg and flour mixtures ready, heat the oil in the pan over medium-high heat. Make sure it is hot when you put the shrimp in, but don't leave the pan unattended for long. Hot oil can burn quickly.

5. Drop about six shrimp into the beaten eggs and toss until each shrimp is completely coated in the egg mixture.

6. Remove shrimp from egg mixture and place into the seasoning bowl. Coat the shrimp completely with the flour and spice mixture.

7. Remove shrimp from flour mixture and place in the hot oil. Fry until lightly golden. Don't stir shrimp. Allow to sit in oil for a minute or so before turning with a spatula; otherwise, the breading will crumble. For small shrimp cooking time will be less. Remove the shrimp with a slotted spoon and place on the plate or baking sheet with paper towels to absorb the excess oil. Repeat for the rest of the shrimp batch. If oil gets thick from flour mixture, clear it out and start with fresh oil. Allow shrimp to cool for several minutes before serving. Serve with Zesty Aioli Dip (page 242) or chipotle-flavored Vegenaise brand vegan mayo.

PREPARATION FOR KICKIN' CHILI SPICE BLEND:
Mix all spices and desired herbs well and set aside until ready to use.

> **NOTE:** For a baked variation of this recipe, preheat oven to 350 degrees F and bake for about two to three minutes on each side. Sometimes I will turn the oven to low broil for just a minute to give it a crispy texture.

> **NOTE:** For low-sodium diet, cut Kickin' Chili Spice Blend or replace salt with substitute.

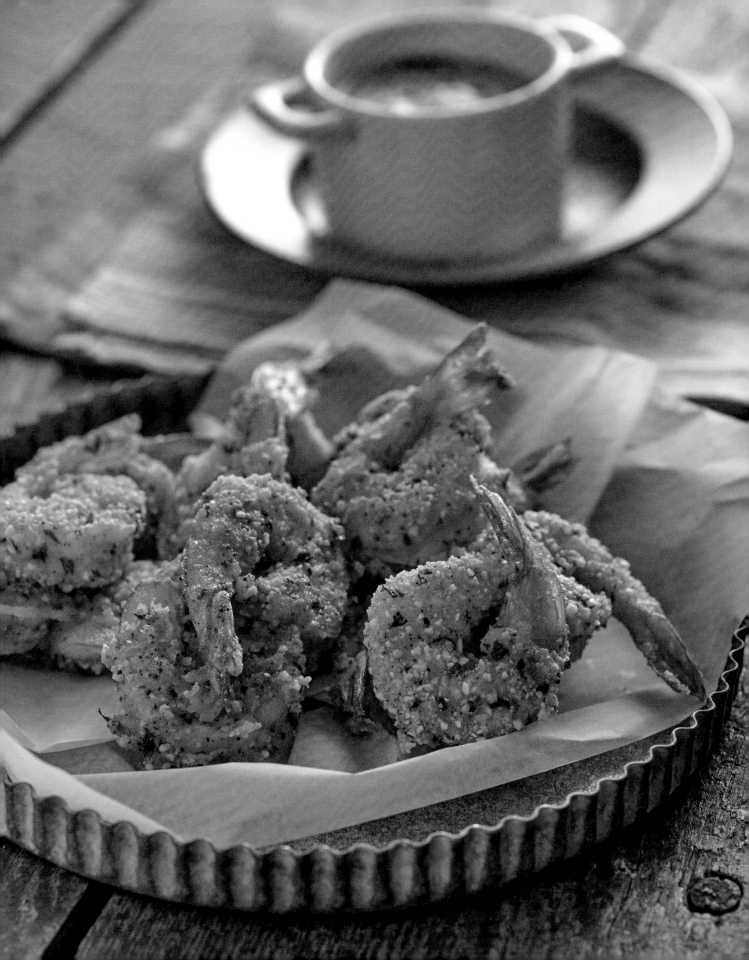

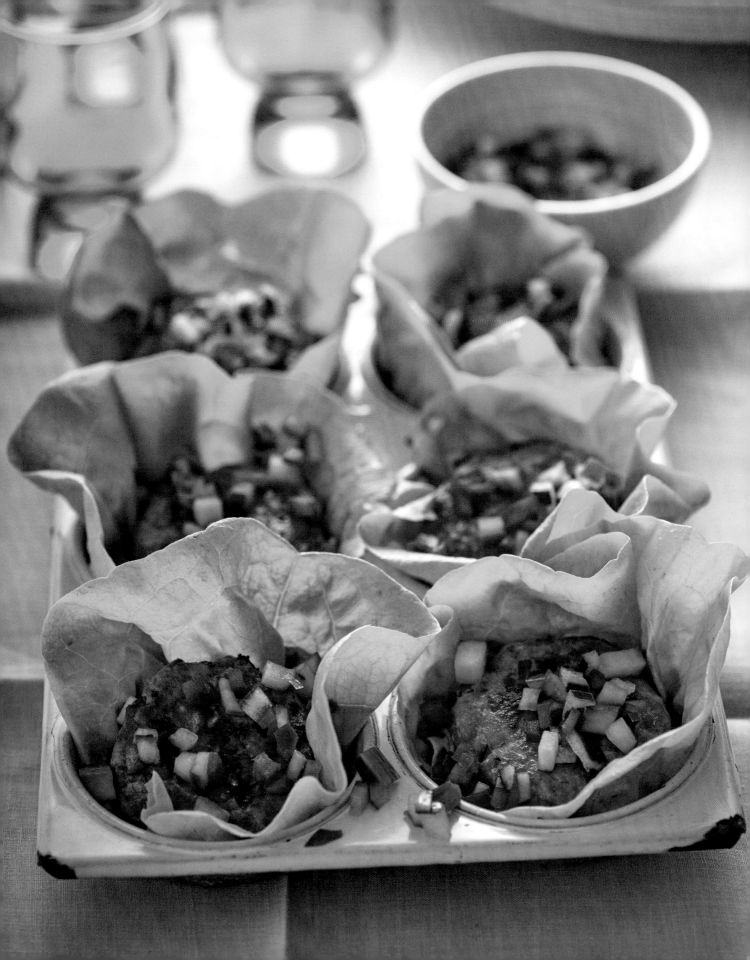

Salmon Sliders

1. To make the light relish, whisk together the vinegar, honey, and salt. Toss with ¼ cup of the onion, ¼ cup of the pepper, and the cucumbers. Place in refrigerator to chill.

2. Place the salmon and the remaining ¼ cup onion and ¼ cup peppers in a food processor and pulse till chopped fine. Add the tamari sauce and pulse again 1 or 2 times. With wet hands remove the mixture from the bowl and make into 8 small slider patties.

3. Heat coconut oil in a sauté pan over medium-high heat. Add the salmon sliders, browning on both sides till cooked through.

4. Place the sliders on lettuce wraps and top with the relish.

NOTE: Curry-flavored coconut wraps are a delicious alternative to lettuce wraps.

SERVES 4 (8 SLIDERS)

INGREDIENTS:

2 tablespoons apple cider vinegar

1 teaspoon raw honey

½ teaspoon salt

½ cup chopped red onion, divided

½ cup chopped red bell pepper, divided

½ cup chopped Persian or hothouse cucumbers

1 pound wild salmon, skin removed, cut into large chunks

2 tablespoons low-sodium tamari sauce

1 tablespoon coconut oil

1 head butter lettuce, leaves separated for wraps

NUTRITIONAL INFORMATION PER SERVING: 111.1 calories, 12.5g protein, 1.7g carbohydrates, 0.3g fiber, 0.9g sugar, 5.8g fat, 2.1g saturated fat, 33.8mg cholesterol, 297.9mg sodium

Lemon Garlic Shrimp
with Noodles

SERVES 4

INGREDIENTS:

SHRIMP:
1 pound shrimp, peeled and deveined

1 to 2 teaspoons minced garlic

1 tablespoon minced fresh parsley or 1 teaspoon dried cilantro

1 teaspoon lemon zest

salt and pepper, to taste

1 tablespoon coconut oil

CREAMY NOODLES:
4 packages shirataki noodles, fettuccine-style (Miracle Noodle brand), or 1 8-ounce box quinoa pasta (corn free)

1 tablespoon coconut oil

1 tablespoon minced white onions

2 teaspoons minced garlic

1 tablespoon arrowroot, rice flour, or other gluten-free flour

1⅓ cups full-fat coconut milk (or a little less plain almond milk)

1 to 2 teaspoons lemon zest (as desired)

1 teaspoon salt

pepper, to taste

OPTIONAL INGREDIENT:
1½ tablespoons fresh minced parsley or cilantro

NUTRITIONAL INFORMATION PER SERVING FOR SHRIMP:
109.9 calories, 18.0g protein, 0.1g carbohydrates, 0.1g fiber, 0.0g sugar, 4.4g fat, 2.9g saturated fat, 165.0mg cholesterol, 550.6mg sodium

NUTRITIONAL INFORMATION PER SERVING FOR QUINOA NOODLES:
186.2 calories, 2.8g protein, 8.2g carbohydrates, 3.2g fiber, 0.3g sugar, 16.2g fat, 11.9g saturated fat, 0.0mg cholesterol, 53.9mg sodium

This recipe is a crowd pleaser, and so simple. Using shirataki noodles makes this dish totally guilt free! If you haven't used shirataki noodles, the preparation may seem a bit different. They come packed in water and "ready to go," so the package amounts are deceptive. Also, there are virtually no digestible calories in shirataki noodles. They are primarily fiber, so they make a great filler. It takes about four packages of shirataki noodles to equal about one eight-ounce package of quinoa pasta after the liquid has been drained. If you choose quinoa pasta, remember that pasta is a "condiment." Even though quinoa pasta is gluten free, it is carbohydrate heavy.

PREPARATION:

1. In large bowl, toss shrimp, garlic, the parsley or cilantro, lemon zest, salt, and pepper. Set aside until ready to sauté.

2. Drain shirataki noodles from solution and boil in medium to large pot of water for about 3 minutes. Leave in water and set aside. If you're using quinoa pasta, prepare according to instructions. While noodles are boiling, prepare sauce.

3. In medium saucepan, add coconut oil and, over medium heat, sauté onions. Add garlic and continue to sauté 15 seconds.

4. Add arrowroot and whisk 30 seconds to create a light sauce and prevent clumping. To ensure arrowroot doesn't clump, you can dissolve it ahead of time in a couple of teaspoons of warm water, but don't make it too thin. While whisking, slowly add coconut milk. Simmer sauce for a couple of minutes over low to medium heat, whisking continuously.

5. Add lemon zest, 1 tablespoon of parsley or cilantro if desired, salt, and pepper. Keep warm on low heat. Set cream sauce aside until you're ready to toss with the noodles.

6. In large sauté pan, cook marinated shrimp in coconut oil over medium heat, about 30 seconds to one minute on each side (less or more depending on the size of the shrimp), until they are just pink on each side and starting to curl up.

7. Toss the noodles with the cream sauce and divide among four plates. Top with shrimp and garnish with remaining parsley or cilantro, if desired. Serve warm.

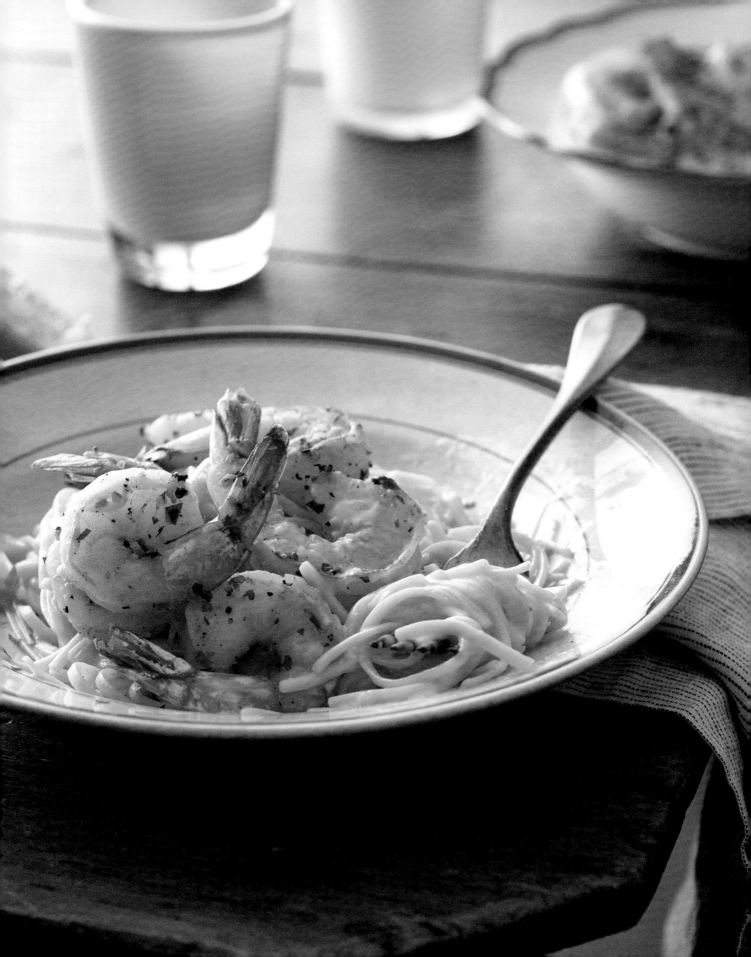

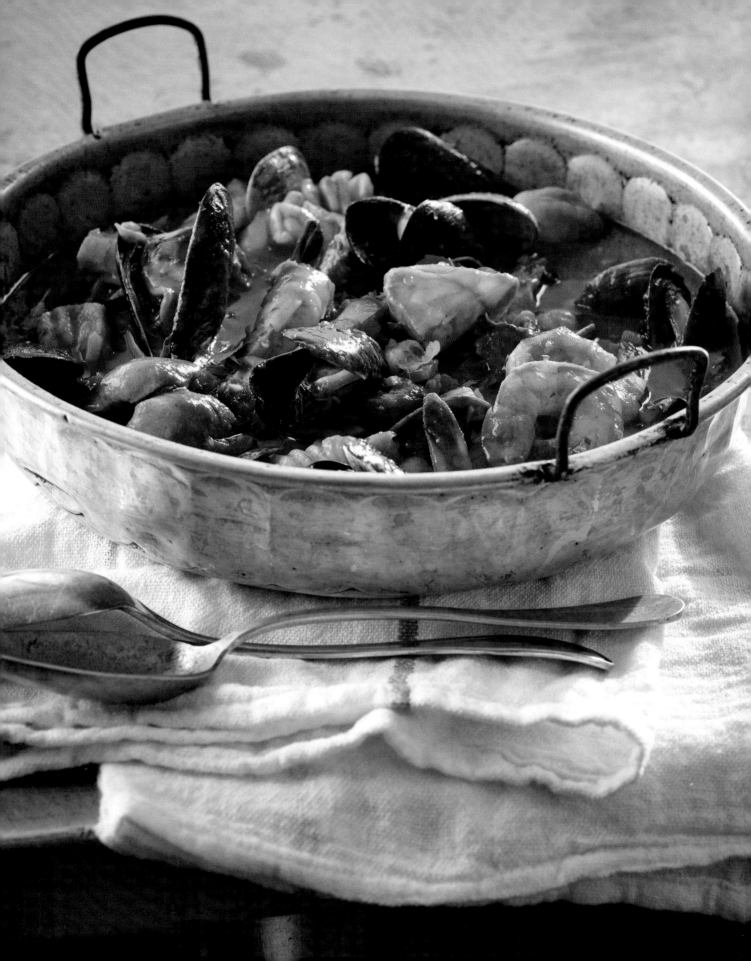

Comforting Fish Stew

1. In a heavy-bottomed pot, heat coconut oil over medium heat. Add onion, celery, shallots, paprika, saffron if desired and bay leaf. Cook for 6 minutes.

2. Add garlic, and cook for 1 more minute.

3. Add tomatoes, tomato sauce, and broth. Bring to a boil. Reduce heat and simmer for 20 minutes.

4. Add the fish, shrimp, clams or mussels, and scallops.

5. Season with salt and pepper. Simmer for 5 minutes or until fish is cooked through and clams open.

6. Sprinkle with parsley if desired, and serve with a large salad and a vegetable dish.

> **NOTE:** For a rich, savory San Francisco–style stew, try blending about ⅓ of the broth and a few chunks of fish in a blender or food processor. Place back in the pot and simmer for 5 minutes.

SERVES 8

INGREDIENTS:
2 tablespoons coconut oil

1 onion, chopped

1 celery stalk, chopped

3 tablespoons chopped shallots

1 teaspoon paprika

1 bay leaf

5 garlic cloves, minced

2½ cups fresh diced tomatoes or 1 (16-ounce) can diced tomatoes with juice, in a pinch

1 (14.5-ounce) can tomato sauce, or fresh (see below) or Simple Fresh Tomato Sauce (page 245)

3 cups vegetable broth or bone broth (page 89)

1 pound firm whitefish (sea bass, halibut, cod), cubed

1 pound large shrimp, peeled and deveined

1 pound clams or mussels

½ pound bay scallops

salt and pepper to taste

OPTIONAL:
pinch of saffron

3 tablespoons chopped parsley

NUTRITIONAL INFORMATION PER SERVING: 327.0 calories, 45.0g protein, 16.0g carbohydrates, 3.0g fiber, 2.6g sugar, 9.0g fat, 4.0g saturated fat, 157.0mg cholesterol, 467.0mg sodium

Curry Shrimp Kebabs

SERVES 4

INGREDIENTS:

1 pound large shrimp, peeled and deveined

1 cup coconut milk

1 tablespoon curry powder

1 tablespoon tomato paste

2 cups cherry tomatoes

½ onion, cut into large chunks

salt and pepper, to taste

½ cup cilantro, chopped

1 lemon, cut in wedges

Marinate for a minimum of 30 minutes, but for best results marinate for 1 hour.

PREPARATION:

1. Place the shrimp in a large self-sealing bag.

2. Stir together the coconut milk, curry powder, and tomato paste. Pour over shrimp and marinate them in the refrigerator for an hour.

3. When shrimp are marinated, preheat grill to medium heat. Place cherry tomatoes and onion pieces on 4 skewers and season with salt and pepper. Divide the shrimp among 4 separate skewers and season with salt and pepper.

4. Vegetables cook slower than shrimp, so put them on the grill 2–3 minutes before putting the shrimp on, depending on desired doneness. Turn several times. Shrimp cooks quickly and should only take 1 or 2 minutes on each side depending on desired doneness and grill temperature. Grill until pink and no longer opaque, but not rubbery.

5. Remove skewers from grill, and divide among 4 plates. Sprinkle cilantro over the top and serve with lemon wedges. This is delicious served with Kale and Quinoa Tabbouleh (page 73)

NUTRITIONAL INFORMATION PER SERVING: 146.9 calories, 19.4g protein, 14.2g carbohydrates, 2.6g fiber, 4.2g sugar, 2.6g fat, 1.3g saturated fat, 165.0mg cholesterol, 583.9mg sodium

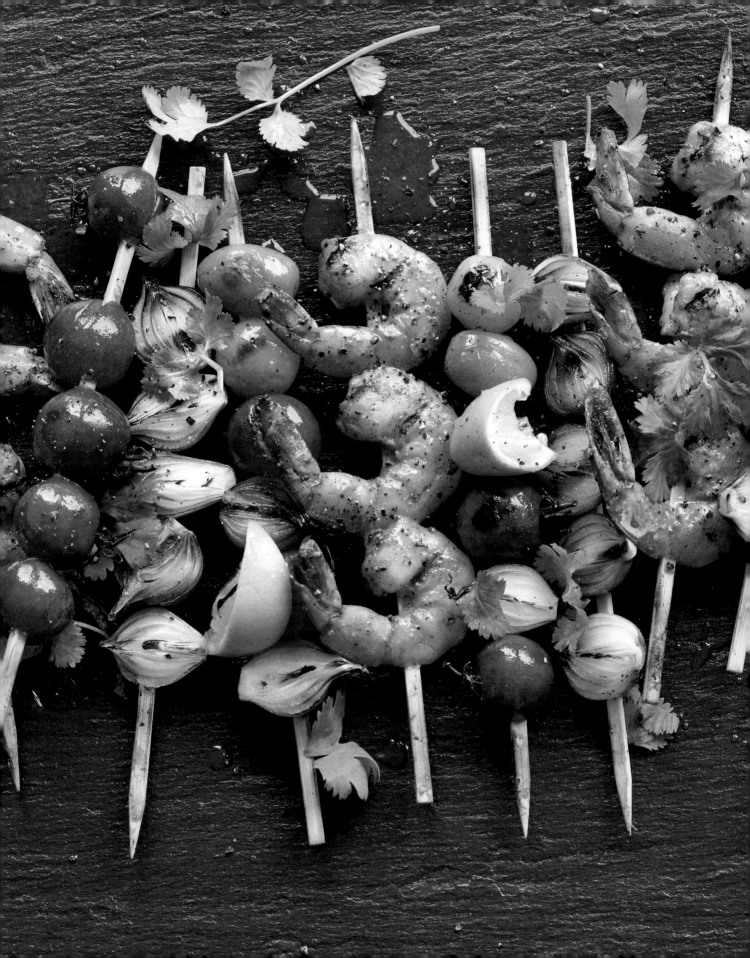

Coconut Cashew Halibut

SERVES 4

INGREDIENTS:

1½ pounds halibut, cut into 4 pieces

salt and pepper, to taste

½ cup finely shredded coconut, unsweetened

½ cup raw cashew pieces, chopped

4 tablespoons coconut oil, divided

PREPARATION:

1. Preheat the oven to 400 degrees F.

2. Rinse fish and pat dry. Season with salt and pepper as desired.

3. Combine the coconut flakes, cashews, and 2 tablespoons of the coconut oil and set aside.

4. Heat the remaining 2 tablespoons coconut oil in a large pan over medium heat. Brown the fish on both sides briefly, then transfer to an oven-safe pan.

5. Divide the coconut mixture evenly, and spread on the tops of each of the fish pieces. Place fish in the oven for 6 to 8 minutes or until cooked through. Cooking time depends on thickness of fish and preferred doneness. If you overcook, the halibut will be dry.

NOTE: Excellent served with Maple-Roasted Brussels Sprouts (page 184).

NUTRITIONAL INFORMATION PER SERVING: 416.1 calories, 18.6g protein, 17.5g carbohydrates, 1.5g fiber, 1.0g sugar, 31.3g fat, 22.0g saturated fat, 23.2mg cholesterol, 114.6mg sodium

Fat Head Fish Sticks

The solid weight of your brain is 60 percent fat. Be happy if someone calls you a fathead! Consuming healthy sources of dietary fat is a critical part of brain health. The fat from fish and plant-based foods that are high in omega-3 fatty acid is the best for brain function. This kid-favorite recipe is a sure way to get your kids to increase their omega-3 fatty acids.

PREPARATION:

1. Place macadamia nuts in a food processor bowl. Grind until nuts are finely chopped, but not to the consistency of flour or meal; mixture should remain coarse. (If you overmix, the natural oils will emerge and the mixture will begin to clump.) Once nuts are finely chopped, place them in a wide, shallow bowl.

2. Mix coconut flour, onion powder, and garlic powder in a separate wide, shallow bowl.

3. In a third bowl, whisk eggs thoroughly.

4. Line bowls up: coconut flour mixture first, then egg, then macadamia nuts.

5. Prepare two baking sheets. Line one baking sheet with parchment paper. Prepare a second sheet with layers of paper towels to place the fish sticks on after cooking. The paper towels will absorb excess oil.

6. Cut halibut into 2-inch strips. Rinse and pat dry with paper towels.

7. Gently place fish strips in coconut flour mixture, lightly dusting on all sides, then dip in egg, covering all sides. Finally, roll in ground macadamia nut and place on baking sheet with parchment paper.

8. When all the fish sticks are prepared, heat 2 tablespoons coconut oil or ghee in large skillet over medium heat. When oil is hot, place fish sticks in skillet and cook for approximately 1 minute on each side. Turn, making sure to cook evenly on all sides. Turn again. Fish sticks should cook for approximately 1½ to 2 minutes per side or until golden brown. Change oil as necessary if solids collect in pan. The thinner the cut of fish, the faster they will cook.

9. Remove fish sticks and place on baking sheet with paper towels to absorb excess oil. Salt and pepper as desired and transfer to serving platter.

SERVES 6

INGREDIENTS:
1 cup macadamia nuts

½ cup coconut flour or almond flour

½ teaspoon onion powder

½ teaspoon garlic powder

2 eggs

1 to 1½ pounds wild halibut or other whitefish, skinned and deboned

½ cup coconut oil or ghee for frying

OPTIONAL INGREDIENT:
½ teaspoon salt
pepper

NUTRITIONAL INFORMATION PER SERVING: 418.7 calories, 16.0g protein, 5.5g carbohydrates, 3.0g fiber, 1.5g sugar, 42.5g fat, 19.4g saturated fat, 77.5mg cholesterol, 51.0mg sodium

Crafty Coconut Shrimp

SERVES 6

INGREDIENTS:

1 pound peeled, deveined extra-jumbo shrimp

1 cup macadamia nuts

1 cup shredded coconut, unsweetened (I like the coarse, long shredded coconut)

¼ cup coconut or almond flour

½ teaspoon onion powder

½ teaspoon garlic powder

2 eggs

3 to 4 tablespoons ghee or coconut oil for frying

OPTIONAL INGREDIENT:

½ teaspoon salt

pepper

This is another kid-friendly favorite I came up with as an alternative to the very unhealthy coconut shrimp recipes served in most restaurants. Because of the coconut and almond meal, coconut shrimp tends to be on the heavy side, so a little goes a long way.

PREPARATION:

1. Rinse shrimp and pat dry with paper towels.

2. Prepare two baking sheets. Line one baking sheet with parchment paper. Prepare second sheet with layers of paper towels to place shrimp on after cooking. The paper towels will absorb excess oil.

3. Place macadamia nuts in a food processor bowl. Grind until nuts are chopped, but not to the consistency of flour or meal; mixture should remain coarse. (If you overmix, the natural oils will emerge and the mixture will begin to clump.) Once nuts are finely chopped, place them in a wide, shallow bowl and mix in coconut. Blend well.

4. In a second wide, shallow bowl, mix coconut flour, onion powder, and garlic powder.

5. In third bowl, whisk eggs thoroughly.

6. Line bowls up: coconut flour mixture first, egg, then the macadamia mixture. One at a time, place each shrimp in coconut flour, lightly coating on all sides. Next, dip shrimp in egg, lightly covering all sides. Add additional egg if necessary. Finally, roll in ground macadamia mixture and place on baking sheet with parchment paper. Do this until all the shrimp are rolled in macadamia nuts and lined up on the parchment paper.

7. In large skillet, heat 2 tablespoons oil or ghee over medium heat. When oil is hot, place shrimp in skillet and cook for approximately 1 minute on each side. Change oil as necessary if solids collect in pan. Turn, making sure to cook evenly on both sides. Turn again. Shrimp should cook for approximately 1½ to 2 minutes per side or until golden brown. The smaller the shrimp, the faster they will cook.

8. Remove shrimp and place on paper towel–lined baking sheet to absorb excess oil. Salt and pepper as desired. Allow to cool for a couple of minutes before serving to children, as the oil gets very hot.

9. Serve this dish with Zesty Aioli Dip (page 242).

> **NOTE:** For a baked variation of this recipe, preheat oven to 350 degrees F and bake for about two to three minutes on each side. Sometimes I will turn the oven to low broil for just a minute to give it a crispy texture.

NUTRITIONAL INFORMATION PER SERVING: 394.0 calories, 11.0g protein, 14.1g carbohydrates, 3.8g fiber, 1.7g sugar, 35.0g fat, 10.7g saturated fat, 110.4mg cholesterol, 190.3mg sodium

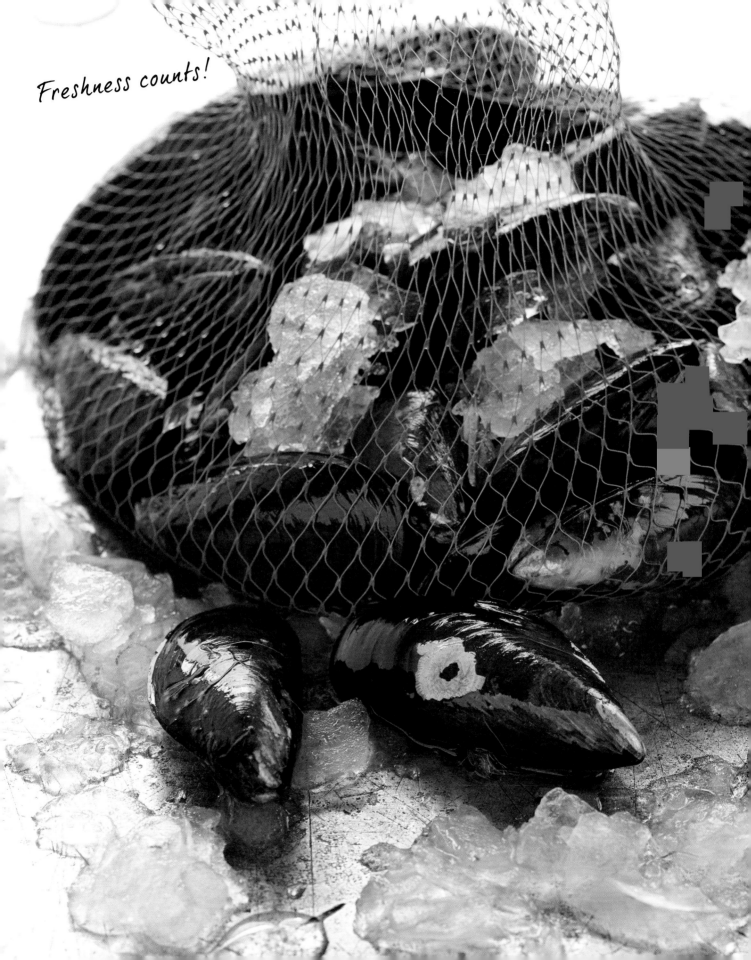
Freshness counts!

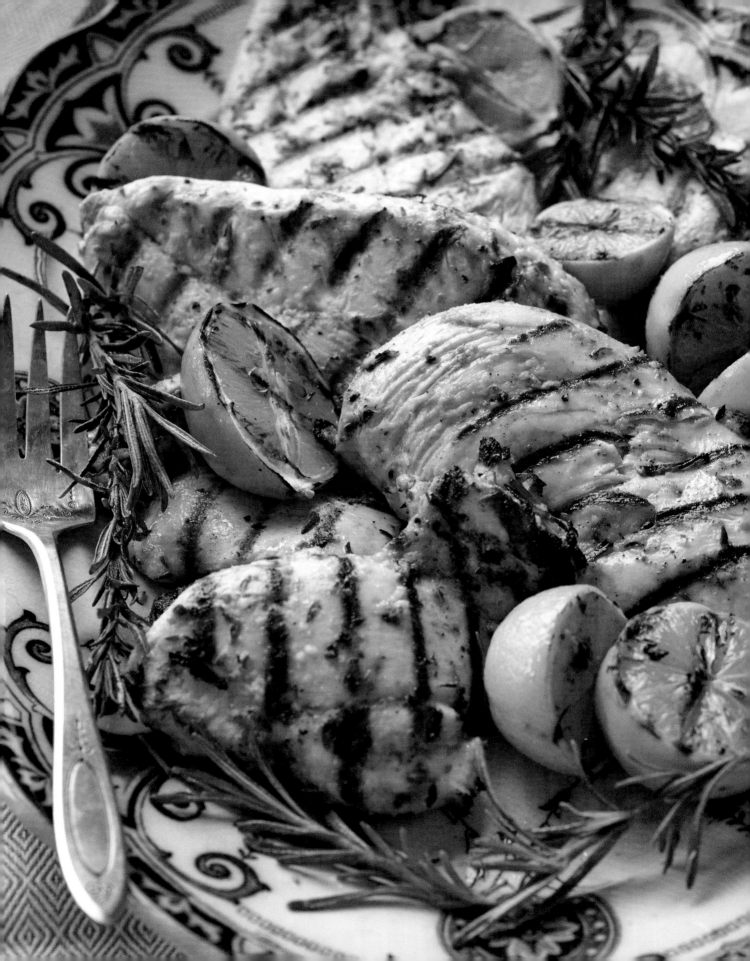

Poultry

■

We are what we repeatedly do. Excellence, therefore, is
not an act but a habit.

—WILL DURANT

When choosing poultry, it's important to choose pasture-raised and
organic, when possible. Yes, it is a bit more expensive, but worth
the effort it may take to be creative with your budget. In this case, quality
is more important than quantity. As a Brain Warrior, protein will no longer
be your staple; it will be your side. So when we tell you the benefits of
purchasing high-quality protein at a higher price, take into account that
you will be eating less protein overall. The budgeting chapter in *The Brain
Warrior's Way* gives detailed suggestions to help you stretch your dollar,
but here are a few additional tips to help boost your budget along with
the quality of your food.

Brain Warrior
Poultry Budgeting Strategies

1. Purchase whole chickens and roast them or cut them yourself.

2. Purchase high-quality chicken on sale and freeze for future use.

3. Leftovers with almost any spices make for great omelets.

4. Diced leftover chicken turns vegetable soup or salad into a hearty meal.

5. Turn leftover chicken into a delicious chicken salad snack by blending meat, Nayonnaise (page 257), and desired spices in a food processor.

■

Shrewd Shepherd's Pie

PREPARATION:

1. Preheat oven to 350 degrees F.

2. Place the yams in a saucepan and add water, just enough to cover the yams, and ½ teaspoon salt if desired, and bring to a boil. Reduce heat to low and cook till soft, 15 to 20 minutes.

3. While yams are cooking, brown the turkey over medium-high heat in a large skillet, season with salt and pepper, and break up the meat into a crumble. Skim the extra fat from the turkey, leaving about 1 to 2 tablespoons.

4. Add carrots, onion, and celery to the meat and cook till tender.

5. In a separate bowl combine the chicken broth, tamari sauce, and the arrowroot powder till well combined. Pour into the turkey and vegetables, and bring back to a boil and cook till the sauce is thick.

6. Add frozen peas to the turkey and vegetables and place in a 4-quart baking dish.

7. When the yams are done, drain off all the water and mash them, season with cinnamon or nutmeg, and salt and pepper to taste. Smooth over the top of the turkey mixture.

8. Bake for 20 minutes. Allow a few minutes for the dish to cool before serving.

SERVES 4

INGREDIENTS:

YAM TOPPING:

2 large yams, peeled and chopped

½ teaspoon salt

½ teaspoon cinnamon or nutmeg

salt and pepper, to taste

FILLING:

1 pound ground turkey

¼ teaspoon pepper

½ cup peeled and chopped carrots

½ cup chopped onion

½ cup chopped celery

1 cup low-sodium chicken broth or bone broth (page 89)

1 tablespoon low-sodium tamari sauce

1 tablespoon arrowroot

1 cup frozen peas

OPTIONAL INGREDIENTS:

½ teaspoon salt (there's a significant amount of salt in broth and tamari sauce)

NUTRITIONAL INFORMATION PER SERVING: 294.0 calories, 26.1g protein, 29.5g carbohydrates, 5.4g fiber, 3.2g sugar, 8.4g fat, 2.7g saturated fat, 81.2mg cholesterol, 305.0mg sodium

Rosemary Thyme Chicken

SERVES 8

INGREDIENTS:

1 tablespoon fresh rosemary, leaves removed from stem

1 tablespoon fresh thyme

1 teaspoon fresh sage

6 garlic cloves, peeled

¼ cup fresh squeezed lemon juice

¼ cup macadamia nut oil or avocado oil

salt, to taste

¼ teaspoon pepper

8 boneless, skinless chicken thighs or breast halves, about 2 pounds

For the tastiest, most tender chicken, I plan ahead for this party favorite and try to marinate the evening before cooking. Marinate for a minimum of 30 minutes, but for best results marinate for 2 to 24 hours.

PREPARATION:

1. Place rosemary, thyme, sage, garlic, lemon juice, and oil in a food processor and set on "chop" until all ingredients are finely minced. If you don't have a food processor, you may chop all ingredients by hand.

2. Transfer mixture to a small mixing bowl and add salt and pepper. Mix well.

3. On a nonporous cutting board, tenderize chicken breasts by lightly pounding them with a meat tenderizer. Do not overpound and make them too thin.

4. Pour marinade mixture into a bowl or baking dish large enough to hold all the chicken. Add the chicken to the mixture, making sure that all chicken is coated with marinade.

5. Cover and refrigerate for 2 hours, up to 24 hours if possible. It will still taste great if you marinate for a shorter period, but the longer the better.

6. Heat grill to medium high.

7. Grill chicken until it is cooked through, turning every two minutes. Cooking time may vary, but is usually 3 to 4 minutes per side. You may use a meat thermometer to test that internal temperature reaches 160 degrees F.

> **NOTE:** Pounding the chicken with a meat tenderizer will help tenderize and infuse the flavor.

> **NOTE:** If you choose to use dried herbs, use 1 teaspoon of dried herbs for each tablespoon of fresh herbs. However, this is one recipe that the flavor will be impacted by not using fresh herbs.

NUTRITIONAL INFORMATION PER SERVING: 148.2 calories, 13.8g protein, 1.6g carbohydrates, 0.2g fiber, 0.2g sugar, 9.7g fat, 1.2g saturated fat, 57.3mg cholesterol, 370.3mg sodium

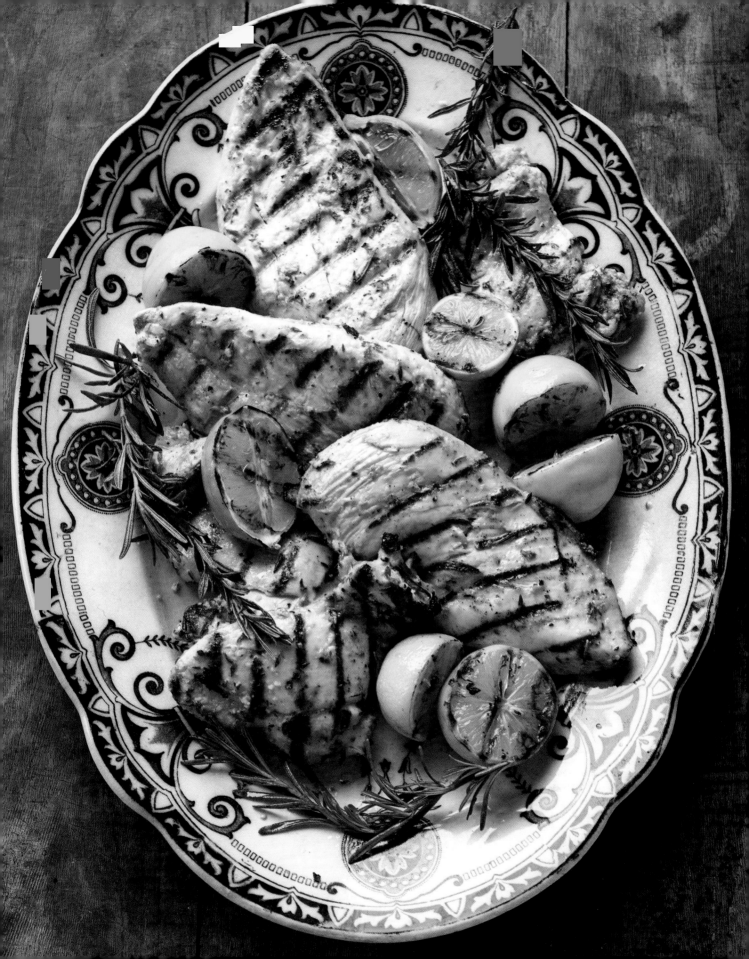

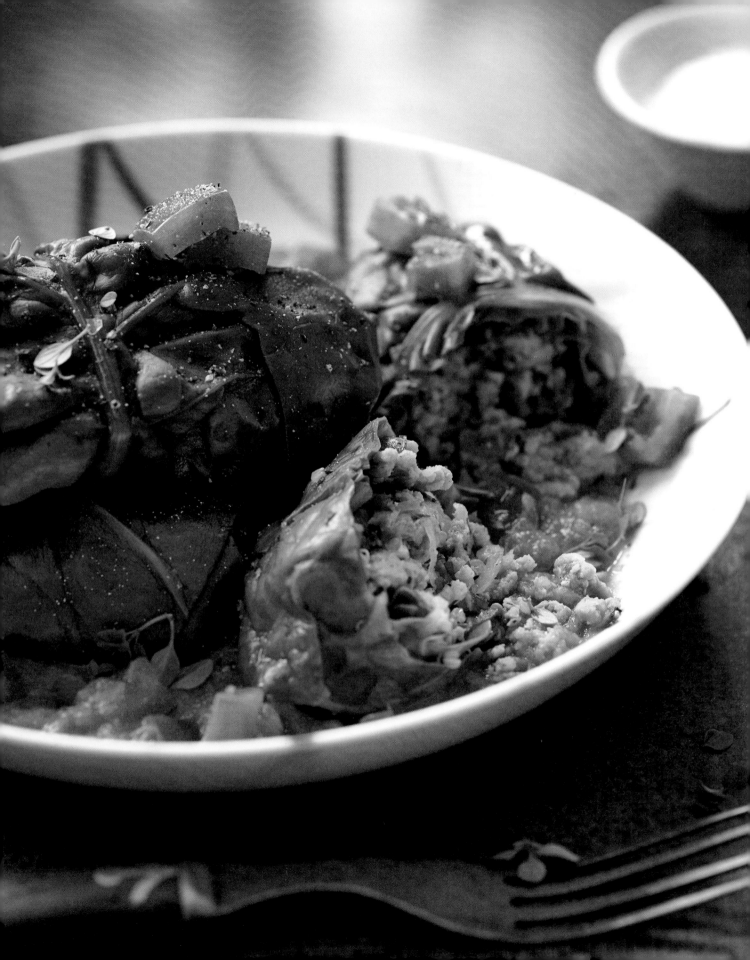

Satisfying Stuffed Chard

PREPARATION:

1. Preheat oven to 400 degrees F, and line a sheet pan with parchment.

2. Toss together the peppers, tomatoes, onion, and garlic with salt and pepper, red pepper flakes if desired, and oil. Spread on the sheet pan, and roast for 20 minutes till soft and slightly browned.

3. Place the roasted vegetables in a blender or food processor with the chicken broth and puree till smooth. Season sauce with salt and pepper to taste.

4. Mix all the ingredients together for the filling.

5. Fill each chard leaf with about ¼ cup filling and roll. Place in baking dish seam side down. Pour sauce over the stuffed leaves, cover with foil, and bake in 400-degree oven for 25 minutes, until the internal temperature is 165 degrees F.

6. Serve warm.

SERVES 4

INGREDIENTS:

SAUCE:
3 red bell peppers, cut into large chunks

2 Roma tomatoes, quartered

½ yellow onion, cut into a few large chunks

3 garlic cloves

salt and pepper, to taste

3 tablespoons macadamia nut oil or avocado oil

½ cup chicken broth or bone broth (page 89)

OPTIONAL INGREDIENT:
pinch of red pepper flakes

FILLING:
1 pound ground turkey

zest of 1 lemon

½ onion, grated

1 garlic clove, minced

3 tablespoons parsley, finely chopped

2 teaspoons fresh thyme

salt and pepper, to taste

½ cup cooked quinoa or brown rice

1 bunch Swiss chard, cleaned and stems removed

NUTRITIONAL INFORMATION PER SERVING: 392.5 calories, 27.6g protein, 28.3g carbohydrates, 4.6g fiber, 6.0g sugar, 20.9g fat, 4.0g saturated fat, 80.6mg cholesterol, 295.0mg sodium

Chicken Thigh "Parmesan" with Spaghetti Squash

SERVES 4

INGREDIENTS:
1 spaghetti squash, quartered, seeds removed

CHICKEN THIGH "PARMESAN":
4 boneless, skinless chicken thighs
½ teaspoon salt
¼ teaspoon pepper
1 cup almond meal
1 teaspoon garlic powder
1 teaspoon onion powder
2 teaspoons Italian seasoning
2 tablespoons nutritional yeast
2 eggs
coconut oil spray

SAUCE:
1 tablespoon olive oil
½ cup chopped onion
2 garlic cloves, minced
1 (28-ounce) can San Marzano crushed tomatoes or 3 large fresh tomatoes
1 tablespoon red wine vinegar
2 tablespoons basil, chopped
salt and pepper, to taste

PREPARATION:

1. Preheat oven to 400 degrees F.

2. Place the quartered squash on a parchment-lined baking sheet and bake till the squash is tender and shreds easily, 40 to 45 minutes. Allow squash to cool, then shred into noodles with fork.

3. Pound chicken thighs to ½ inch thick with a meat tenderizer. Season them with salt and pepper.

4. Combine the almond meal, garlic and onion powders, dried herbs, and nutritional yeast in a shallow bowl.

5. Place the beaten eggs in another shallow bowl, and season with salt and pepper.

6. Dip the chicken in the eggs, then in the almond meal mixture, pressing to coat the thighs.

7. Place the thighs on a parchment-lined sheet pan, sprayed lightly with the coconut oil, and bake for 20 minutes.

8. In a saucepan heat the olive oil, then add the onion and cook till soft, add garlic, and cook for 30 seconds.

9. Add the tomatoes, vinegar, and basil, and simmer for 10 minutes. Season with salt and pepper.

10. Serve chicken thighs over spaghetti squash, then ladle sauce over the dish.

NUTRITIONAL INFORMATION PER SERVING FOR CHICKEN: 388.6 calories, 28.8g protein, 36.1g carbohydrates, 22.1g fiber, 2.3g sugar, 14.1g fat, 9.7g saturated fat, 150.3mg cholesterol, 247.4mg sodium

NUTRITIONAL INFORMATION PER SERVING FOR SAUCE: 75.5 calories, 1.4g protein, 10.3g carbohydrates, 2.4g fiber, 4.0g sugar, 3.4g fat, 0.5g saturated fat, 0.0mg cholesterol, 125.1mg sodium

NUTRITIONAL INFORMATION FOR ½ CUP SPAGHETTI SQUASH: 21.0 calories, 0.5g protein, 5.0g carbohydrates, 1.1g fiber, 2.0g sugar, 0.2g fat, 0.5g saturated fat, 14.0mg sodium

Ginger Chicken Meatballs and Broccoli Pasta with Almond Coconut Sauce

PREPARATION:

1. Preheat oven to 350 degrees F.

2. Combine all meatball ingredients and mix well.

3. Shape into walnut-sized meatballs.

4. Place on a parchment-lined sheet pan and bake for 20 minutes.

5. While meatballs are baking, combine all sauce ingredients in a blender, and blend till smooth. Warm over very low heat until ready to serve. Stir occasionally.

6. For the Broccoli Pasta, bring a large pot of water to boil. Add broccoli slaw and cook for 2 minutes. Drain, and season with salt and pepper to taste.

7. Toss the meatballs with the sauce, and serve over broccoli pasta.

INGREDIENTS:

MEATBALLS:
1 pound ground chicken

1 garlic clove, minced

2 teaspoons minced fresh ginger

1 to 2 tablespoons low-sodium tamari sauce

4 green onions, white and light green parts only, chopped

¼ cup coconut milk

SAUCE:
½ cup almond butter

1 cup coconut milk

juice of 1 lemon

1 tablespoon low-sodium tamari sauce

1 teaspoon sriracha sauce

BROCCOLI PASTA:
4 cups broccoli slaw (shredded broccoli, usually sold preshredded)

salt and pepper, to taste

NUTRITIONAL INFORMATION PER SERVING FOR MEATBALLS:
217.6 calories, 21.7g protein, 3.8g carbohydrates, 0.2g fiber, 2.1g sugar, 13.1g fat, 5.1g saturated fat, 84.4mg cholesterol, 131.25mg sodium (for 1 tablespoon low-sodium tamari sauce)

NUTRITIONAL INFORMATION PER SERVING FOR SAUCE: 209.3 calories, 6.0g protein, 12.1g carbohydrates, 5.3g fiber, 3.5g sugar, 17.3g fat, 2.8g saturated fat, 0.0mg cholesterol, 180.3mg sodium

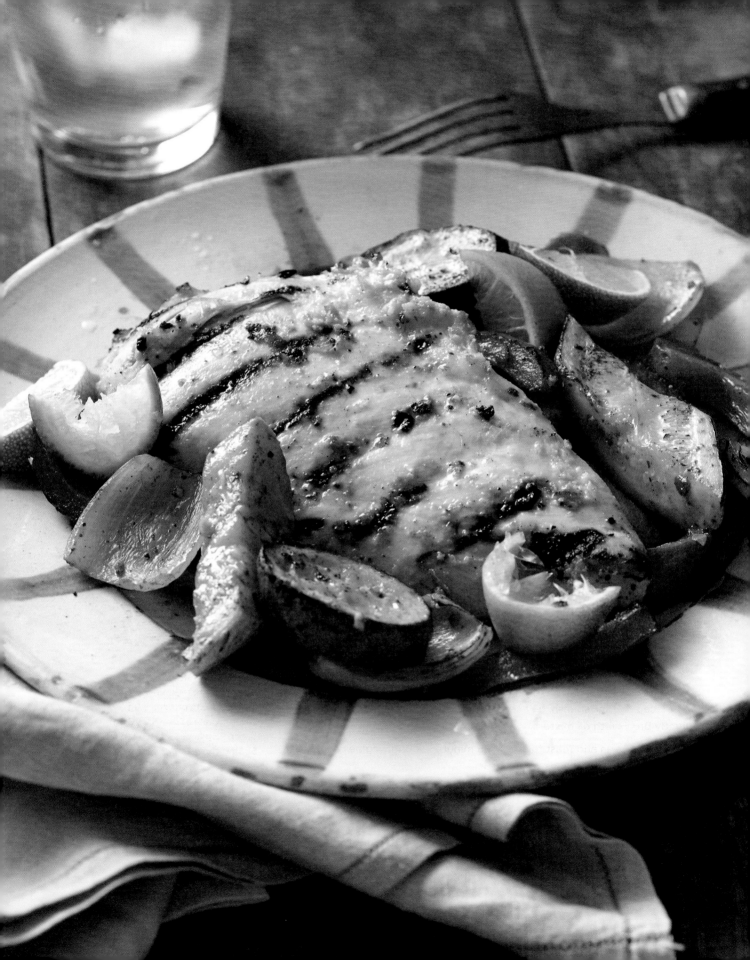

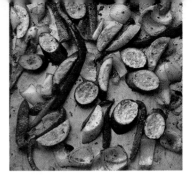

Chicken Asada with Fajita-Style Veggies

Marinate for a minimum of 30 minutes, but for best results, marinate for 2 to 24 hours. Planning ahead and marinating the night before will yield amazingly moist and flavorful chicken.

PREPARATION:

CHICKEN ASADA:

1. For the most tender chicken, lightly pound the chicken on both sides with a meat tenderizer. Be sure to put chicken on nonporous surface and don't overpound or chicken will become mushy.

2. Place all ingredients except chicken in a food processor or blender and run till smooth.

3. Place chicken and marinade in a bowl or self-sealing bag, making sure chicken is covered with marinade, and refrigerate for 2 to 24 hours (minimum of 30 minutes).

4. After chicken has marinated, be sure you prepare the veggies and preheat the oven so veggies and chicken will be finished at about the same time.

5. Heat grill to medium high when ready and grill for 4 to 5 minutes per side. Thighs will cook faster than breasts. You may want to use a meat thermometer to ensure internal temperature is 165 degrees F. Or make a small cut in the thickest piece. Chicken will be white in the center and no longer look opaque or pink when it is cooked.

FAJITA-STYLE ROASTED VEGGIES:

1. Preheat oven to 400 degrees F.

2. In a small bowl mix together oil (may need to be melted), cumin, paprika, chili powder, salt, pepper, and garlic.

3. Place zucchini, squash, bell pepper, and onion on baking sheets and lightly brush with oil mixture.

4. Place in oven and roast for 20 to 25 minutes or until veggies are tender. Be sure to turn vegetables at least once.

5. Remove veggies from oven and serve together, with diced avocado and fresh Restaurant-Style Salsa (page 235).

SERVES 4

INGREDIENTS:

CHICKEN ASADA:
½ cup chopped onion
2 garlic cloves
zest and juice of 1 lime
2 tablespoons olive oil
1 teaspoon salt
½ teaspoon pepper
4 boneless, skinless chicken thighs or breast halves, about 1 pound

OPTIONAL INGREDIENT:
¼ teaspoon cayenne pepper for heat

FAJITA-STYLE VEGGIES:
2 tablespoons macadamia nut oil or melted ghee
½ teaspoon cumin
½ teaspoon paprika
1 teaspoon chili powder
½ teaspoon salt
¼ teaspoon pepper
2 garlic cloves, minced
1 zucchini, sliced
1 yellow squash, sliced
1 red bell pepper, sliced
1 yellow onion, diced large
1 avocado, diced

NUTRITIONAL INFORMATION PER SERVING FOR CHICKEN: 156.7 calories, 14.0g protein, 4.0g carbohydrates, 0.9g fiber, 0.3g sugar, 9.5g fat, 1.6g saturated fat, 57.3mg cholesterol, 99.3mg sodium

NUTRITIONAL INFORMATION PER SERVING FOR VEGETABLES: 97.2 calories, 1.6g protein, 8.5g carbohydrates, 2.4g fiber, 2.2g sugar, 7.4g fat, 1.0g saturated fat, 0.0mg cholesterol, 51.6mg sodium

Mini Turkey Meat Loaves

SERVES 8

(1 LARGE MEAT LOAF OR 4 MINI MEAT LOAVES)

MEAT LOAF INGREDIENTS:

2 pounds ground turkey

3 eggs

1½ cups finely chopped (or pulsed in a food processor) white mushrooms

1 cup grated onion

¼ cup fresh parsley, chopped, or 1 tablespoon dried

¼ cup fresh basil, chopped, or 1 tablespoon dried

2 tablespoons tomato paste

1 tablespoon Dijon mustard

¾ teaspoon salt

¼ teaspoon pepper

SAUCE INGREDIENTS:

4 tablespoons tomato paste

2 tablespoons low-sodium tamari sauce

PREPARATION:

1. Preheat oven to 375 degrees F.

2. Mix all the meat loaf ingredients and shape into 4 mini meat loaves. Place them on a parchment-lined baking sheet, or put into a 9 x 5-inch oiled loaf pan.

3. In a separate bowl, mix together tomato paste and tamari sauce and spread the sauce over the tops of the meat loaves.

4. Bake 4 mini loaves for 30 minutes or large loaf for 1 hour, or until cooked through. Using a meat thermometer, the internal temperature should read 165 degrees F.

5. Allow dish to cool for a few minutes before serving.

> **NOTE:** If you prefer, substitute a jar of your favorite sugar-free, organic pasta sauce instead of the tomato paste and tamari sauce recipe.

NUTRITIONAL INFORMATION PER SERVING: 199.5 calories, 24.8g protein, 2.6g carbohydrates, 0.6g fiber, 0.4g sugar, 9.9g fat, 3.1g saturated fat, 149.8mg cholesterol, 200.8mg sodium

Simple Citrus Chicken

Citrus chicken is an excellent choice to serve at parties due to the mild and universally loved flavor. It's fresh and light, and there are no intense flavors that stand out.

Be sure to use low-sodium tamari sauce and go light with salt when serving this recipe to large groups. Guests on low-sodium diets won't tolerate the excess salt. Tamari sauce may be skipped altogether if necessary.

Marinate for a minimum of 30 minutes, but for best results marinate for 2 to 24 hours. Planning ahead and marinating the night before will yield amazingly moist and flavorful chicken.

PREPARATION:

1. Place chicken on a nonporous surface and pound lightly with meat tenderizer on both sides. Set aside.

2. Place all ingredients except chicken in a food processor or blender. Include garlic if desired. Blend or pulse to a coarse puree to form a marinade.

3. Transfer chicken and marinade into gallon-sized self-sealing bag or baking dish. Cover chicken completely with marinade. If necessary, turn bag, or turn chicken in bowl to be sure all sides have been covered. Refrigerate for 2 to 24 hours (minimum 30 minutes).

4. Preheat grill to medium high or set oven to broil. If broiling, place chicken on broiling pan and put about six inches under broiler heat. Be sure to turn once or twice. Broiling time is 10 to 12 minutes depending on size of chicken pieces. Breasts take longer than thighs. For grilling, be sure to turn every two minutes. Grill for a total of 4 to 5 minutes each side or until internal temperature reaches 165 degrees F.

5. Remove and cover with foil for five minutes before serving.

SERVES 4

INGREDIENTS:

4 chicken breasts, halved, or 8 chicken thighs

¼ cup orange juice or pink grapefruit juice

¼ cup lime juice

¼ cup olive oil

1 to 2 tablespoons low-sodium tamari sauce

1 to 2 teaspoons salt

½ bunch cilantro, finely chopped

OPTIONAL INGREDIENT:
2 garlic cloves, minced

NUTRITIONAL INFORMATION PER SERVING: 304.7 calories, 28.2g protein, 3.0g carbohydrates, 0.1g fiber, 0.2g sugar, 19.7g fat, 3.3g saturated fat, 114.5mg cholesterol, 621.8mg sodium (using 1 teaspoon salt and 1 tablespoon low-sodium tamari sauce)

Turkey-Stuffed Peppers

SERVES 4

INGREDIENTS:

¼ cup extra-virgin olive oil, divided

2 medium onions, finely chopped, divided

6 garlic cloves, divided

1 teaspoon dried Italian seasoning

1 (28-ounce) can San Marzano whole tomatoes

salt and pepper, to taste

1 pound ground turkey

½ cup cooked quinoa or brown rice (according to package)

1 tablespoon crushed red pepper flakes

2 teaspoons dried marjoram

4 bell peppers, red and yellow

¼ cup low-sodium chicken or vegetable broth or bone broth (page 89)

¼ cup canned tomato sauce or Simple Fresh Tomato Sauce (page 245)

PREPARATION:

1. Preheat oven to 375 degrees F.

2. Heat 2 tablespoons of the olive oil in a saucepan over medium-high heat, add half the onion, and cook till soft, then add half the garlic and cook for 30 seconds.

3. Add Italian seasoning and the tomatoes, and simmer for about 20 minutes.

4. Puree the sauce with an immersion blender or in a regular blender. Season to taste with salt and pepper. Set aside.

5. Heat the remaining 2 tablespoons olive oil in a large sauté pan over medium-high heat, add the remaining onion and cook till soft, then add remaining garlic and cook for 30 seconds.

6. Add the ground turkey, breaking it up with a wooden spoon till cooked through. Add the rice or quinoa and 1 cup of the tomato sauce. Season to taste with red pepper flakes and marjoram. Set aside to allow the filling to cool. Cut tops off the bell peppers and remove seeds. Cut a small slice of pepper off the bottom to help them stand up.

7. Stuff the peppers with the filling.

8. Mix broth and canned tomato sauce and pour on the bottom of a baking dish. Place the peppers in the pan and cover with remaining sauce.

9. Cover with foil. Bake for 15 to 20 minutes until peppers are soft.

10. Allow to cool for a few minutes before serving. (Internal temperature will be very hot.)

NOTE: This recipe also tastes great with lamb, bison and grass-fed beef.

NUTRITIONAL INFORMATION PER SERVING: 341.0 calories, 26.2g protein, 26g carbohydrates, 4.7g fiber, 7.0g sugar, 15.9g fat, 3.6g saturated fat, 80.3mg cholesterol, 383.0mg sodium

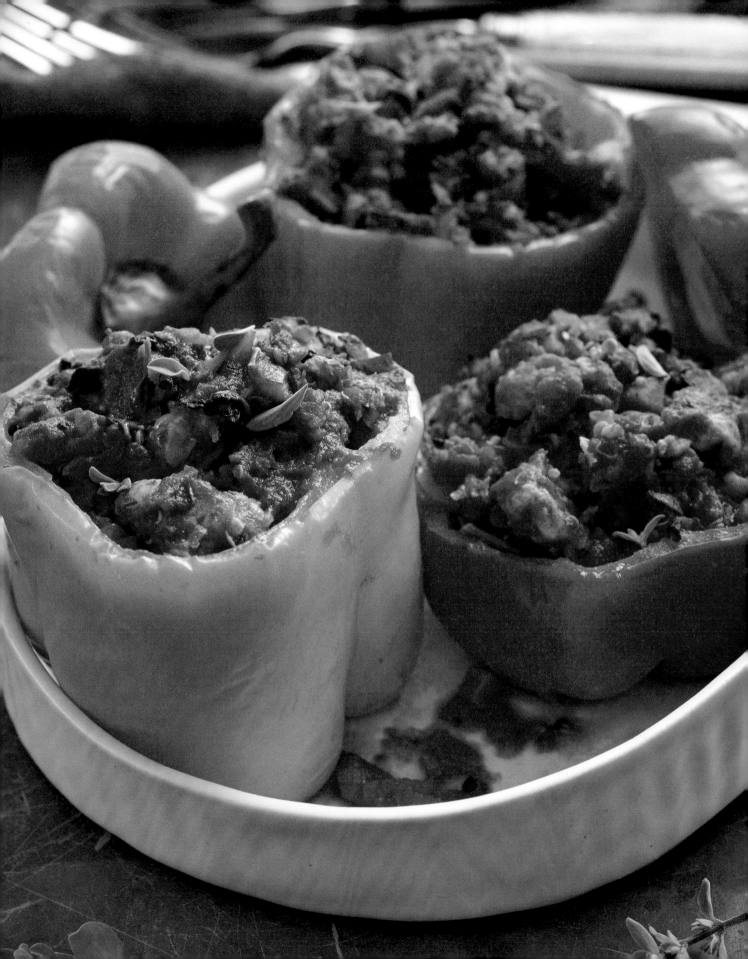

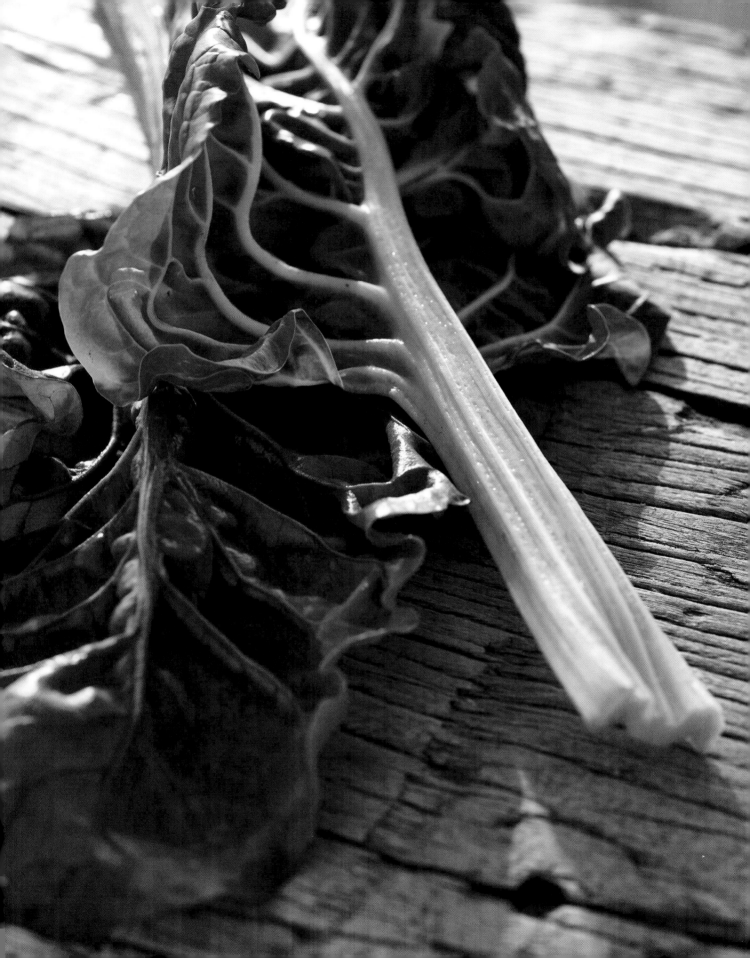

Tomato Basil Chicken Breast Rolls

PREPARATION:

1. Preheat oven to 375 degrees F, and coat a shallow baking dish with coconut oil nonstick cooking spray.

2. Place chicken on nonporous surface and pound to ½-inch thickness with meat tenderizer.

3. Season the chicken with salt and pepper.

4. Evenly divide the spinach, basil, Italian seasoning, and sun-dried tomatoes on top of the chicken pieces. Roll up the chicken, starting at the short end and secure with toothpicks.

5. Beat eggs together in a shallow bowl and season with salt and pepper.

6. Season the almond meal with salt and pepper and place in a separate shallow bowl.

7. Dip the chicken in the eggs, and then roll in the almond meal to coat.

8. Place in the baking dish and bake for 30 minutes or until the internal temperature reaches 165 degrees F.

9. While chicken is cooking, make Simple Fresh Tomato Sauce. The sauce should be a little chunky.

10. Allow chicken to cool, and serve with Simple Fresh Tomato Sauce.

SERVES 6

INGREDIENTS:

coconut oil nonstick cooking spray

1½ pounds boneless chicken breasts or thighs

salt and pepper

½ cup chopped spinach

¼ cup basil, chopped, or 1 tablespoon dried

5 tablespoons Italian seasoning

¼ cup sun-dried tomatoes

2 eggs

1 cup almond meal

Simple Fresh Tomato Sauce (page 245)

NUTRITIONAL INFORMATION PER SERVING, INCLUDING SAUCE: 448.1 calories, 52.3g protein, 14.9g carbohydrates, 7.6g fiber, 1.6g sugar, 22.2g fat, 3.0g saturated fat, 198.4mg cholesterol, 289.5mg sodium

Savory Chicken Masala

SERVES 4

INGREDIENTS:

10 garlic cloves, peeled

½ cup (about 2 ounces) fresh ginger, peeled and chopped

1 (13½-ounce) can coconut milk, divided

1 teaspoon salt

½ teaspoon pepper

1 pound boneless, skinless chicken thighs

2 tablespoons coconut oil or macadamia nut oil

½ onion, chopped

1 jalapeño pepper, minced (add the seeds and ribs if you prefer more heat)

2 tablespoons tomato paste

1½ teaspoons garam masala

2 (14-ounce) cans chopped tomatoes, or 4 cups fresh chopped tomatoes with 1 cup chicken broth

OPTIONAL INGREDIENT:
chopped cilantro, for garnish

Marinate for a minimum of one hour and up to 24 hours.

PREPARATION:

1. Combine the garlic and ginger in a food processor and pulse till smooth.

2. Mix half of the garlic-and-ginger paste, 1 cup coconut milk, salt, and pepper in a self-sealing bag. Add the chicken thighs and marinate in the fridge for at least 1 hour and up to overnight.

3. In a large saucepan over medium-high heat, add the oil, the onion, and the jalapeño pepper, and cook till soft, 2 to 3 minutes.

4. Add the remaining garlic and ginger paste, and cook till fragrant, about 2 minutes.

5. Add the tomato paste and the garam masala, cooking till the tomato paste is a little browned.

6. Add the chopped tomatoes (and broth if you're using fresh tomatoes), stirring to loosen anything stuck on the bottom of the pan. Let the sauce simmer for 10 to 15 minutes.

7. Add in ½ cup coconut milk, stir and continue simmering.

8. Heat your indoor grill pan, or outdoor grill. Remove the chicken from the marinade and grill till cooked through, about 6 minutes per side. Internal temperature should be 165 degrees F with a meat thermometer.

9. Let the chicken cool, dice, and fold into the sauce.

10. Serve over Cauliflower Rice Pilaf (page 187), and garnish with cilantro, if desired.

NOTE: Remember to cut salt in half or eliminate it for low-sodium diet.

NUTRITIONAL INFORMATION PER SERVING: 343.7 calories, 30.3g protein, 22.5g carbohydrates, 1.0g fiber, 3.9g sugar, 15.2g fat, 9.9g saturated fat, 114.5mg cholesterol, 646.8mg sodium

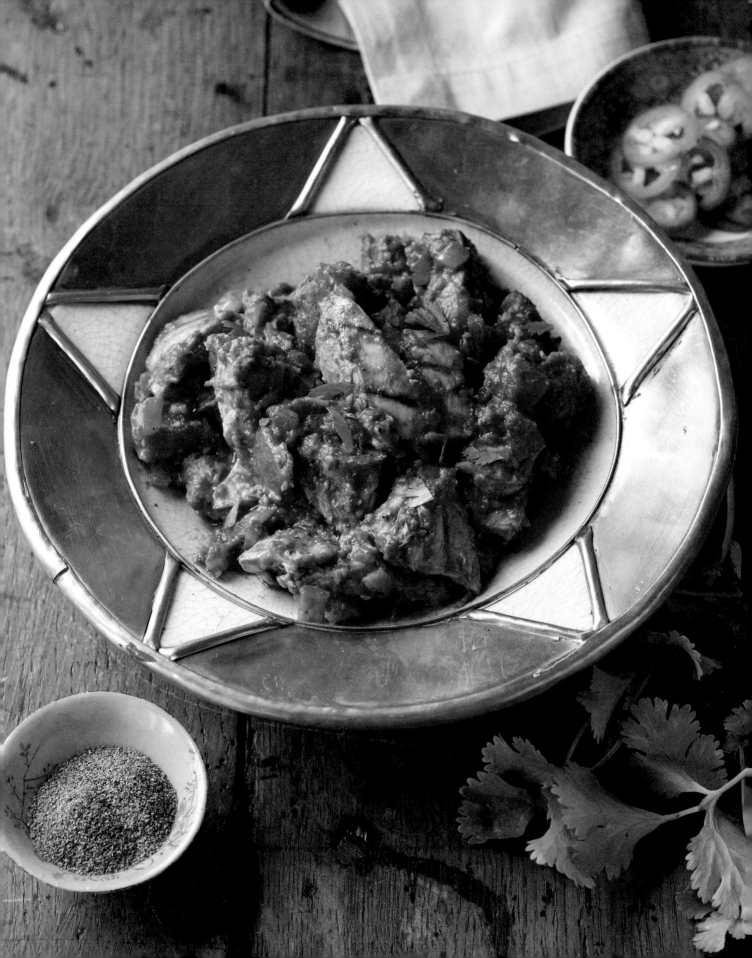

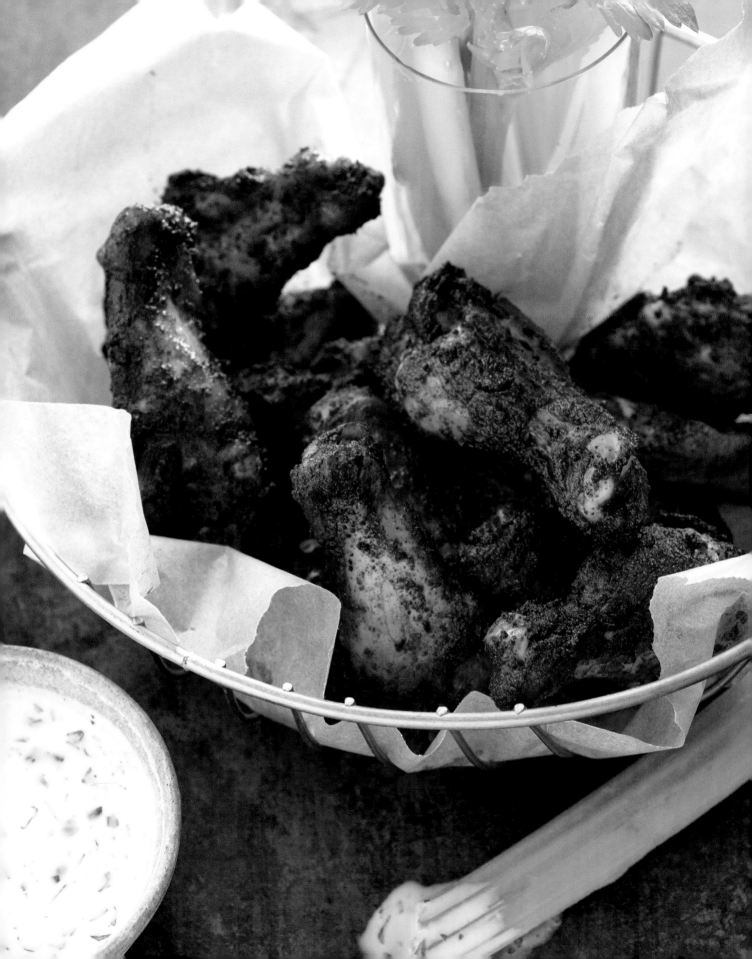

Chloe's Favorite Chicken Wings

This recipe was originally called "Party Favorite Chicken Wings." They became such a hit with our daughter that she insisted we change the name to "Chloe's Favorite Chicken Wings." This is also one of my favorite recipes because it's so simple and makes great leftovers for school lunch.

PREPARATION:

1. Preheat oven to 375 degrees F.

2. Blend spices together in a small mixing bowl.

3. Place chicken wings in a large mixing bowl and coat all pieces thoroughly with oil.

4. Toss chicken with spice blend. Be sure to cover all pieces lightly and evenly with the spice blend.

5. Place chicken in a baking dish and bake for approximately 30 minutes. Serve hot.

> **NOTE:** Try serving chicken wings with Zesty Aioli Dip (page 242) or Ranch-Style Dressing (page 239).

SERVES 8

INGREDIENTS:

1 teaspoon onion powder

1 teaspoon garlic powder

1 teaspoon ancho or chipotle chile powder, to desired spiciness

2 tablespoons smoked paprika

2 dozen chicken wings or mini drumsticks

2 tablespoons macadamia nut oil or avocado oil

OPTIONAL INGREDIENTS:

¼ teaspoon cinnamon

½ teaspoon pepper

salt, to taste

NUTRITIONAL INFORMATION PER SERVING FOR CHICKEN WINGS AND SPICE BLEND: 162.0 calories, 19.3g protein, 0.6g carbohydrates, 0.0g fiber, 0.2g sugar, 6.5g fat, 3.1g saturated fat, 58.3mg cholesterol, 70.7mg sodium

Smarty-Pants Chicken Fingers

SERVES 6

INGREDIENTS:

1 pound chicken breast tenders

pinch of salt, if desired

½ teaspoon garlic powder

3 eggs

¾ cup almond meal or coconut flour

OPTIONAL INGREDIENT:

1–2 tablespoons coconut oil (see note below)

PREPARATION:

1. Preheat oven to 375 degrees F and line a baking sheet with parchment paper.

2. Sprinkle chicken with salt and garlic powder.

3. Lightly beat the eggs in a shallow medium-sized bowl.

4. Dip the chicken pieces in the egg, coating both sides.

5. Place chicken in the almond meal or coconut flour, lightly covering both sides.

6. Place chicken on parchment-lined baking sheet. Bake for about 12 minutes, being sure to turn chicken over after 6 minutes.

7. Allow to cool for several minutes if serving to children. Serve with Ranch-Style Dressing (page 239).

> **NOTE:** Chicken tenders will not be crispy when baked. If you prefer a crispier texture, finish off cooking process by panfrying. To do this, simply remove chicken from oven after about 8 minutes of baking time. Heat a couple of tablespoons of coconut or macadamia nut oil in a skillet over medium-high heat. When skillet is hot, add half the baked tenders to the skillet. Cook for 30 to 60 seconds on each side, depending on desired crispiness. Remove tenders and repeat process for remaining chicken tenders. Slice one tender in the middle to be certain they are cooked through. Chicken will be white inside, not opaque or pink, when done. Or internal temperature should be 165 degrees using a meat thermometer.

NUTRITIONAL INFORMATION PER SERVING: 224.0 calories, 29.6g protein, 2.7g carbohydrates, 1.5g fiber, 0.7g sugar, 10.8g fat, 1.1g saturated fat, 81.2mg cholesterol, 118mg sodium

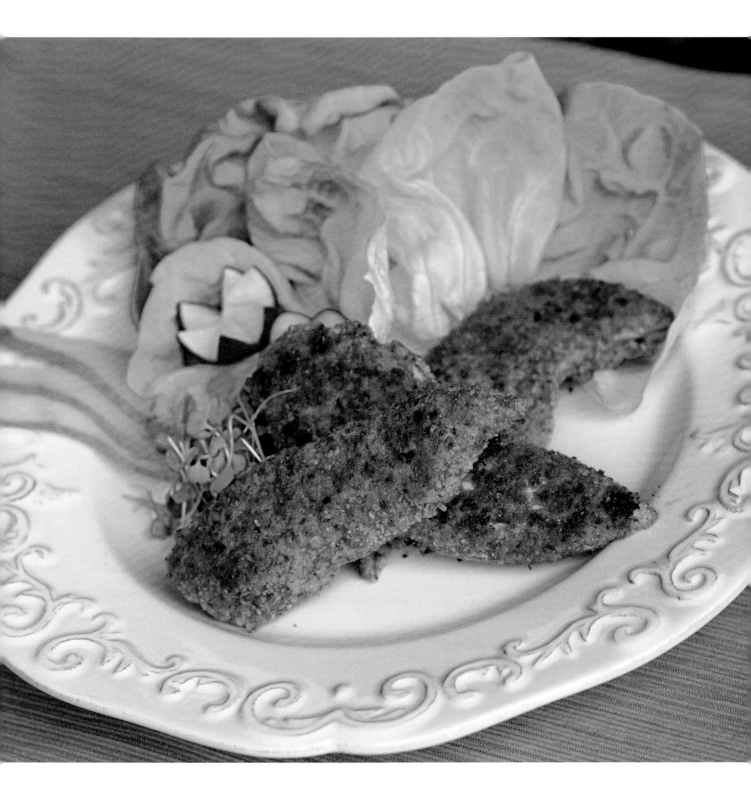

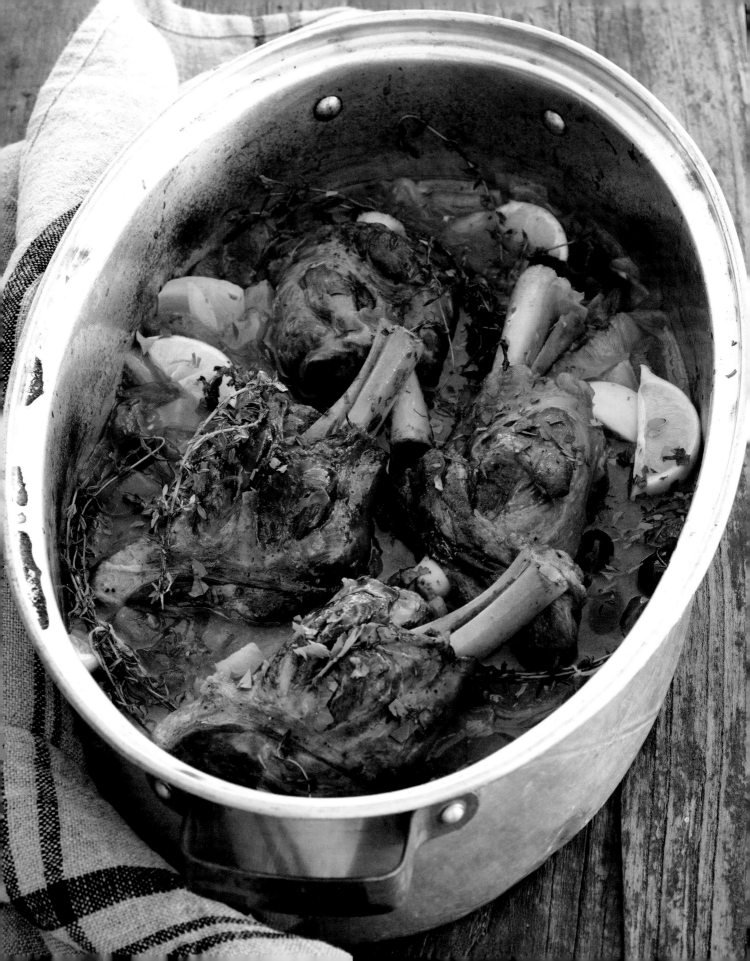

Meat, Lamb, and Pork

■

Do not let what you can't do interfere with what you can
do.

—JOHN WOODEN

Brain Warriors often ask us how much meat, if any, belongs in a
brain-healthy diet. We work with serious, meat-eating "cavemen"
and completely meat-free vegans and the answer is always the same:
Your body doesn't care about your food philosophy and neither do we.
We want to help you optimize your important health numbers and feel
amazing. Some people do very well without any form of animal protein, as
long as they focus on getting all the appropriate nutrients. Other people
show up to our clinics feeling and looking miserable on a vegan diet, and
their important lab numbers reflect that, which we discuss thoroughly
in *The Brain Warrior's Way*. There are many reasons that the exact same
program doesn't work for everyone.

Our recommendation is to eat red meat no more than once or twice
a week. Choose lamb or bison when you have the option. Make sure it's
grass fed, hormone free, and antibiotic free as much as you can. And eat
small portions—no larger than the palm of your hand at one meal. Studies
have shown that too much protein at once can burden the body and
create oxidative stress, like the way rust forms on a car. So think of protein
like medicine and take it in small doses throughout the day.

Brain Warrior
Meat Mastery Strategies

1. Save time by having the butcher dice or cube your meat for soups or stews. There's usually no extra charge.

2. Purchase directly from ranchers who farm completely cage-free, naturally raised animals. Meat is guaranteed to be antibiotic and hormone free, and it's far more humane. Meat comes overnight on dry ice and can be kept in the freezer.

3. Plan your menu in advance so you can marinate meat overnight for best results.

4. Use a Crock-Pot to slow cook meals while you work. Add all ingredients in the morning and by evening you'll have a delectable meal.

5. Pack unused cooked meat into airtight packaging and freeze, and add small unused portions to salads, stews, and soups.

■

Lamb and Quinoa Stuffed Cabbage

We love this healthy twist on traditional stuffed cabbage, which can be very heavy. By swapping lamb for beef and quinoa for rice, you gain more omega-3 fatty acids and lose some of the starchy carbs.

PREPARATION:

1. Preheat oven to 375 degrees F.

2. In a large saucepan or stockpot, bring water to a boil and boil cabbage leaves for 2 to 3 min. Keep leaves separated and do not allow to bunch. Remove from water and lay leaves flat on paper towel to dry out.

3. In a medium-sized bowl combine quinoa, lamb, egg, rosemary, marjoram, onion, salt, pepper, and 2 tablespoons of the tomato sauce.

4. In a small mixing bowl, combine tomato sauce, red wine vinegar, and erythritol or maple syrup. Set aside.

5. Lay cabbage leaves out on a cutting board or clean cooking space. Divide the lamb mixture evenly among the cabbage leaves. Roll and secure them burrito-style.

6. Pour half of the tomato sauce mixture in a 9 x 11 baking dish. Lay the stuffed cabbage rolls side by side in the sauce so they are placed snugly together. Drizzle the remainder of the sauce on top of the cabbage rolls.

7. Bake for 30 minutes, uncovered. Remove from oven and allow cabbage rolls to cool for a few minutes, as internal temperature gets very hot. Serve with Cruciferous Cold Slaw (page 67)

> **NOTE:** Ground turkey, chicken, or bison can be substituted in place of lamb.

INGREDIENTS:

8 full-sized green cabbage leaves

¾ cup cooked and cooled quinoa, prepared according to package directions

¾ pound ground lamb

1 egg

2 teaspoons finely chopped fresh rosemary or ½ teaspoon dried

1 tablespoon fresh marjoram or 1¼ teaspoons dried

¼ cup finely minced onion

½ teaspoon sea salt or as desired

¼ teaspoon pepper

1½ cups canned tomato sauce, or Simple Fresh Tomato Sauce (page 245)

3 tablespoons red wine vinegar

¼ teaspoon erythritol or maple syrup

NUTRITIONAL INFORMATION PER SERVING: 313.0 calories; 30.1g protein; 28.5g carbohydrates; 4.9g fiber; 5.2g sugar; 8.5g fat, 2.5g saturated fat; 77.0mg cholesterol; 788.0mg sodium

Herb-Roasted Rack of Lamb

SERVES 4

INGREDIENTS:

2 tablespoons macadamia nut oil or avocado oil, plus 2 teaspoons

1 tablespoon fresh rosemary, no need to chop

1 tablespoon fresh thyme, no need to chop (you may include the fine stems, but discard the thick stems)

2 whole sage leaves

3 garlic cloves, whole

1 teaspoon coarse pepper

1 teaspoon salt

1½ pounds rack of lamb

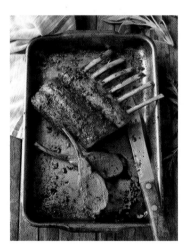

NUTRITIONAL INFORMATION PER SERVING: 240.0 calories, 143.0 calories from fat, 21.6g protein, 1.1g carbohydrates, 0.3g fiber, 0.0g sugar, 16.1g fat, 3.4g saturated fat, 68.0mg cholesterol, 626.0mg sodium

You're sure to impress guests at the most formal of dinner parties with this surprisingly simple recipe. Daniel claims he has never eaten lamb as flavorful as the lamb I make for him at home. I believe it's the marinating process that makes the difference.

Marinate for a minimum of 30 minutes, but for best results marinate for 2 hours to 24 hours. Planning ahead and marinating the night before will yield amazingly moist and flavorful lamb.

PREPARATION:

1. Place 2 tablespoons of the oil, and the rosemary, thyme, sage, garlic, pepper, and salt in a small food processor. Chop until herbs and garlic are minced to a fine consistency and there are no large pieces.

2. Rub or brush lamb with the oil mixture.

3. Wrap lamb in plastic wrap or a self-sealing bag, eliminating as much air as possible. Place on a small tray and refrigerate for at least 2 hours, up to 24 hours.

4. When you are ready to cook, preheat oven to 400 degrees F. Remove lamb from plastic wrap. Allow meat to reach room temperature before cooking.

5. Heat the remaining 2 teaspoons of the oil in a small roasting pan with oven-safe handles over medium-high heat. Make sure pan is hot before introducing lamb. Place the lamb in the pan and brown on both sides, 3 to 4 minutes on each side.

6. When lamb is browned, turn meaty side up. Place pan in oven, on middle rack. Roast for 20 minutes for medium rare, 22 minutes for medium, or until meat reaches desired doneness.

7. Remove from oven and cover with foil for 5 to 10 minutes, allowing lamb to rest to seal in juices before serving.

NOTE: Cut salt in half for a low-sodium diet.

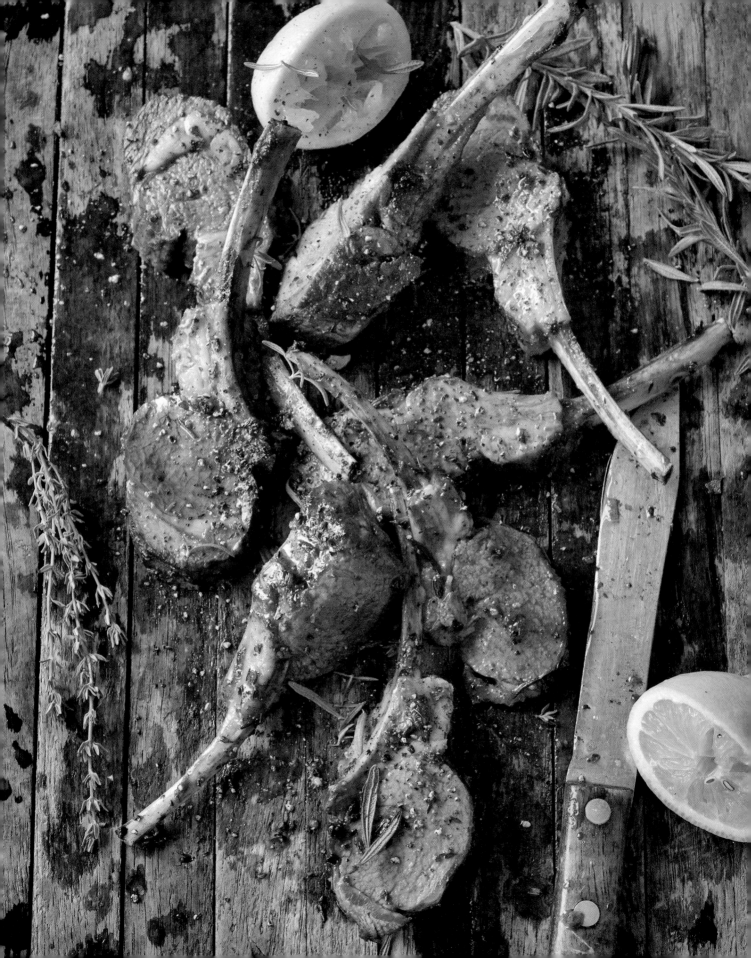

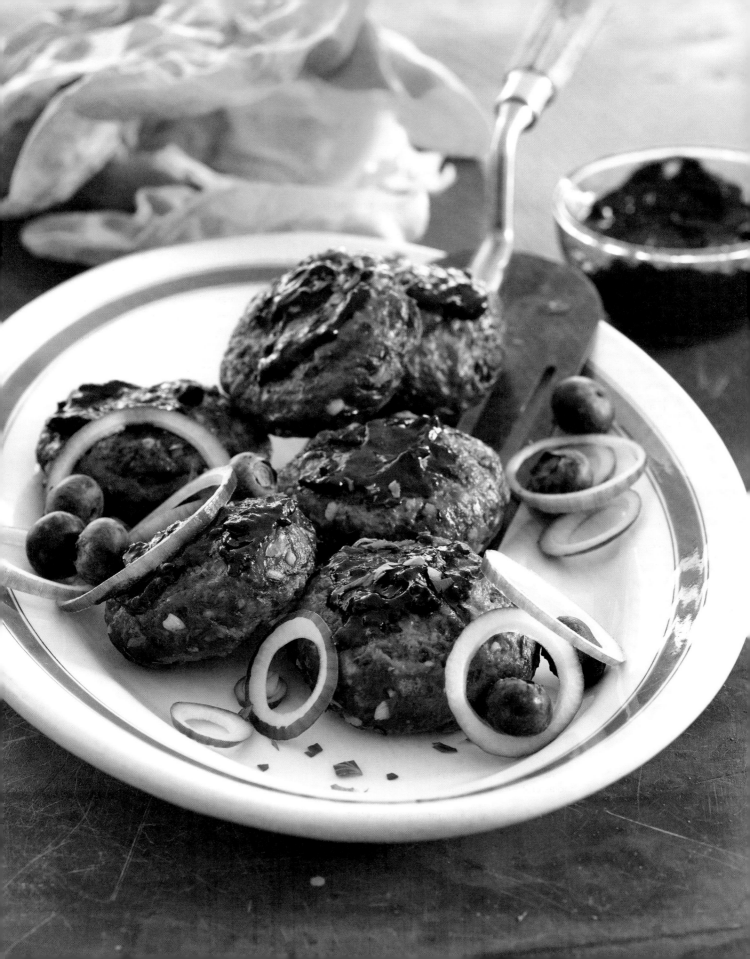

Herbed Bison Sliders with Blueberry Barbecue Sauce

The blueberry barbecue sauce in this recipe gives it a unique and fresh twist, and it's surprisingly low glycemic for barbecue sauce.

PREPARATION:

BURGERS:

1. In a mixing bowl, combine meat, oil, garlic, parsley, and seasoning.

2. Form 8 small biscuit-sized patties.

3. Grill burgers to desired doneness (for medium rare, about 3 minutes per side).

SAUCE:

1. In a heavy saucepan, cook onion and jalapeño in oil until soft, 2 to 3 minutes.

2. Add vinegar, water, honey, mustard, and tomato paste, and bring to a simmer.

3. Add blueberries and cook for 5 to 10 minutes till the sauce is very purple. Cool to room temperature.

4. Blend till mostly smooth, and season to taste with hot sauce and salt.

5. Wrap each burger in lettuce, then top with onions and a drizzle of Blueberry Barbecue Sauce.

SERVES 4 (8 SLIDERS)

INGREDIENTS:

SLIDERS:
1 pound ground bison, free range, all natural

2 tablespoons extra-virgin olive oil

1 tablespoon minced garlic

2 tablespoons parsley, minced

1 teaspoon salt

¼ teaspoon pepper

½ red onion, sliced very thin and set in a bowl of salted ice water

1 head butter lettuce, washed, and leaves separated for wraps

BLUEBERRY BARBECUE SAUCE:
¼ cup chopped red onion

1 tablespoon chopped jalapeño (add the seeds and ribs if you prefer more heat)

1 tablespoon olive oil

2 tablespoons red wine vinegar

2 tablespoons water

1 tablespoon raw honey

2 tablespoons Dijon mustard

2 tablespoons tomato paste

1 cup fresh blueberries

hot sauce, to taste

salt, to taste

NUTRITIONAL INFORMATION PER SERVING FOR SLIDERS: 318.8 calories, 25.6g protein, 1.2g carbohydrates, 0.4g fiber, 0.0g sugar, 23.1g fat, 7.9g saturated fat, 88.2mg cholesterol, 118.1mg sodium

NUTRITIONAL INFORMATION PER SERVING FOR BARBECUE SAUCE: 39.6 calories, 0.4g protein, 5.7g carbohydrates, 0.8g fiber, 4.4g sugar, 1.7g fat, 0.5g saturated fat, 0.0mg cholesterol, 69.9mg sodium

Bison London Broil

SERVES 8

INGREDIENTS:

4 garlic cloves

2 tablespoons fresh oregano, not chopped

2 tablespoon fresh basil (about 8 leaves)

1 tablespoon fresh rosemary

2 tablespoons macadamia nut oil or avocado oil

3 tablespoons red wine vinegar

4 tablespoons fresh lemon juice

2 tablespoons Dijon mustard

1 tablespoon low-sodium tamari sauce

2 pounds bison, top or rump roast, free range, all natural

½ teaspoon pepper

OPTIONAL INGREDIENT:

¼ teaspoon cayenne pepper (for more kick)

London broil refers to a method of preparation, not a cut of meat. Look for a top roast or rump roast for this recipe. Buffalo, elk, and other wild meats are much lower in saturated fat than industrial beef and other farm-raised meats. They tend to overcook quickly and should be cooked for less time.

Marinate for a minimum of 30 minutes, but for best results marinate for 2 hours to 24 hours. Planning ahead and marinating the night before will yield amazingly moist and flavorful meat.

PREPARATION:

1. In small food processor, place garlic, oregano, basil, rosemary, oil, vinegar, lemon juice, mustard, and tamari sauce. Process on "chop" setting until herbs and garlic are finely minced and blended with liquid. If you prefer, you can chop herbs finely by hand and blend ingredients thoroughly in a bowl.

2. Place meat in a large self-sealing bag with marinade. Cover meat completely with marinade. Refrigerate for at least 2 hours, up to 24 hours.

3. When ready to prepare meat, preheat oven to broil. Place meat on broiler tray with pan to catch juices.

4. Broil for about 7 minutes per side for medium rare or until meat reaches an internal temperature of 135 degrees F. Allow internal temperature to reach 140 degrees if you like your meat cooked medium.

5. Remove from oven, transfer to a cutting board, and let stand for a few minutes before cutting diagonally across the grain in thin slices.

NOTE: This is great served as a main entrée or over fresh greens as a "steak salad" for lunch.

NUTRITIONAL INFORMATION PER SERVING (APPROXIMATE BASED ON SIZE OF ROAST): 245.0 calories, 29.2g protein, 2.2g carbohydrates, 0.2g fiber, 2.0g sugar, 13.3g fat, 4.3g saturated fat, 81.0mg cholesterol, 261.0mg sodium

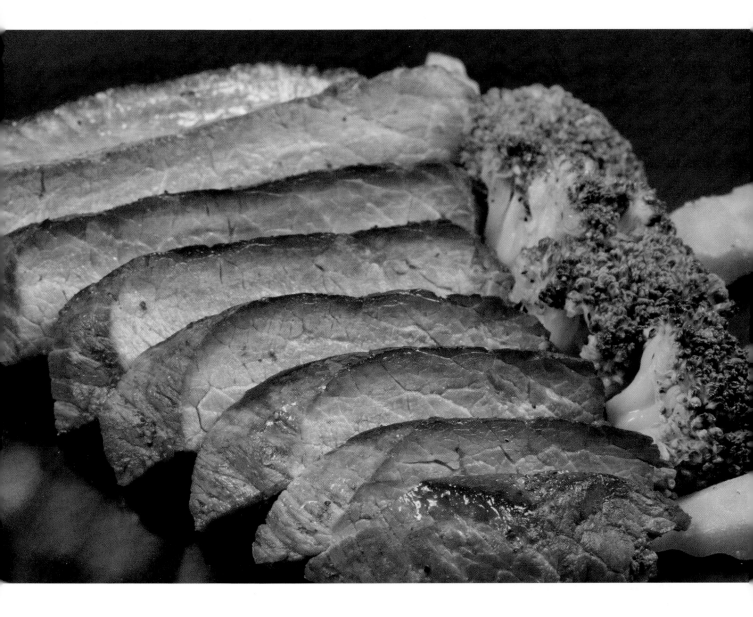

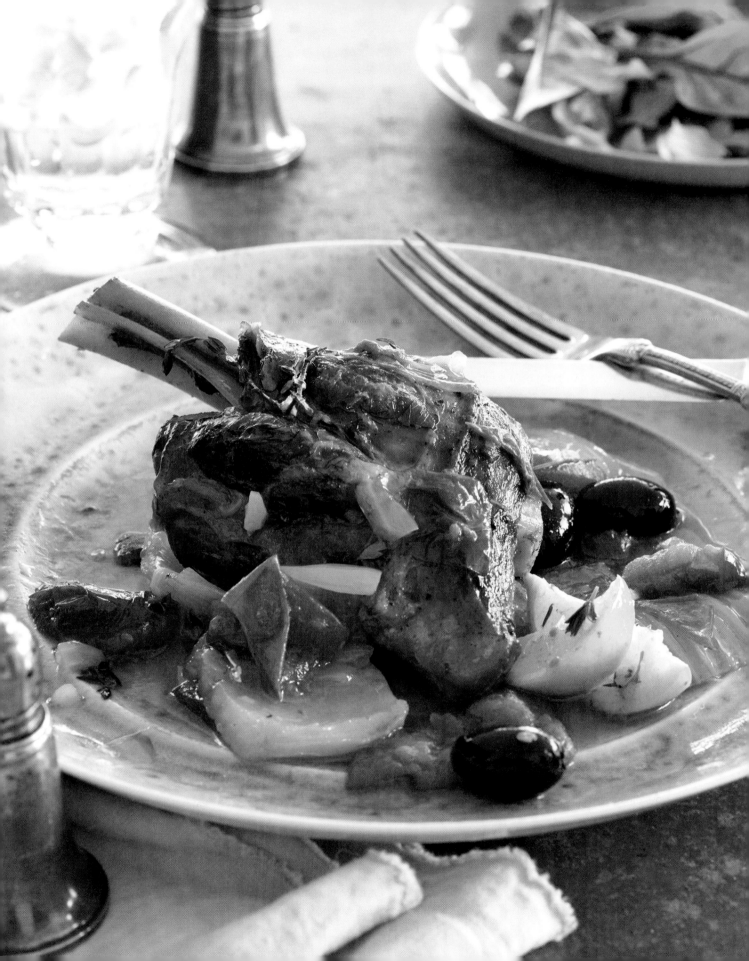

Braised Lamb Shanks

If you really love to cook, try this recipe the traditional way by braising, but my preference is to cook this in the Crock-Pot. It's just as tasty, and much simpler. Put it in before leaving for the day, and you'll have a perfectly cooked, healthy meal when you get home. I have included preparation instructions for both cooking methods below.

PREPARATION:

TRADITIONAL METHOD:

1. Preheat oven to 400 degrees F.

2. Heat oil in a Dutch oven or large, heavy pot over medium-high heat. Salt and pepper the shanks. Sear lamb until browned on all sides (a couple of minutes per side), then remove from pan and place on a separate plate.

3. Add the fennel and onion and sauté till soft, about 3 or 4 minutes. Then add garlic and sauté for 30 seconds. Add the tomatoes and thyme.

4. Place the shanks back in the pot with any accumulated juices. Add the chicken broth until it covers about ¾ of the meat—it should not be covered completely with liquid.

5. Bring to a boil, then reduce heat to simmer. Cover loosely with a piece of parchment paper that has been cut to fit as a lid.

6. Place in the oven and cook for 1½ hours.

7. Check after 1 hour to make sure there is still enough liquid in the pan. If necessary, add ½–1 cup broth to the pot. The meat should be very tender when finished cooking. Remove the thyme.

8. Remove the shanks and vegetables from the pan and serve with the lemon, olives, and parsley.

SLOW-COOKER METHOD:

1. Sear the shanks, and sauté the fennel, onion, and garlic as above.

2. Transfer to a Crock-Pot with the tomatoes, thyme, and chicken broth.

3. Cook on high for 3 hours, or on low for 6 hours.

4. Remove the shanks and vegetables from Crock-Pot and serve with the lemon, olives, and parsley.

SERVES 4

INGREDIENTS:

1 tablespoon macadamia nut oil, avocado oil, or almond oil

salt and pepper

4 lamb shanks

1 fennel bulb, chopped

1 onion, chopped

2 garlic cloves, minced

6 Roma tomatoes, chopped

1 small bunch thyme, tied together with kitchen string

2 cups low-sodium chicken broth or bone broth (page 89)

zest and juice of 1 lemon

¼ cup (about 16) pitted Kalamata olives, chopped

¼ cup parsley, chopped

NUTRITIONAL INFORMATION PER SERVING (APPROXIMATE BASED ON SIZE OF SHANKS):
337.0 calories, 9.2g protein, 16.6g carbohydrates, 5.4g fiber, 6.3g sugar, 14.2g fat, 3.6g saturated fat, 102mg cholesterol, 319.0mg sodium

Apple-Infused Pork Medallions with Onions

SERVES 6

INGREDIENTS:

1 uncured pork tenderloin, about 1½ pounds

salt and pepper, to taste

½ cup low-sodium chicken broth or bone broth (page 89)

1 tablespoon apple cider vinegar

1 tablespoon Dijon mustard

2 teaspoons maple syrup

1½ tablespoons coconut oil

1 onion, sliced thin

1 Granny Smith apple, cored and sliced thin

PREPARATION:

1. Remove the tendon from the pork tenderloin, and cut into 4 pieces. Using the heel of your hand, press the pork pieces into medallions ½ inch thick. Season with salt and pepper and set aside.

2. In a small bowl, whisk together the chicken broth, vinegar, mustard, and maple syrup and set aside.

3. Heat 1 tablespoon of the coconut oil in a large sauté pan over medium-high heat. Add the pork and brown on both sides. Remove from pan and set aside on a plate.

4. Add remaining ½ tablespoon coconut oil and the onion and apples to the pan, and start to brown. Add the broth mixture and scrape the bottom of the pan to remove any browned bits. Return the pork to the pan and continue cooking for 5 to 10 minutes, until the pork reaches 145 degrees F internal temperature.

5. When the pork is finished cooking, remove it from the pan and place on a cutting board to rest for several minutes before slicing. Meanwhile, spoon apple and onions from the pan onto a serving platter, reserving most of the juice.

6. Slice pork into ½-inch-thick medallions and layer over the apple and onion mixture. Using a spoon, drizzle the remaining juice from the pan evenly over the pork.

> **NOTE:** This recipe is great served with Shredded Brussels Sprout Sauté (page 201).

NUTRITIONAL INFORMATION PER SERVING (APPROXIMATE BASED ON SIZE OF TENDERLOIN): 345.1 calories, 22.7g protein, 8.8g carbohydrates, 1.2g fiber, 5.2g sugar, 24.3g fat, 17.3g saturated fat, 60.1mg cholesterol, 274.6mg sodium

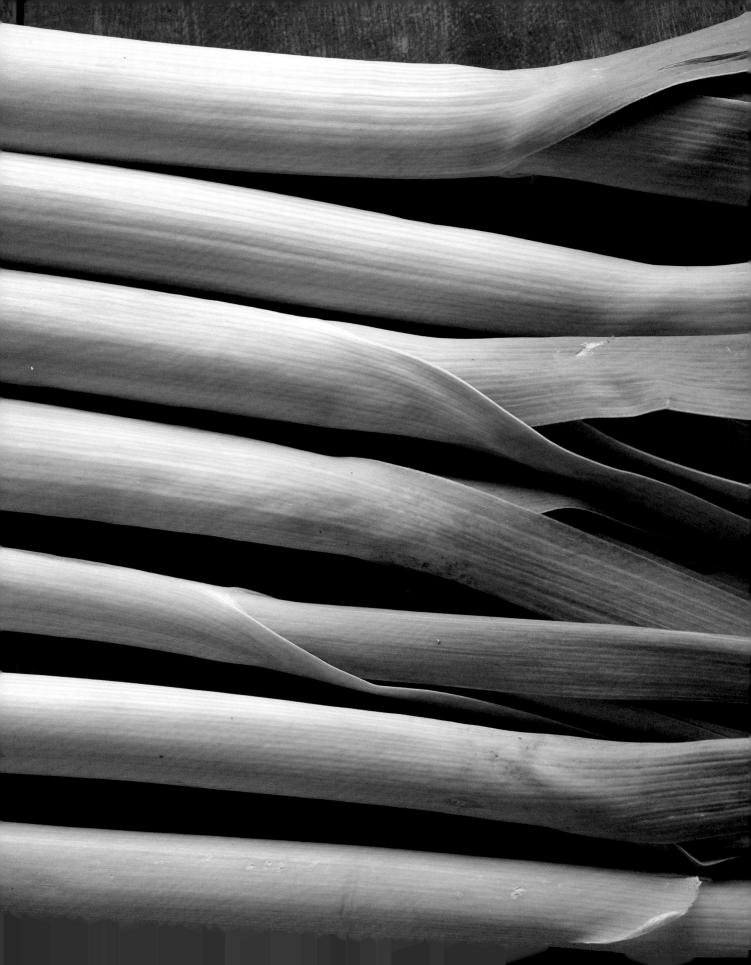

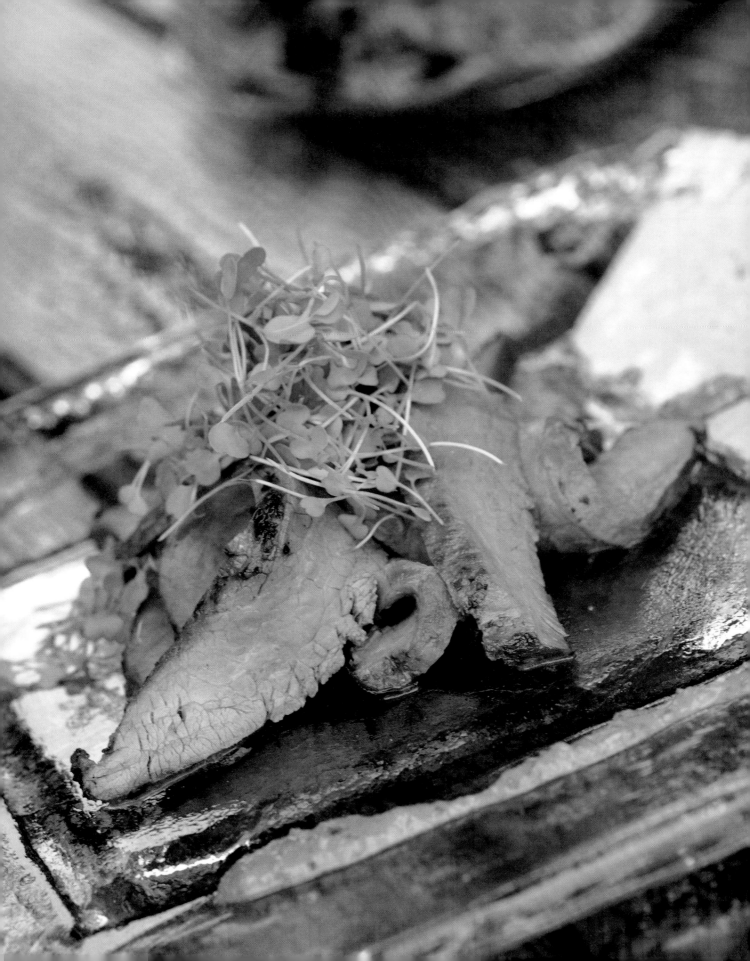

Cinnamon Spice Flank Steak

Being of Lebanese heritage, Daniel and I both have a love for meat spiced with cinnamon and nutmeg, which are favorites in Mediterranean dishes. Cinnamon has been shown to improve focus, and it has historically been used as an aphrodisiac for men. When we told my mother-in-law this bit of information, she playfully slapped her head and said, "That's why I have seven children!"

PREPARATION:

1. Preheat grill to medium-high heat.

2. Rub the steak all over with the avocado oil.

3. Combine the rest of the ingredients and rub all over the steak. Allow to rest for 15 minutes if possible.

4. Grill meat to desired doneness. For medium rare, this is usually 4 to 5 minutes per side. Medium usually requires 5 to 7 minutes per side.

5. Remove meat from grill, cover with foil, and allow to rest for 5 to 10 minutes before slicing. Remove foil and cut into thin slices. Slicing against the grain of flank steak (diagonally) will often make it more tender.

6. Layer slices on a serving platter and serve with Shredded Rainbow Salad (page 77).

SERVES 4

INGREDIENTS:
20-ounce grass-fed beef or bison flank steak, or tri-tip sirloin, free range, all natural

1 tablespoon avocado oil or macadamia nut oil

1 teaspoon cinnamon

1 teaspoon smoked paprika

1 garlic clove, crushed or minced

1 teaspoon salt

½ teaspoon pepper

OPTIONAL INGREDIENTS:
1 teaspoon ancho chile powder (for spicier flavor)

¼ teaspoon nutmeg

NUTRITIONAL INFORMATION PER SERVING: 235.2 calories, 22.2g protein, 1.0g carbohydrates, 0.5g fiber, 0.1g sugar, 17.6g fat, 6.0g saturated fat, 69.0mg cholesterol, 296.0mg sodium

Rosemary Maple Pork Tenderloin

SERVES 4

INGREDIENTS:

1 tablespoon plus 1 teaspoon macadamia nut oil or avocado oil

2 tablespoons apple cider vinegar

1 tablespoon pure maple syrup

2 garlic cloves

1 tablespoon fresh rosemary, not chopped

¼ teaspoon pepper

salt, to taste

1 pound pork tenderloin

OPTIONAL INGREDIENT:

4 whole sage leaves

Marinate for a minimum of 30 minutes, but for best results marinate for 2 hours to 24 hours.

PREPARATION:

1. In a small food processor, place 1 tablespoon oil, vinegar, maple syrup, garlic, rosemary, pepper, salt, and sage leaves, if desired. Process until all ingredients are finely chopped and thoroughly mixed.

2. Place tenderloin in self-sealing bag and pour marinade over the tenderloin inside the bag, being sure to cover the entire piece of meat.

3. Press all air out of the bag. Place bag with meat in a bowl or small pan and refrigerate for 2 to 24 hours if possible.

4. Preheat oven to 425 degrees F when ready to cook.

5. Over medium-high heat on the stove top, heat remaining 1 teaspoon of oil in a small roasting pan that can easily transfer from the cooktop to the oven. Remove tenderloin from bag and place it in the roasting pan. Discard remainder of marinade. Turn slightly after 45 seconds to 1 minute.

6. Continue browning and turning the tenderloin all the way around every 45 seconds to 1 minute. After you have turned the tenderloin all the way around once (this should take 3 to 4 minutes), transfer pan to the oven on the top rack.

7. Roast tenderloin for 10 minutes for medium rare, 12 minutes for medium, or 14 minutes for well done. Be sure to turn the tenderloin at least once in the middle of cooking.

8. Slice in medium-thin slices against the grain, and serve warm.

NUTRITIONAL INFORMATION PER SERVING: 208.0 calories, 86.0 calories from fat, 24.5g protein, 4.2g carbohydrates, 0.1g fiber, 3.0g sugar, 9.6g fat, 2.2g saturated fat, 75.0mg cholesterol, 65.0mg sodium

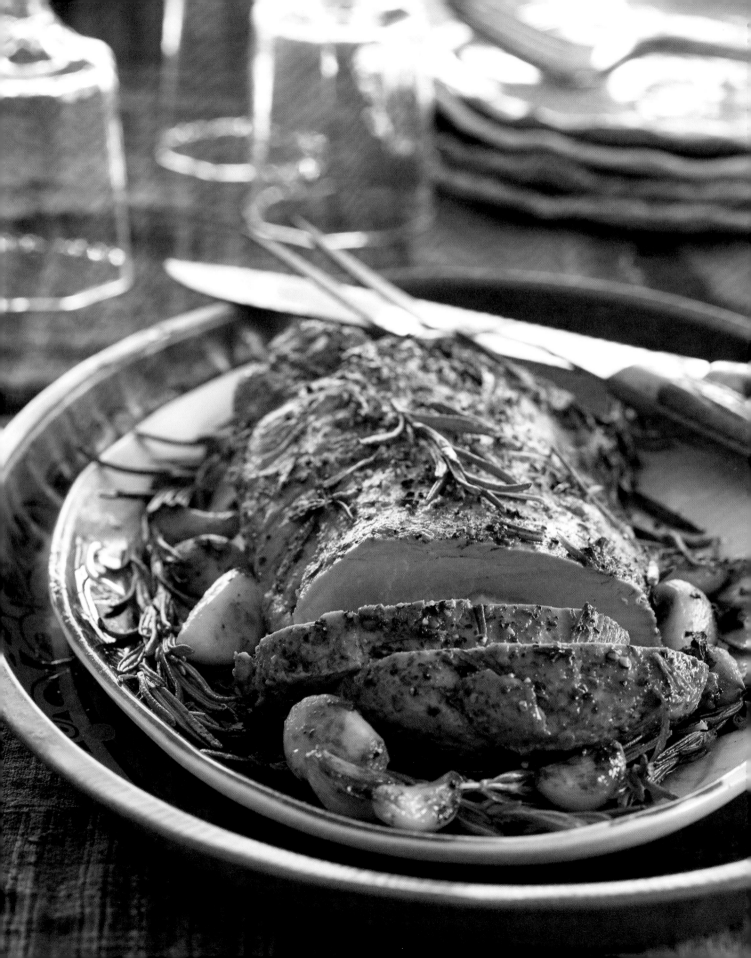

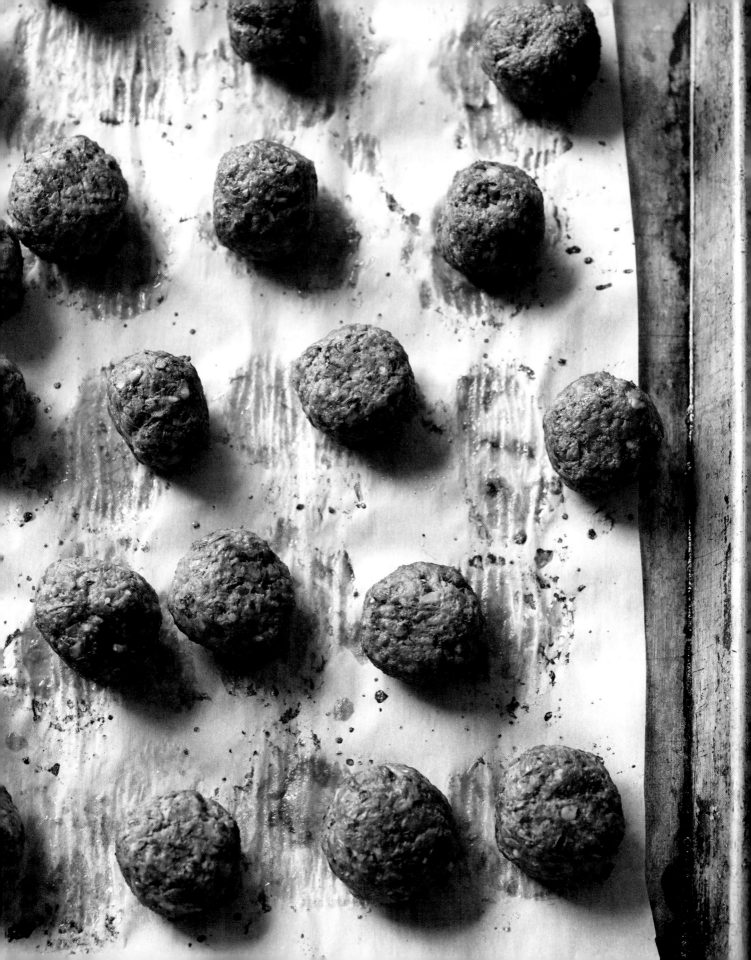

Fortifying Bison Meatballs

Swapping out traditionally used bread crumbs for vegetables and nuts dramatically boosts the nutritional value, and the meatballs themselves come out surprisingly moist. This is a simple, tasty way to get your kids to eat more vegetables.

PREPARATION:

1. Preheat oven to 375 degrees F. Line baking sheet with parchment paper.

2. In a food processor, add the almonds and carrots and pulse until finely chopped. Add remaining ingredients except bison, and pulse until well blended and finely chopped but not mushy.

3. Place vegetable mixture in a bowl and mix in the ground meat.

4. Using wet hands, form the mixture into balls, and place on baking sheet.

5. Bake for 20 minutes total. After 10 minutes, roll them around so they do not get too dark on one side.

> **NOTE:** Serve with Simple Fresh Tomato Sauce (page 245) or Creamy Fettuccine-Style Noodles (page 203).

SERVES 6 (20 TO 25 MEATBALLS)

INGREDIENTS:
¼ cup raw almonds
½ cup carrot, roughly chopped
1 cup chopped zucchini
1 cup chopped kale, thick stems removed
¼ cup chives, chopped
1 garlic clove
1 tablespoon macadamia nut oil
1½ teaspoons dried Italian seasoning
1 teaspoon salt
¼ teaspoon pepper
1 pound ground bison (other options: chicken, turkey, or grass-fed beef)

NUTRITIONAL INFORMATION PER SERVING: 390.5 calories, 29.8g protein, 8.9g carbohydrates, 3.5g fiber, 2.6g sugar, 26.8g fat, 7.9g saturated fat, 88.2mg cholesterol, 136.7mg sodium

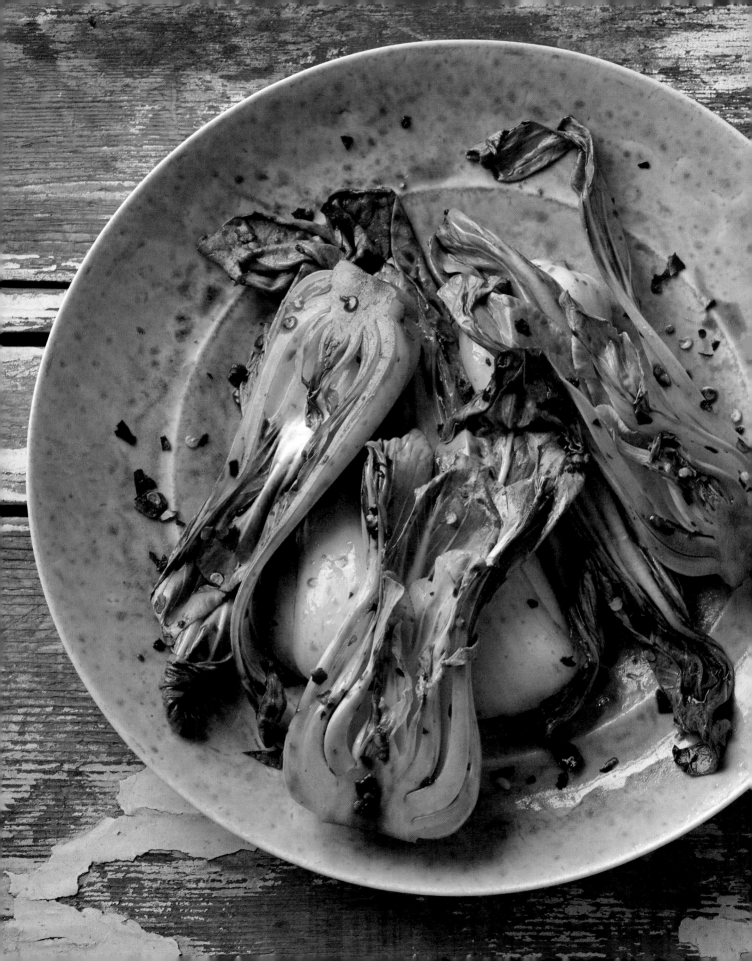

Staples, Not Sides

∎

The difference in winning and losing is most often not quitting.

—WALT DISNEY

Instead of thinking of these primarily plant-based dishes as "sides," begin to think of them as the focus of your meal. Brain Warriors strive to consume at least 70 percent plant-based foods. The remaining 30 percent should be high-quality protein. However, animal protein is not the only source of high-quality protein. We advocate plant-based protein powder and other high-protein plant foods to supplement as well. If you're vegetarian, focus on this section, along with smoothies, soups, salads, and desserts.

These simple tips will help you focus on the antioxidant benefits that colorful plant-based foods provide, while getting enough protein to keep your focus and blood sugar stable.

Brain Warrior Suggestions for Eating a 70/30 Ratio

1. Serve a big salad or bowl of soup and a vegetable-based side with every meal.

2. Serve protein over a bed of pureed cauliflower or sweet potato.

3. Use the palm of your hand as the guide for protein portions. The rest of your meal should consist of colorful plant-based foods.

4. Vegans can add protein powder to breakfast and organic tofu to dinner recipes. Vegetarians can supplement with protein from eggs.

5. Use lettuce wraps and coconut wraps in place of bread, and avocado in place of cheese.

■

Butternut Squash Puree

PREPARATION:

1. Fill a large pot with about 6 cups of water and bring to a boil. Add squash to boiling water, making sure there is enough water to cover the squash. Add more if necessary. Boil uncovered for about 20 minutes or until squash is tender. Drain water.

2. In a food processor or high-powered blender, or with a handheld electric mixer, combine the cooked butternut squash, ¼ cup almond milk, erythritol, and nutmeg. Blend until smooth. (Add additional almond milk for thinner puree.)

3. Keep mixture warm in saucepan over medium-low heat if necessary and set aside until ready to serve. Stir occasionally.

4. Try serving halibut or trout on a bed of Butternut Squash Puree.

SERVES 4

INGREDIENTS:
2 cups peeled and chopped butternut squash
¼ to ½ cup plain, unsweetened almond milk
¼ teaspoon erythritol
¼ teaspoon nutmeg

NUTRITIONAL INFORMATION PER SERVING: 48.8 calories, 1.1g protein, 12.8g carbohydrates, 3.3g fiber, 0.2g sugar, 0.7g fat, 0.2g saturated fat, 0.0mg cholesterol, 27.1mg sodium

Maple-Roasted Brussels Sprouts

SERVES 4

INGREDIENTS:

1 pound brussels sprouts, trimmed and halved

2 tablespoons ghee or coconut oil

2 large garlic cloves, minced

2 tablespoons low-sodium tamari sauce

2 teaspoons maple syrup

PREPARATION:

1. Remove loose, flyaway leaves from brussels sprouts, and set leaves aside.

2. Boil water in a medium pot. Place halved brussels sprouts into boiling water for 4 to 5 minutes. Drain water and set aside brussels sprouts.

3. Heat 1 tablespoon of the oil in a large pan over medium-high heat. Place flyaway leaves in skillet and cook for a couple of minutes, until crisp. Remove leaves with a slotted spoon, leaving oil in the pan. Repeat the process until all leaves have been added and crisped.

4. Reduce heat to medium, add garlic to pan, and stir for about 30 seconds. Add tamari sauce, maple syrup and halved brussels sprouts.

5. Cook until liquid is nearly evaporated, which could take up to 10 minutes.

6. Add cooked flyaway leaves back in to heat for 2 to 3 minutes.

7. Remove from heat and serve warm.

NUTRITIONAL INFORMATION
PER SERVING: 131.3 calories, 4.1g protein, 11.0g carbohydrates, 3.0g fiber, 3.5g sugar, 7.5g fat, 7.5g saturated fat, 16.5mg cholesterol, 129.5mg sodium

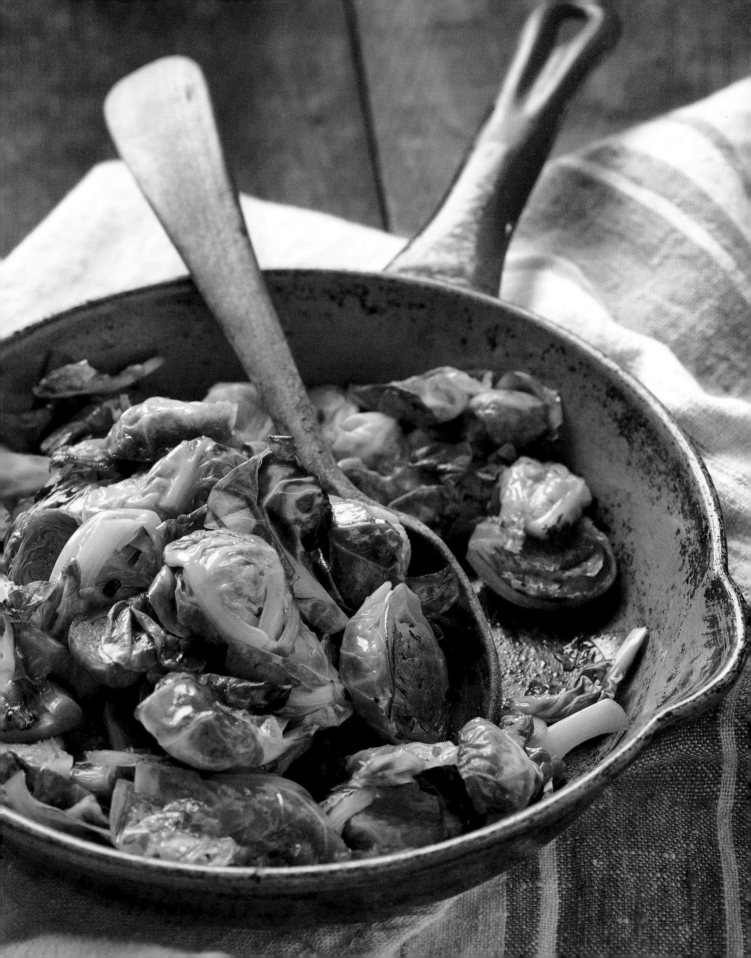

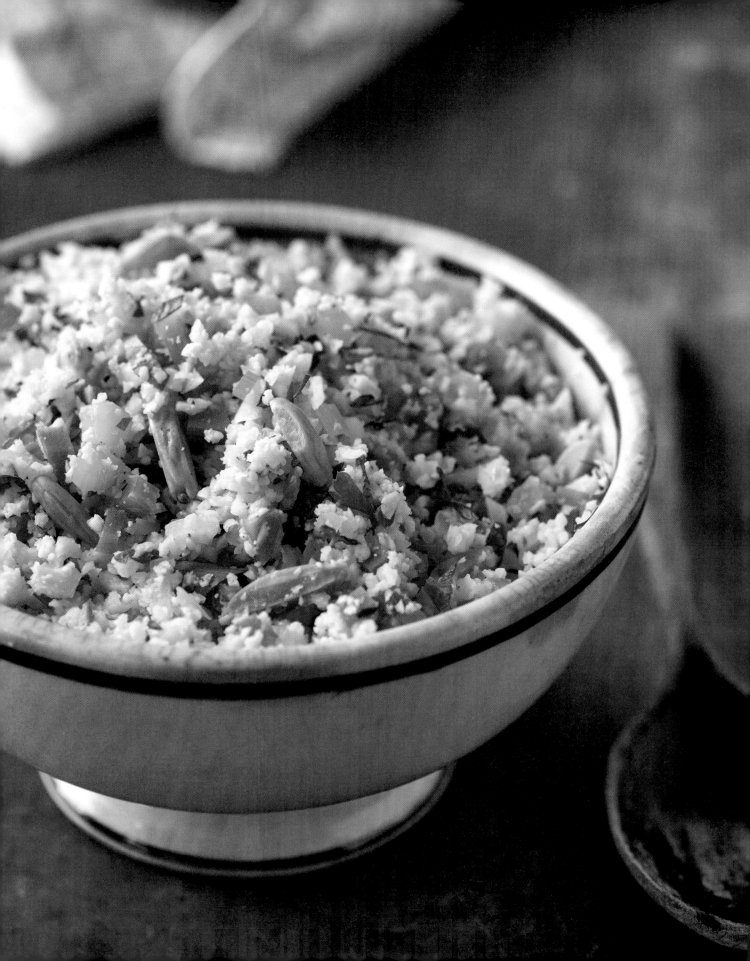

Cauliflower Rice Pilaf

I served this at a family gathering and, amazingly, not one person realized they were eating cauliflower in place of rice! Even the pickiest of kids usually love this dish.

PREPARATION:

1. Put cauliflower florets in a food processor and pulse until coarsely shredded but not mushy. Set aside.

2. In a large pan, sauté the carrot, celery, and onion in the oil or ghee for 3 to 5 minutes.

3. Add the garlic and sauté another 3 to 5 minutes.

4. Add the shredded cauliflower and stir while slowly adding the chicken or vegetable broth. You will want to cook until tender but still a little firm, like rice. If you overcook, it will be mushy.

5. Stir in fresh herbs, a little salt and pepper, if desired, and almond slivers before removing from heat.

> **NOTE:** For best results, dice the carrot, celery, and onion to a brunoise-sized dice, about $1/16$ inch if possible. In other words, really small. Also, be sure the cauliflower is fine but not mushy. In this way you'll fool everyone into thinking this really is rice pilaf!

SERVES 8

INGREDIENTS:

1 head cauliflower, florets only

1 large carrot, finely diced

1 to 2 stalks celery, finely diced

½ large white or sweet onion, finely diced

2 tablespoons macadamia nut oil, coconut oil, or ghee for sautéing

1 to 2 tablespoons minced garlic

1 cup low-sodium chicken broth or vegetable broth

2 to 3 tablespoons favorite minced herbs such as parsley and/ or thyme

½ cup slivered almonds, lightly toasted

OPTIONAL INGREDIENTS:

pinch of salt and pepper

NUTRITIONAL INFORMATION PER SERVING: 48.6 calories, 0.8g protein, 3.0g carbohydrates, 0.8g fiber, 1.1g sugar, 3.8g fat, 3.8g saturated fat, 8.3mg cholesterol, 37.5mg sodium

Goji Curry Broccoli

SERVES 6

INGREDIENTS:

1 tablespoon coconut oil, macadamia nut oil, or ghee

2½ cups finely chopped broccoli

1 cup cooked quinoa, prepared according to package directions

½ cup pine nuts

2 tablespoons goji berries or ½ cup halved grapes

OPTIONAL INGREDIENTS:

1 teaspoon curry powder

1 teaspoon lemon juice

½ teaspoon white pepper

salt to taste

You have the option of keeping this recipe simple, which goes over better with children. However, I strongly suggest trying it with the optional spices listed below. It is a unique and flavorful twist, and loaded with antioxidants.

I consider quinoa a "condiment," so I use only 1 cup of cooked quinoa. Vegetarians can increase the amount of quinoa to make this dish more substantial.

PREPARATION:

1. Heat oil in a large pan over medium-high heat. Add broccoli and sauté for 2 to 3 minutes. Add curry, lemon juice, pepper, and salt, if desired. Stir to mix in spices.

2. Add precooked quinoa to broccoli and stir. Mix in pine nuts and goji berries or grapes and heat through for about 2 minutes. Remove from heat and serve warm.

3. This dish is excellent with Rosemary Thyme Chicken (page 140).

> **NOTE:** Adding the curry powder to this recipe creates a wonderful contrast of sweet and savory flavors, along with a burst of powerful, healing antioxidant nutrition.

NUTRITIONAL INFORMATION PER SERVING: 232.0 calories, 6.8g protein, 26.2g carbohydrates, 3.4g fiber, 3.2g sugar, 12.1g fat, 2.7g saturated fat, 0.0mg cholesterol, 14.0mg sodium

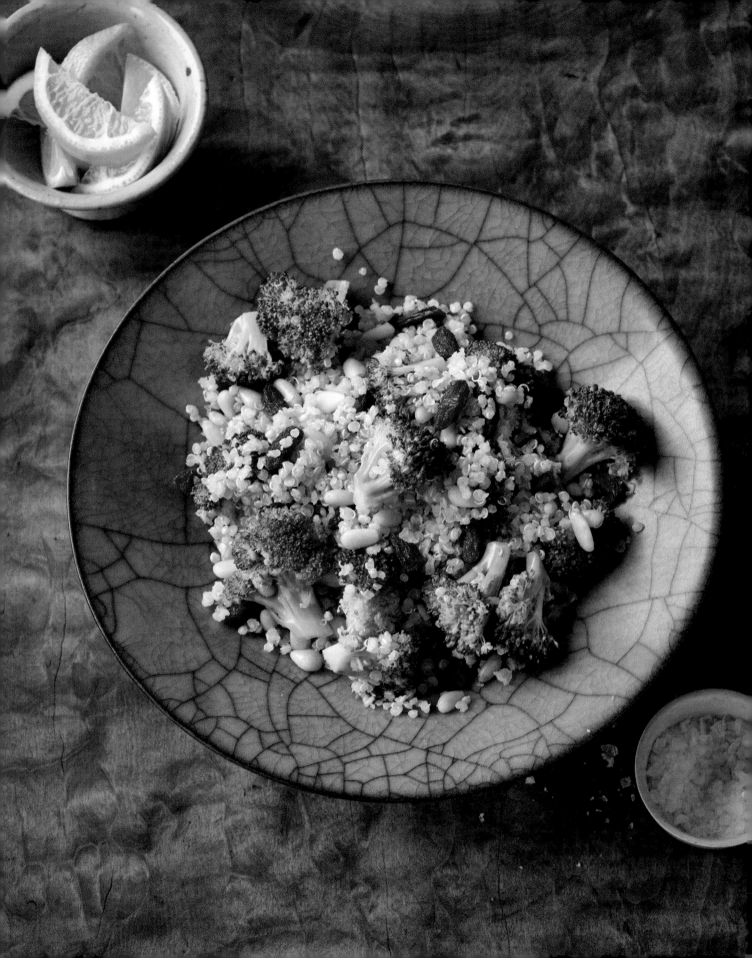

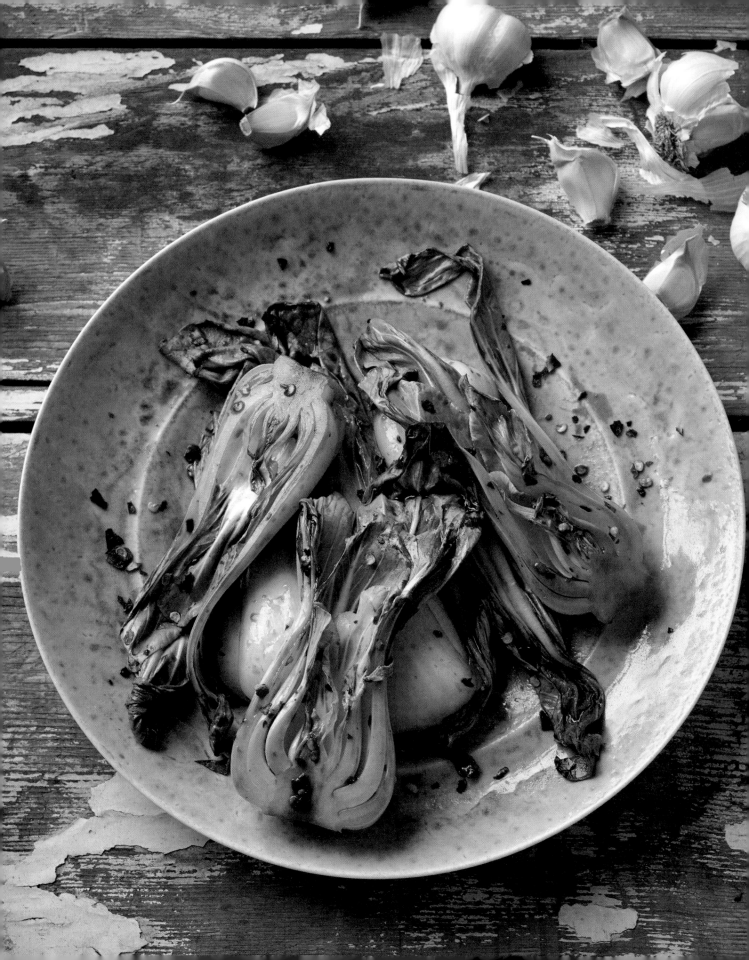

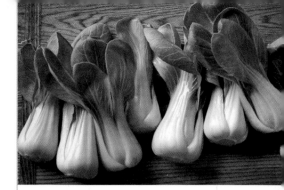

Peppery Bok Choy

PREPARATION:

1. Heat oil in a large skillet over medium heat. Add garlic and ginger for about a minute. Add red pepper flakes if desired.

2. Add tamari sauce to skillet. If you'd like a bit more moisture for sautéing, add 2 tablespoons chicken or vegetable broth instead of more oil.

3. Add bok choy to oil or hot broth and cook for about 5 minutes. Leaves should turn bright green. Add salt and pepper to taste. Serve hot.

SERVES 4

INGREDIENTS:

1 tablespoon macadamia nut oil or coconut oil

2 to 3 garlic cloves

1 tablespoon finely minced fresh ginger

1 tablespoon low-sodium tamari sauce

8 heads bok choy, sliced or chopped large (use both base and leafy portion)

salt and pepper

OPTIONAL INGREDIENTS:

1 to 2 teaspoons crushed red pepper flakes

2 tablespoons low-sodium chicken or vegetable broth

NUTRITIONAL INFORMATION PER SERVING: 143.9 calories, 7.1g protein, 11.8g carbohydrates, 6.1g fiber, 1.0g sugar, 10.4g fat, 5.3g saturated fat, 11.0mg cholesterol, 133.3mg sodium

Sautéed Spinach with Sun-Dried Tomatoes

SERVES 6

INGREDIENTS:

2 tablespoons macadamia nut oil, coconut oil, or ghee

2 pounds fresh spinach

2 garlic cloves, minced

¼ cup sun-dried tomatoes, chopped

¼ cup pine nuts

salt and pepper, to taste

OPTIONAL INGREDIENT

1 small onion, finely chopped

PREPARATION:

1. Heat oil or ghee in large skillet over medium heat. Sauté spinach in batches until wilted, 3 to 5 minutes. Set spinach aside.

2. Add garlic, and onion if desired, to the same pan. Add a touch more oil if necessary. Sauté for 3 minutes.

3. Add spinach, tomatoes, and pine nuts to garlic and onion. Mix well, distributing tomatoes, onions, garlic, and pine nuts evenly through the spinach. Heat through and remove from heat. Add salt and pepper as desired.

NUTRITIONAL INFORMATION PER SERVING: 39.4 calories, 0.7g protein, 1.5g carbohydrates, 0.2g fiber, 1.1g sugar, 3.6g fat, 0.5g saturated fat, 0.0mg cholesterol, 185.7mg sodium

Sweet Potato Hash

Sweet potatoes are an example of a smart carbohydrate that helps to elevate serotonin, the "feel good" neurotransmitter. If you need a boost after a tough day, give yourself a boost by adding a side of sweet potatoes to a meal. Sweet Potato Hash is one of my favorite preworkout recipes. By topping it with a poached egg, I have the perfect combination of fat, protein and carbohydrates.

PREPARATION:

1. In a large sauté pan, heat the macadamia nut oil, coconut oil, or ghee. Add the onion and bell pepper and sauté 2 minutes.

2. Add the potatoes, paprika, salt and pepper to the pan. Mix well and spread the potatoes flat.

3. Let the potatoes cook until browned on the bottom, 4 to 5 minutes. Then carefully turn the potatoes over and continue cooking until tender. If you prefer a crispier hash, turn the potatoes again for about a minute on each side, allowing potatoes to become lightly browned.

SERVES 6

INGREDIENTS:

2 tablespoons macadamia nut oil, coconut oil, or ghee

½ yellow onion, diced

½ red bell pepper, diced

2 sweet potatoes, peeled and grated on a box grater

1 teaspoon smoked paprika

½ teaspoon salt

¼ teaspoon pepper

NUTRITIONAL INFORMATION
PER SERVING: 110.5 calories, 1.4g protein, 16.2g carbohydrates, 3.8g fiber, 1.5g sugar, 5.3g fat, 0.4g saturated fat, 0.0mg cholesterol, 194.0mg sodium

Sautéed Cauliflower with Lemon Basil Dressing

SERVES 4

INGREDIENTS:

2 tablespoons ghee or coconut oil

1 large head cauliflower, cut into florets

2 tablespoons dried basil or 6 tablespoons fresh, chopped

¼ cup olive oil

1 tablespoon lemon juice

salt and pepper

PREPARATION:

1. In large skillet, heat ghee or coconut oil over medium heat. Sauté cauliflower, stirring often, until light golden brown.

2. Place basil, olive oil, and lemon juice in a food processor or blender and puree. Season with salt and pepper to taste. Drizzle basil sauce over cauliflower and serve hot.

NUTRITIONAL INFORMATION PER SERVING FOR 1 CUP CAULIFLOWER FLORETS: 25.0 calories, 0.0g protein, 5.1g carbohydrates, 2.5g fiber, 2.4g sugar, 0.1g fat, 0.0g saturated fat, 0.0mg cholesterol, 30.0mg sodium

NUTRITIONAL INFORMATION FOR 1 TABLESPOON DRESSING: 84.0 calories, 0.0g protein, 0.1g carbohydrates, 0.0g fiber, 0.0g sugar, 9.7g fat, 3.9g saturated fat, 0.0mg cholesterol, 0.0mg sodium

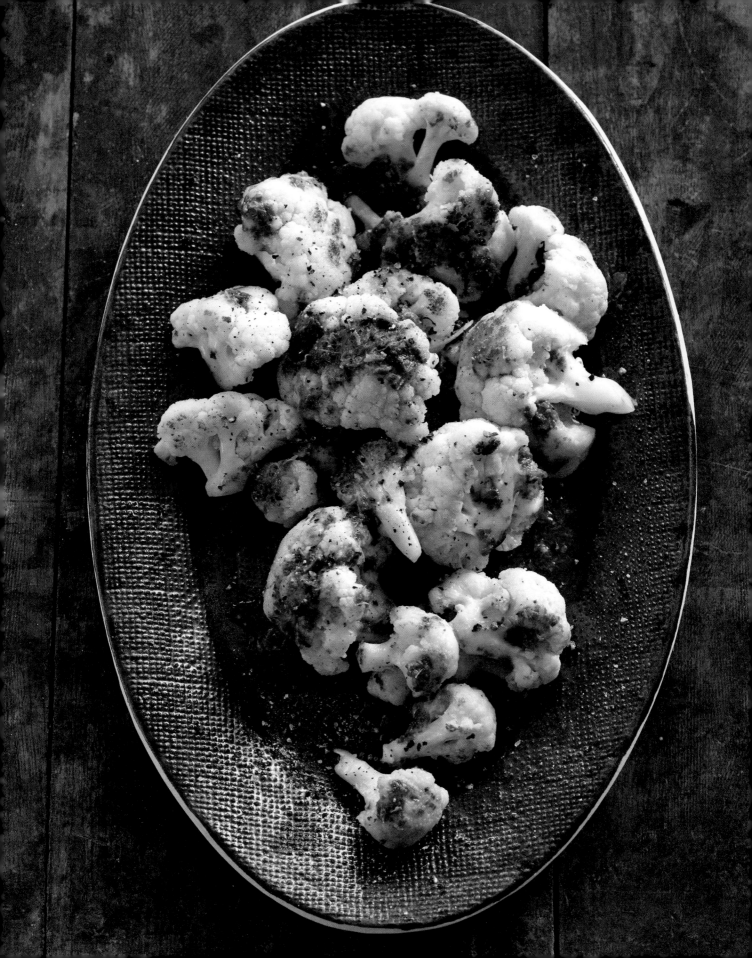

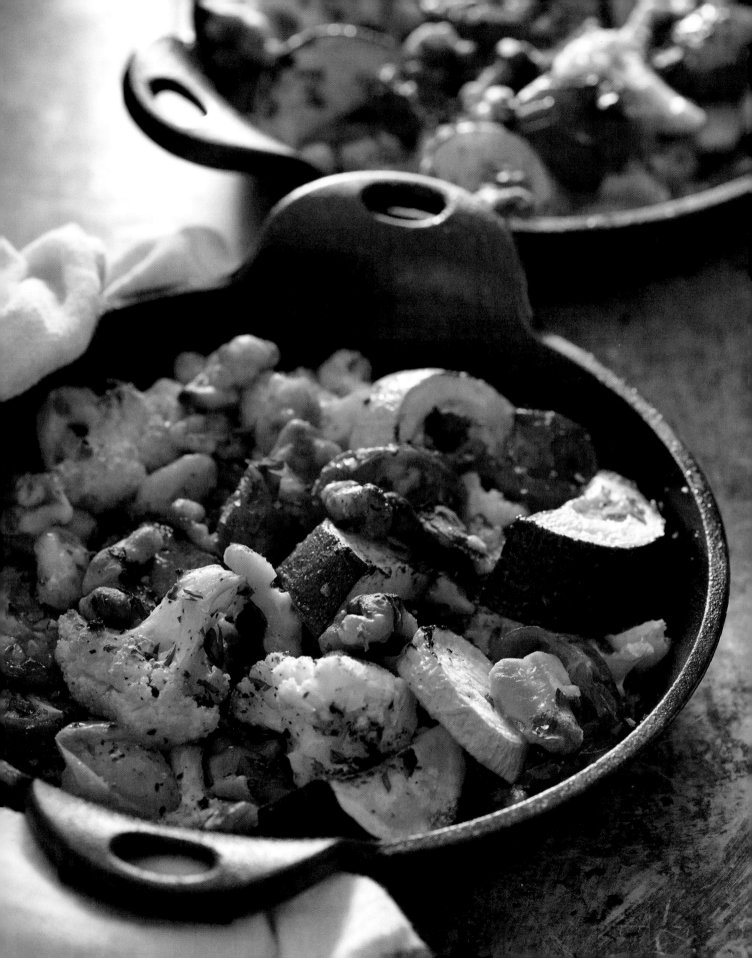

Veggie Gratin

This wonderful vegetarian option is loaded with nutrition and a decent amount of protein.

PREPARATION:

1. Preheat oven to 375 degrees F.

2. Combine tomatoes, cauliflower, squash, zucchini, beans, and garlic in a large bowl.

3. Stir in the oil, salt, and pepper.

4. Place the mixed vegetables in a 2-quart casserole pan, and sprinkle the walnuts and parsley on top.

5. Bake for 40 minutes or till veggies are tender.

SERVES 6

INGREDIENTS:

2 cups cherry tomatoes, halved

1 cup chopped cauliflower

1 cup chopped yellow squash

1 cup chopped zucchini

1 (15-ounce) can white beans, drained and rinsed

5 garlic cloves, minced

2 tablespoons macadamia nut oil or avocado oil

1 teaspoon salt

½ teaspoon pepper

½ cup walnuts, chopped

2 tablespoons flat-leaf parsley, chopped

NUTRITIONAL INFORMATION PER SERVING: 237.0 calories, 8.7g protein, 28.1g carbohydrates, 6.0g fiber, 3.1g sugar, 11.3g fat, 1.3g saturated fat, 0.0mg cholesterol, 39.4mg sodium

Wide Veggie Noodles with Sesame Tahini Sauce

SERVES 8

INGREDIENTS:

2 zucchini

2 yellow squash

2 carrots

¼ cup tahini

zest and juice of 1 lemon

1 teaspoon dark sesame oil

2 tablespoons black sesame seeds

OPTIONAL INGREDIENT:

salt to taste

This colorful, tangy dish is one of my favorites. It's not only beautiful but makes an excellent replacement for pasta as well. You may also try the "noodles" without the tahini sauce for other dishes. This dish is awesome warm or cold. It makes a great salad on a hot summer day.

PREPARATION:

1. Using a vegetable peeler, shred the zucchini, squash and carrots lengthwise into large, wide veggie noodles. Try to get a thicker noodle, rather than very thin, as they will fall apart easier. Just apply a bit more pressure while shredding for thicker noodles.

2. Bring a large pot of water to a boil. Add in veggie noodles and cook for 1 to 2 minutes, just long enough for them to soften slightly. Drain veggies completely. If you oversteam, the noodles will fall apart.

3. Combine remaining ingredients with enough water to make a light sauce.

4. Toss sauce with the veggie noodles. Serve as a side or as a colorful bed beneath Simple Citrus Chicken (page 149)

NUTRITIONAL INFORMATION
PER SERVING: 97.0 calories, 2.5g protein, 6.8g carbohydrates, 2.1g fiber, 1.9g sugar, 7.2g fat, 0.5g saturated fat, 0.0mg cholesterol, 94.1mg sodium

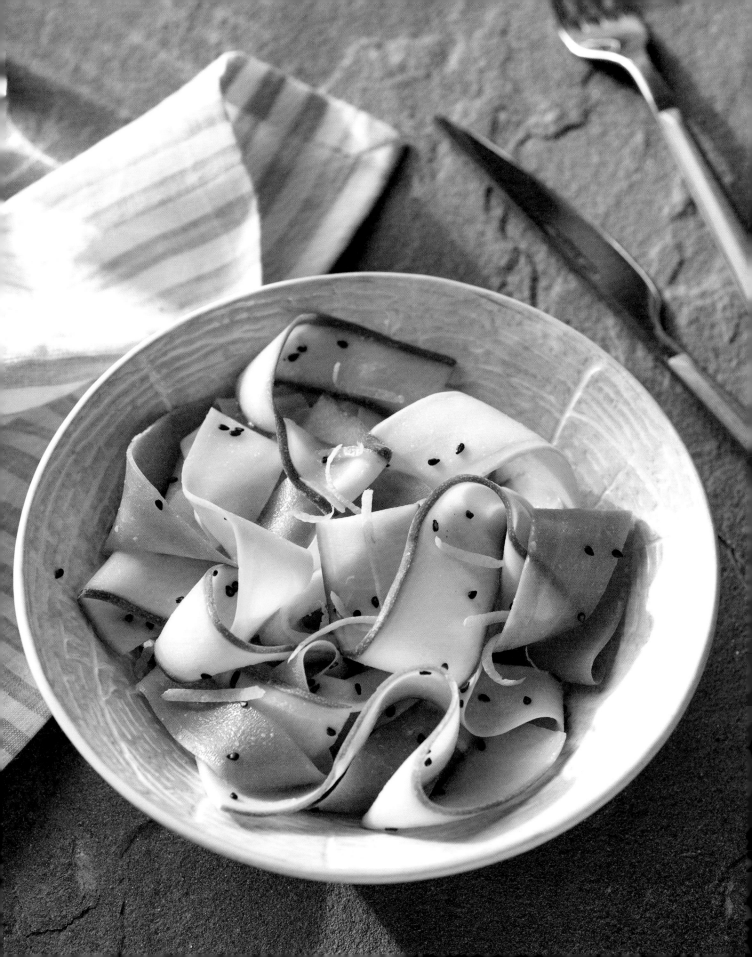

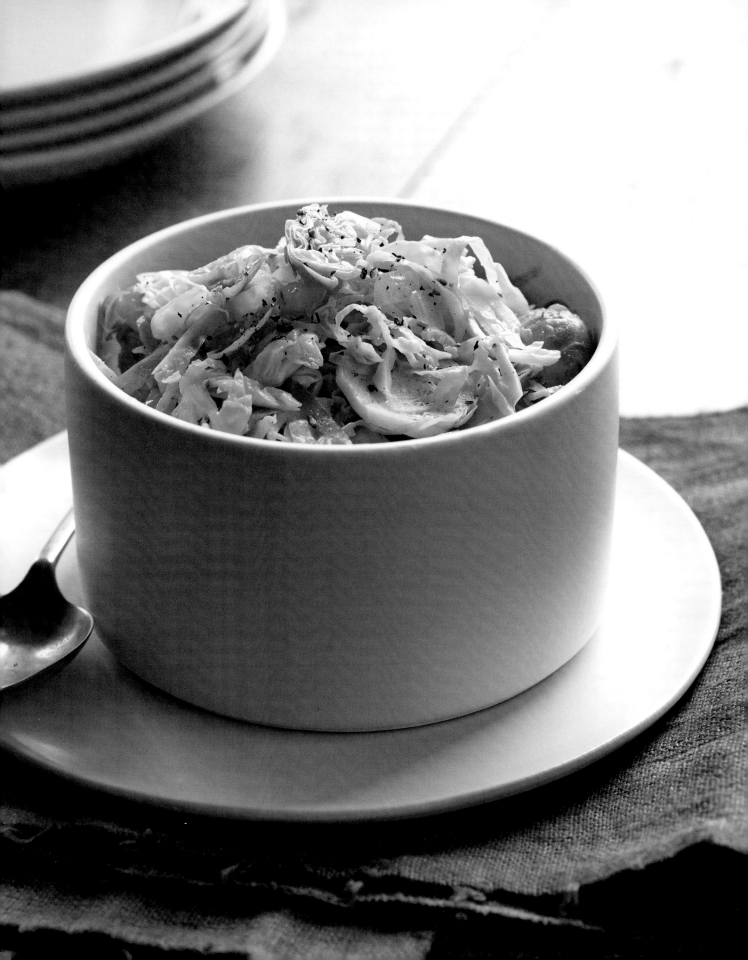

Shredded Brussels Sprout Sauté

One reason people often resist eating nutrient-dense brussels sprouts is due to their tough texture. The shredded texture is not only more palatable, but it makes a wonderful pasta replacement. Buy them preshredded, or use a food processor or mandoline to shred.

PREPARATION:

1. Heat the oil in a large frying pan over medium-high heat.

2. Add the onion and cook till soft, 1 to 2 minutes.

3. Add the shredded brussels sprouts and cook till they wilt, about 5 minutes.

4. Add the vinegar, and season to taste with salt and pepper.

SERVES 4

INGREDIENTS:
2 tablespoons coconut oil

½ cup chopped onion

1 pound brussels sprouts, shredded

2 tablespoons apple cider vinegar

salt and pepper

**NUTRITIONAL INFORMATION
PER SERVING:** 117.6 calories, 3.2g protein, 9.7g carbohydrates, 3.4g fiber, 2.0g sugar, 7.0g fat, 6.5g saturated fat, 0.0mg cholesterol, 15.6mg sodium

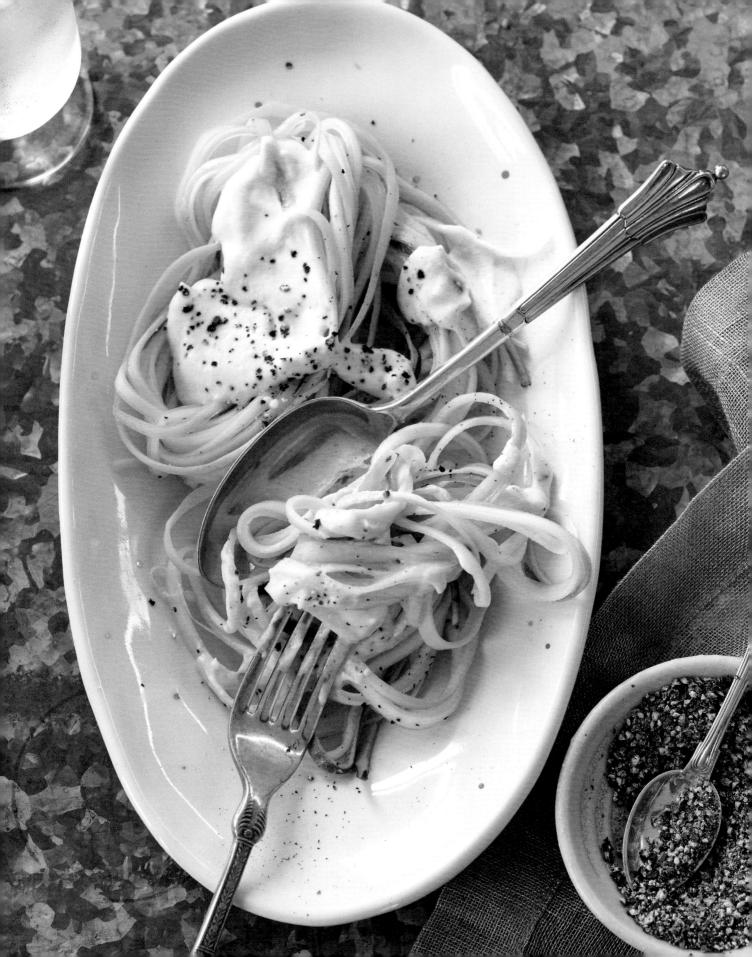

Creamy Fettuccine-Style Noodles

When making this dish for children, I will often omit the onion and garlic. However, there's nothing like sautéed onion and garlic to add rich flavor to almost any sauce.

Our first choice for pasta is "Zoodles," which are zucchini and squash noodles. They are colorful, nutritious, and simple to make. For thin Zoodles, you can purchase a simple tool for making zucchini pasta. I prefer wide Zoodles, which are easy enough to create with a vegetable peeler.

Other pasta options include soy-free shirataki noodles or quinoa pasta. Quinoa pasta tastes very similar to regular pasta so many children won't notice the difference. While quinoa pasta is gluten free, it will increase your carb intake significantly.

PREPARATION:

SAUCE:

1. Steam cauliflower florets in steamer basket until soft, 5 to 7 minutes.

2. While cauliflower is steaming, heat vegetable broth or ghee in small sauté pan. Sauté onion and garlic for 2 to 3 minutes or until soft. Remove from heat.

3. Remove cauliflower from heat and drain thoroughly.

4. In a large food processor or high-powered blender, add cauliflower and milk. Pulse or blend until cauliflower is smooth.

5. Add remaining ingredients to processor or blender. Blend until all ingredients are thoroughly mixed and sauce resembles a creamy Alfredo sauce. Serve sauce over your choice of noodles.

VEGETABLE ZOODLES:

1. Shred 3 zucchini and 3 yellow squash lengthwise with a vegetable peeler. Try to get a thicker noodle, rather than very thin, as they will fall apart easier. Just apply a bit more pressure while shredding for thicker noodles.

2. Boil a couple of inches of water in the bottom of a medium pot. Add Zoodles to a steamer basket and steam for 1 to 2 minutes. If you over-steam, the noodles will fall apart.

(RECIPE CONTINUES)

SERVES 4

INGREDIENTS:

SAUCE:

1 head cauliflower, cut into small florets

2 tablespoons low-sodium vegetable broth or 1 tablespoon ghee for sautéing

¼ sweet onion, diced

2 garlic cloves

¾ cup unsweetened coconut milk or almond milk

1 cup cashews, presoaked for 30 to 60 minutes

¼ cup nutritional yeast

1 to 2 garlic cloves

2 tablespoons lemon juice

¼ teaspoon white pepper

salt to taste

ZOODLES:

3 zucchini and 3 yellow squash or 4 packages shirataki noodles

NUTRITIONAL INFORMATION PER SERVING: 258.0 calories, 11.4g protein, 20.1g carbohydrates, 5.4g fiber, 3.3g sugar, 17.1g fat, 3.3g saturated fat, 0.0mg cholesterol, 77.0mg sodium

3. Gently remove noodles from steamer basket and drain completely.

4. Place Zoodles in colorful circles on each plate and spoon sauce over the top.

SHIRATAKI NOODLES:

1. Place noodles in a strainer and rinse thoroughly to remove all liquid they came packed in.

2. Boil in water for 3 minutes.

3. Drain well (they hold a lot of water), and divide among four plates.

4. Spoon sauce over the top.

FOR QUINOA PASTA:

1. Prepare pasta according to directions on package.

2. Put about ½ cup pasta on each plate, and spoon sauce over the top.

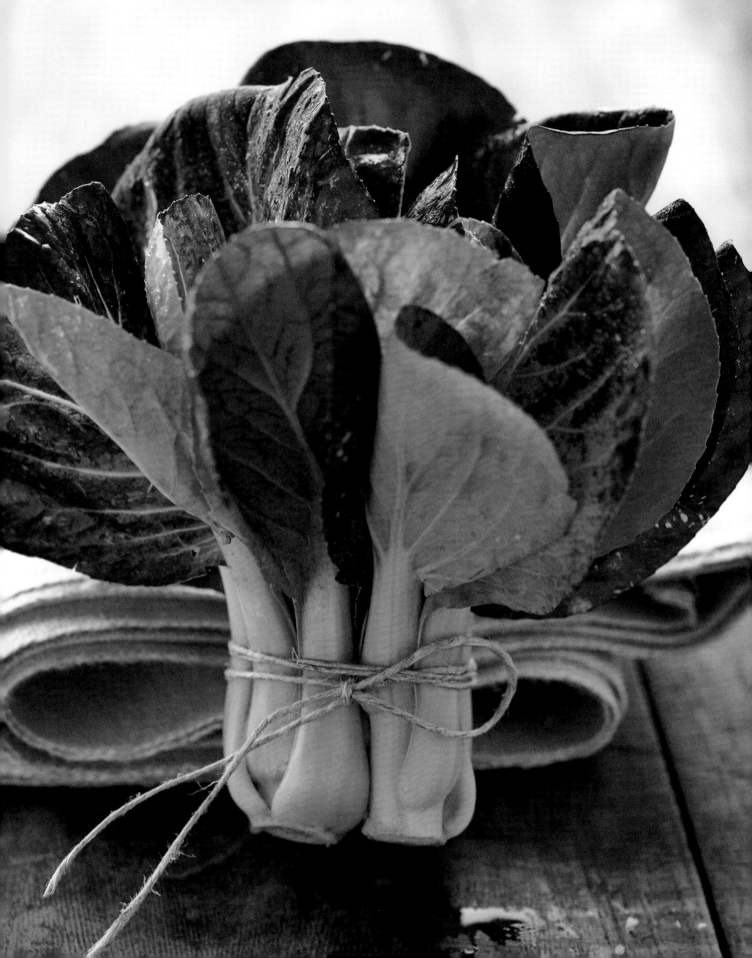

"Great health is always about abundance—of what serves you. Food that makes you sick—that's deprivation."

Snacks

■

If you really want to do something, you'll find a way. If you don't, you'll find an excuse.

—JIM ROHN

I f you fail to plan, you plan to fail. Having healthy snacks on hand *everywhere* you go is critical in winning the war for your health. When people talk to me about "white-knuckling it" and using "willpower" and simply not eating the lousy food, I know it's only a matter of time before they give in. It sounds exhausting just listening to them. Using willpower is the equivalent of setting a boat on autopilot and trying to manually turn the boat around, against the direction that the autopilot has been set. The second you let go, the boat will turn back around to what it was programmed for. You have to have a plan that takes your biology and psychology into account. Get your body working for you. Great health is about abundance. Save your energy for the real fight.

Brain Warriors do not engage in extreme calorie restriction programs that destroy their metabolism and set them up for failure. We don't want you feeling hungry, having low blood sugar, and sabotaging your program with unhealthy bingeing because you "white-knuckle it" so long that you finally cave to temptation. We want you making healthy choices that will fuel your success. Having delicious, healthy snacks will dramatically improve your success and your satisfaction.

Brain Warrior Snack Prep

1. Take one day each week to prepare. Boil a dozen eggs, chop several days of snack veggies, and prepare several of these snack recipes in advance.

2. Measure out proper portions of nuts and seeds in snack bags.

3. Keep plenty of healthy snacks ready for the family to grab and go.

4. Keep healthy snacks with you in your briefcase or purse, at the office, and when you travel.

■

Refreshing Salmon Salad

This is a delicious way to make use of leftover salmon. Using your pre-cooked salmon, skip the poaching instructions and start at step 2.

PREPARATION:

1. Quickly poach salmon by simmering it in ½ cup lightly salted water for 10 minutes. Keep covered until finished cooking. Drain water and gently remove fish. Pat dry.

2. Whisk together the lemon zest, juice, and mayonnaise.

3. Combine salmon carefully with the remaining ingredients, being careful not to break up the salmon too much.

4. Season with salt and pepper, and chill.

5. Serve on lettuce cups or in a coconut wrap.

SERVES 4

INGREDIENTS:

1 pound salmon

salt and pepper

zest and juice of 1 lemon

¼ cup Nayonnaise (page 257) or vegan mayonnaise

1 cup diced hothouse-style cucumber

½ cup diced celery

2 tablespoons fresh chives, chopped

2 tablespoons fresh dill, chopped

OPTIONAL INGREDIENTS:

4 butter lettuce leaves for serving or 4 curry-flavored coconut wraps

NUTRITIONAL INFORMATION PER SERVING: 234.0 calories, 30.1g protein, 5.3g carbohydrates, 0.9g fiber, 0.1g sugar, 10.1g fat, 0.8g saturated fat, 75.9mg cholesterol, 216.6mg sodium

One-Minute Avocado
Egg Basket

SERVES 2

INGREDIENTS:

1 avocado

2 eggs

salt and pepper, to taste

OPTIONAL INGREDIENTS:

1 tablespoon cilantro, finely chopped

¼ teaspoon chili powder

salsa

This is a great snack to eat on the run. You can bake this in the oven if you have time. If not, better to microwave than choose a chemical-laden fast-food concoction. You can have a healthy breakfast cooked within a minute.

PREPARATION:

1. If you prefer to use a toaster oven, preheat oven to 350 degrees F. Otherwise no oven prep is needed for the microwave.

2. Leaving the skin intact, cut avocado in half and remove the seed.

3. Using a spoon, increase the size of the hole where the seed was, just enough for a whole raw egg to fit. Do this to both avocado halves.

4. Crack eggs, and gently dump one into each opening you created in the avocado halves. Be careful not to break the yolks.

5. Place each avocado half in either the toaster oven or the microwave. Bake in the toaster oven for 12–15 minutes or until egg whites are opaque. If you're using the microwave, cook for approximately 1 minute. The whites should be cooked, while the yolks should remain runny. If you choose to cook both halves at the same time, you may need to add 5 to 10 seconds of cooking time.

6. Remove from the toaster oven or microwave, and sprinkle the avocados with salt and pepper. Top with cilantro, chili powder, and salsa if desired.

BAKING METHOD:

1. Place avocado half with egg on a baking sheet and bake for approximately 12 to 15 minutes or until egg whites are opaque.

2. Remove from oven, and sprinkle with salt and pepper. Top with cilantro, chili powder, and salsa, if desired.

NUTRITIONAL INFORMATION PER SERVING: 216.4 calories, 8.0g protein, 7.9g carbohydrates, 5.9g fiber, 0.5g sugar, 18.1g fat, 3.4g saturated fat, 186.0mg cholesterol, 77.8mg sodium

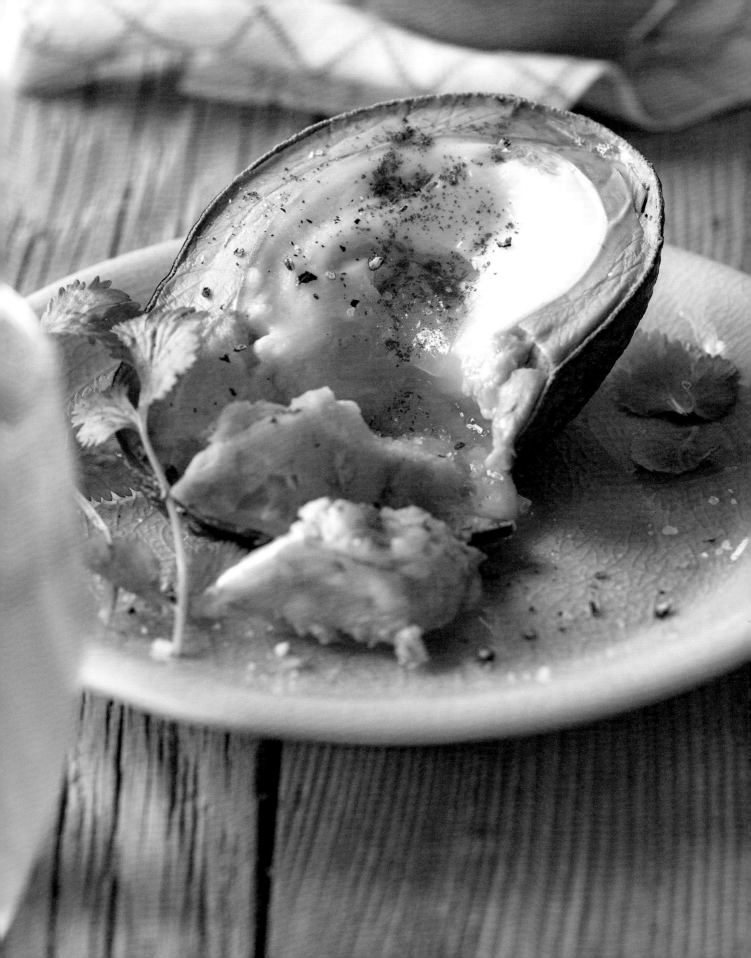

Chia Protein Pudding

SERVES 2

INGREDIENTS:

1 tablespoon chia seeds

1 tablespoon hemp seed or flaxseed

1 scoop chocolate or vanilla protein powder (plant based, sugar free)

1 cup unsweetened almond milk or coconut milk

½ cup berries or ½ banana, sliced

PREPARATION:

1. Mix chia seeds, hemp seed or flaxseed, protein powder, and milk until protein powder is thoroughly blended. Divide between two small bowls and cover.

2. Refrigerate 3 to 8 hours.

3. Top with berries or bananas.

> **NOTE:** You may also try spicing this dish up with cinnamon, nutmeg, or cardamom.

NUTRITIONAL INFORMATION PER SERVING: 169.5 calories, 14.6g protein, 16.75g carbohydrates, 6.0g fiber, 5.1g sugar, 7.0g fat, 0.5g saturated fat, 0.0mg cholesterol, 91.0mg sodium

Pumpkin Spice Smoothie

PREPARATION:

Blend all ingredients in a high-powered blender until smooth. Pour into a large glass or shake container to go.

INGREDIENTS:

1 cup organic canned pumpkin

½ banana

2 scoops chocolate or vanilla protein powder (plant based, sugar free)

1 to 2 teaspoons pumpkin pie spice *or* combine 1 teaspoon cinnamon, ¼ teaspoon ginger and ½ teaspoon nutmeg

1 tablespoon coconut oil

10 ounces unsweetened almond or coconut milk

10 ounces cold water

Pumpkin spice–flavored stevia to taste (about a dropperful)

1 cup ice, approximately

OPTIONAL INGREDIENTS:

2 tablespoons flaxseed meal

1 cup spinach

NUTRITIONAL INFORMATION PER SERVING: 252.0 calories, 22.8g protein, 20.6g carbohydrates, 7.3g fiber, 5.7g sugar, 11.2g fat, 6.0g saturated fat, 0.0mg cholesterol, 113.7mg sodium

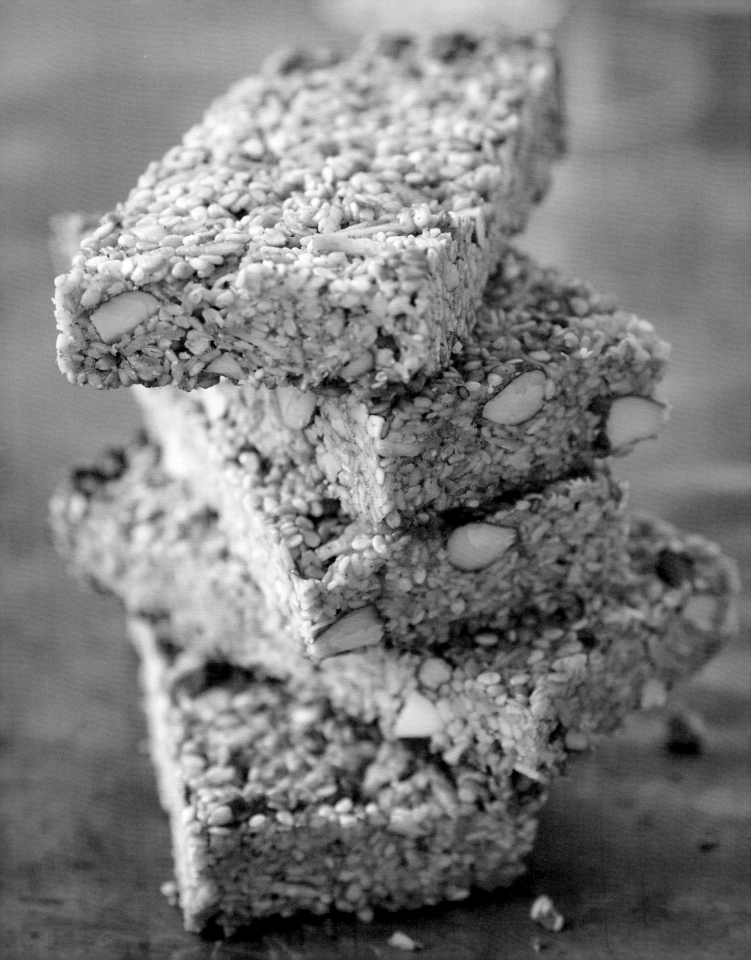

Sesame Almond Bars

PREPARATION:

1. Preheat oven to 350 degrees F.

2. Combine all ingredients till well mixed, except cooking spray.

3. Line an 8 x 8-inch square pan with parchment paper, so the paper comes above the sides of the pan. Spray the parchment with coconut oil spray.

4. Spray your hands with the coconut oil spray and push the seed mixture evenly into the pan, flattening the top.

5. Bake for 25 minutes.

6. Let cool completely, then lift out of the pan and cut into 16 bars. Keep in an airtight container.

> **NOTE:** Bars will keep for about a week in an airtight container in the refrigerator. To preserve longer, store in the freezer.

INGREDIENTS:

1¼ cups sesame seeds

¾ cup shredded coconut, unsweetened

¼ cup raw almonds, chopped

¼ cup almond butter

2 tablespoons raw honey

½ teaspoon pure vanilla extract

¼ teaspoon salt

coconut oil nonstick cooking spray

NUTRITIONAL INFORMATION PER SERVING: 149.1 calories, 3.8g protein, 7.6g carbohydrates, 3.0g fiber, 3.0g sugar, 12.3g fat, 1.1g saturated fat, 0.0mg cholesterol, 12.9mg sodium

Mac-N-No Cheese

SERVES 8

INGREDIENTS:

1 cup (about 9 ounces) raw cashews

6 cups (about 1½ pounds) diced yams

1 tablespoon lemon juice

3 tablespoons nutritional yeast

¼ teaspoon garlic powder

½ teaspoon Dijon mustard

½ teaspoon apple cider vinegar

1 tablespoon avocado oil

1 to 2 tablespoons water

½ teaspoon salt

2 8-ounce boxes quinoa pasta (corn free)

Dairy-free kids and vegans will love this recipe because the nutritional yeast makes it taste like real "Mac-n-Cheese." Nutritional yeast is an inactive form of yeast (usually a strain of Saccharomyces cerevisiae) with a rich cheesy flavor. Unlike active yeast, it doesn't cause bread to rise. It's gluten free, loaded with B vitamins—including vitamin B_{12}—and is a complete protein. Nutritional yeast is a delicious, healthy supplement to a vegan diet. The only caution is the high phosphorus content, which can deplete calcium if overconsumed without the addition of a calcium supplement. This is only a concern when nutritional yeast is consumed on a regular basis.

PREPARATION:

1. Soak the cashews in cold water overnight in the refrigerator. Rinse and drain.

2. Boil yams in water for approximately 20 minutes, or until soft.

3. Blend all ingredients except yams and pasta in a food processor until smooth, scraping down sides every couple of minutes. It will take about 8 minutes total to get a smooth consistency.

4. Add boiled yams and blend. Taste and adjust ingredients as desired.

5. Heat the mixture in a small saucepan over very low heat, whisking often. The sauce should be thick. Add more water if needed, but be very careful, because once you add the hot pasta, the sauce thins.

6. Meanwhile, cook quinoa pasta per package directions.

7. Toss hot pasta with warmed "cheese" sauce. This is delicious served with Rosemary Thyme Chicken (page 140).

NUTRITIONAL INFORMATION PER SERVING: 337.0 calories, 8.25g protein, 59.1g carbohydrates, 5.9g fiber, 3.2g sugar, 8.8g fat, 1.2g saturated fat, 0.0mg cholesterol, 387.0mg sodium

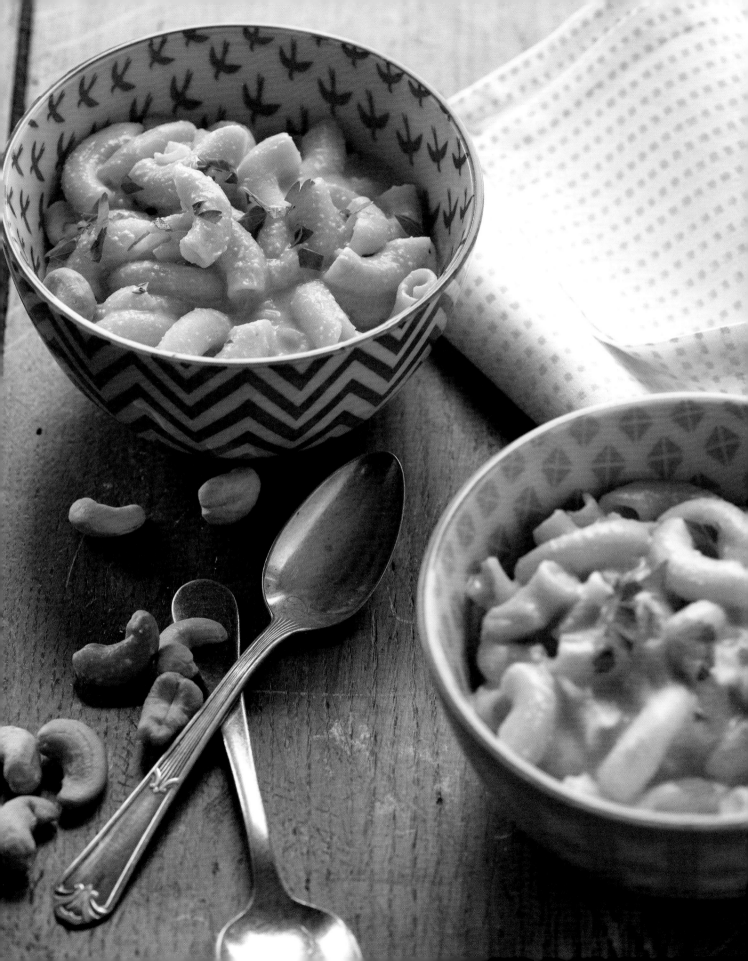

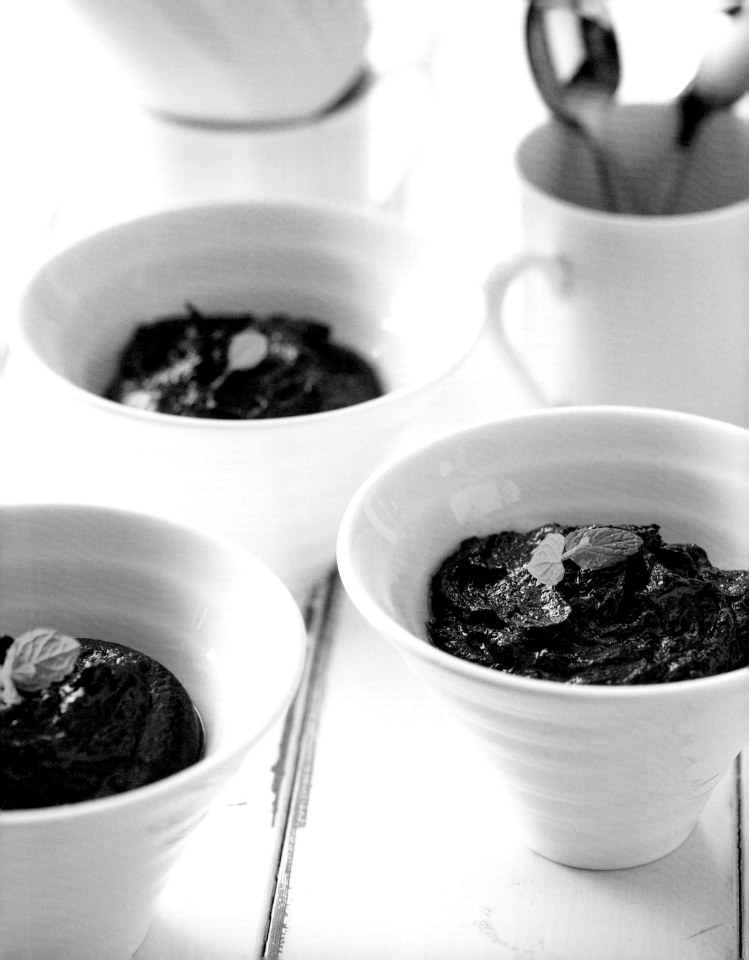

Coconut Avocado Protein Pudding

Try serving this to your kids or grandkids before telling them that it is made of avocado. It's unlikely they will have any idea. The rich chocolaty flavor is deliciously satisfying.

PREPARATION:

1. Put all ingredients in a high-powered blender and start on low. Increase speed of blender as mixture begins to blend. Mixture should be very thick. Start with ¼ cup coconut milk and add more if necessary.

2. If your blender doesn't have a tamping tool to stir as the blender is running, you may need to stop the blender and use a spoon to scrape the mixture away from the sides if it gets stuck.

3. When mixture reaches a smooth puddinglike consistency, remove from blender and place in an airtight container. Refrigerate for one hour or until ready to eat.

> **NOTE:** For fudge pops, spoon contents into ice pop molds and place a wooden stick into the center of each. Freeze for about 2 hours and serve frozen.

SERVES 8

INGREDIENTS:

2 large or 3 small avocados, peeled and pitted

½ cup coconut butter

½ cup chocolate protein powder (plant based, sugar free)

¼ to ½ cup coconut milk (depending on desired thickness)

10 to 15 drops liquid stevia, chocolate flavored

OPTIONAL INGREDIENTS:

2 to 3 tablespoons raw honey or maple syrup

2 to 3 tablespoons raw cacao (for a really chocolaty flavor and darker color)

NUTRITIONAL INFORMATION PER SERVING: 214.5 calories, 9.8g protein, 10.4g carbohydrates, 7.0g fiber, 1.5g sugar, 17.1g fat, 9.2g saturated fat, 0.0mg cholesterol, 15.2mg sodium

Smoked Salmon Curry Roll-Up

SERVES 1

INGREDIENTS:

1 coconut wrap, plain or curry flavor

2 ounces smoked, nitrate-free lox, cold, or canned wild salmon

1 slice of cucumber, sliced lengthwise

¼ avocado, sliced

OPTIONAL INGREDIENT:

1 teaspoon vegan mayonnaise or Nayonnaise (page 257)

A word of caution: these snacks are simple and delicious, and they have been my teenage daughter's favorite since she was a toddler. However, they are high in sodium, so make alterations if you're on a low-sodium diet. You can substitute lox for low-sodium canned wild salmon or use leftover salmon from the previous night's dinner.

PREPARATION:

1. Spread vegan mayonnaise, if desired, on coconut wrap.

2. Add lox, cucumber, and avocado.

3. Roll tightly with a fold at the bottom so contents don't spill.

4. If necessary, wrap with parchment paper or paper towel for transport.

NOTE: The curry-flavor wraps add a lot of flavor to this snack. Also, the avocado makes it so creamy, you really don't need vegan mayonnaise. Since I usually make these on the road, I don't have a lot of condiments on hand, and they still taste great.

NUTRITIONAL INFORMATION PER SERVING: 300.0 calories, 14.1g protein, 17.6g carbohydrates, 9.1g fiber, 3.3g sugar, 21.0g fat, 6.9g saturated fat, 13.0mg cholesterol, 1143.8mg sodium

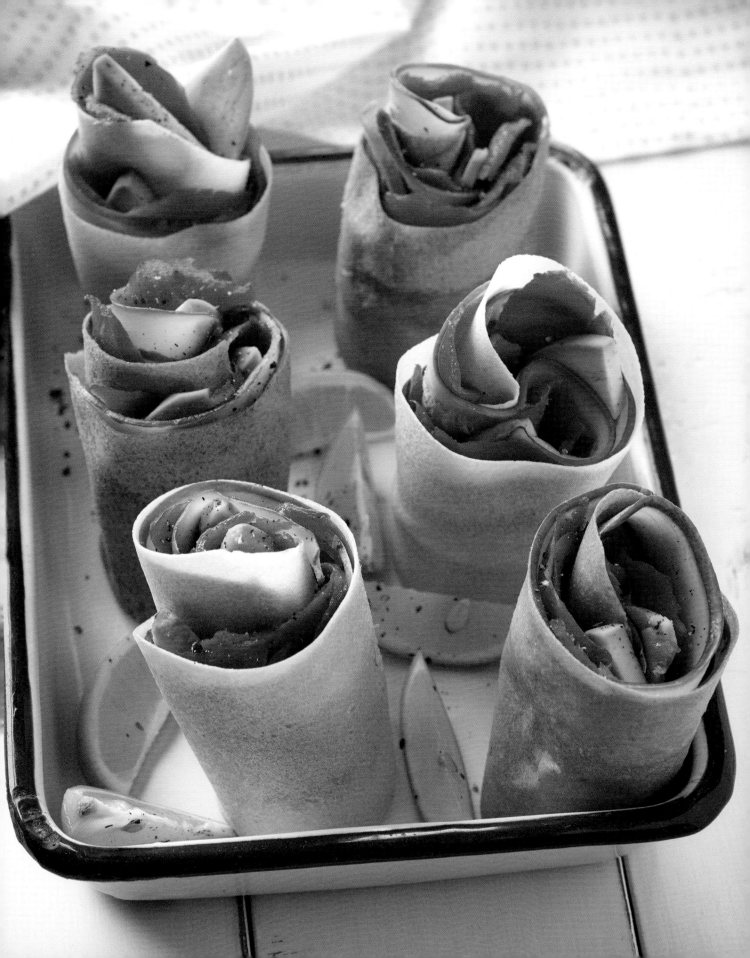

Quick Egg Salad Wrap

SERVES 4

INGREDIENTS:

8 hard-boiled, peeled eggs

1 to 2 tablespoons vegan mayonnaise or Nayonnaise (page 257)

OPTIONAL INGREDIENTS:

½ teaspoon salt

½ teaspoon curry powder or paprika

One of the tricks to being a Brain Warrior is always being prepared. One of the ways I do this is by preparing simple staples once a week and keeping the refrigerator stocked with healthy options ready to grab and go. Boiling a dozen eggs once a week can make life easy for families on the run. Hard-boiled eggs and egg salad are some of the easiest healthy options that I have found that kids like in a variety of ways.

While eggs contain significant amounts of cholesterol, it may come as a surprise that cholesterol-containing foods have less of a negative effect on blood cholesterol for most people than foods with sugar and simple carbohydrates. Excess sugar is converted to palmitic acid in your liver, which then floods the bloodstream with triglycerides. Excessive triglycerides are what's required for the processing of VLDL (very low density lipoprotein), which ultimately contributes to increased production of LDL—the worst, most dangerous kind of blood cholesterol.

PREPARATION:

1. In a food processor, blend eggs with vegan mayonnaise and spices of your choice. Pulse a few times and check for consistency. Don't overblend or egg salad will become mushy. You can mash eggs by hand if you wish. Mashing by hand usually yields a chunkier textured egg salad.

2. Seal in an airtight container until ready to serve.

> **NOTE:** This recipe is great on coconut-flavored coconut wraps or butter lettuce wraps. Also great as a dip for chopped veggies.

NUTRITIONAL INFORMATION
PER SERVING: 111.7 calories, 8.6g protein, 0.8g carbohydrates, 0.0g fiber, 0.8g sugar, 7.8g fat, 2.3g saturated fat, 253.0mg cholesterol, 90.0mg sodium

Snappy Chicken Salad Snacks

Here's a great way to make use of leftover chicken scraps. It's super simple and makes a great healthy lunch option for kids, although they seem to prefer it without the celery. In a pinch I sometimes buy a precooked chicken for this recipe, but any leftovers work: breast, whole roasted, etc.

PREPARATION:

1. Put chicken, vegan mayonnaise, and spices in a food processor bowl and pulse several times until chicken salad reaches desired consistency. Be careful not to overprocess or it turns out mushy.

2. Transfer chicken salad to a bowl, mix in celery and add more spices if necessary.

3. Slice cucumbers in half lengthwise and scoop ¼ of contents out to create cucumber boats.

4. Fill each cucumber boat with equal amounts of chicken salad and serve cold.

> **NOTE:** If preferred, serve in coconut wraps or even on top of slices of raw red bell pepper instead of in cucumber boats.

SERVES 4

INGREDIENTS:
2 cups cooked chicken, off the bone

1 to 2 tablespoons Nayonnaise (page 257) or Wholesome Hummus (page 236)

1 teaspoon paprika

½ cup finely diced celery

4 large cucumbers

OPTIONAL INGREDIENTS:
½ teaspoon curry

other spices of your choice

NUTRITIONAL INFORMATION PER SERVING: 159.8 calories, 25.7g protein, 0.0g carbohydrates, 0.0g fiber, 0.0g sugar, 5.3g fat, 0.9g saturated fat, 70.2mg cholesterol, 81.9mg sodium

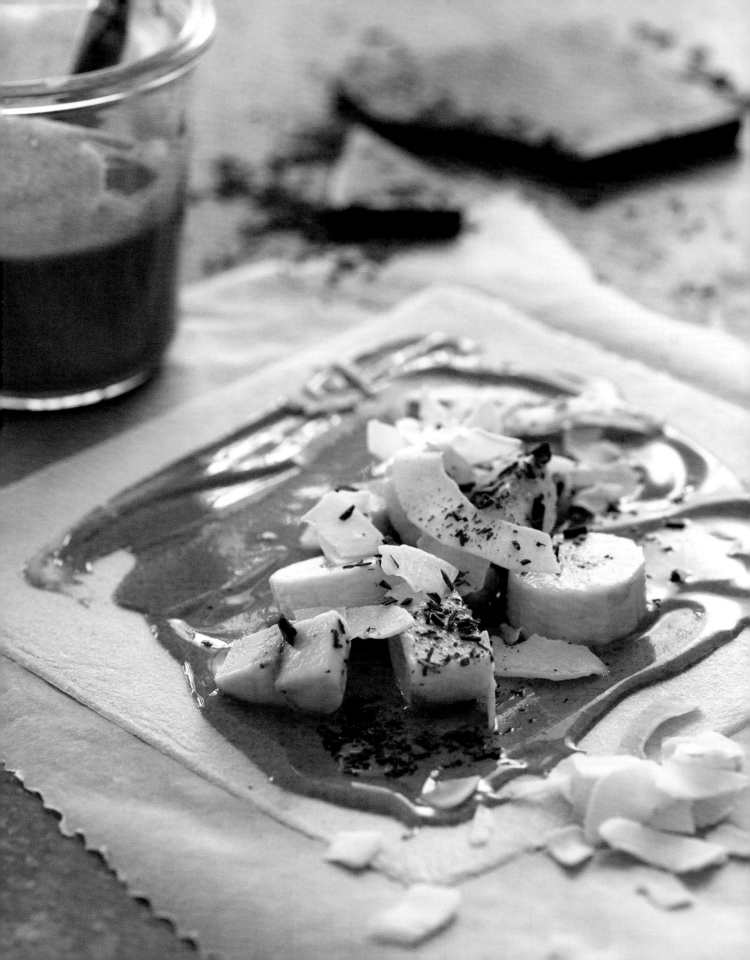

Banana Nut Roll

This is one of my favorite go-to snacks on the road because it can be made anywhere and is deliciously satisfying. I carry travel-sized packs of nut butter and coconut wraps. Bananas can be purchased at nearly any store, coffee shop or fruit stand.

PREPARATION:

1. Spread almond butter on wrap.

2. Cut banana into small bite-sized pieces and arrange over almond butter. Sprinkle cinnamon and hemp seeds if desired.

3. Roll wrap with the almond butter and banana inside.

SERVES 1

INGREDIENTS:
1 tablespoon almond butter

1 coconut wrap

⅓ banana

OPTIONAL INGREDIENTS:
cinnamon

1 teaspoon shelled hemp seeds

NUTRITIONAL INFORMATION PER SERVING: 116.2 calories, 2.2g protein, 14.0g carbohydrates, 3.1g fiber, 6.7g sugar, 6.5g fat, 2.7g saturated fat, 0.0mg cholesterol, 5.5mg sodium

Luscious Green Ice

INGREDIENTS:

16 ounces Detoxifying Green Juice (page 27) or your favorite green drink, frozen into cubes

1 frozen banana (should be halved before freezing)

½ green apple, quartered

½ cup ice

¼ cup coconut cream or almond milk

2 tablespoons cacao nibs

OPTIONAL INGREDIENTS:

2 dates or a few drops of stevia for sweetness

2 tablespoons dark chocolate squares or chips

hemp seeds

This dessert is inspired by my teenage daughter, Chloe. After years of pushing back, she suddenly jumped on the health bandwagon full steam ahead. As she developed a passion for green juice and lost her desire for sugary desserts, she asked if I could make a healthy option for the occasions that she wanted a "clean treat." It's surprisingly sweet from the little bit of fruit, but you can increase the sweetness for little ones, if necessary, by adding a few sugar-free chocolate chips or a few drops of stevia.

I order a green drink to take home and freeze while I'm at the grocery store. For best results, pour the juice into an ice tray and make green juice cubes for the near future. We usually have frozen bananas in the freezer as well.

My favorite green drink blend for this recipe, and what this recipe is based on, is Detoxifying Green Juice. Feel free to experiment with your own favorite juices.

PREPARATION:

1. A few hours before you plan to serve this recipe, prepare Detoxifying Green Juice, or your favorite green drink, and pour juice into ice cube trays. Freeze the juice until solid.

2. Place green drink cubes, frozen banana, apple, ice, coconut cream or milk, and cacao nibs and dark chocolate, if desired, in a high-powered blender. Start on the low setting. Ingredients will be difficult to mix. It should be very thick. If your blender has a tamping tool, you may need to use it to keep the mixture moving.

3. Blend until mixture is smooth and cacao nibs are thoroughly blended, not chunky. However, don't allow the mixture to become overliquefied. It should remain somewhere between the consistency of soft serve and a slushy.

4. Scoop into four dessert bowls and sprinkle with hemp seeds or a bit of shaved chocolate as desired.

5. If time allows, place in freezer for 10 to 15 minutes to give mixture time to chill and set before serving.

NOTE: Refrigerate a can of coconut milk and skim the thicker cream off the top to get the coconut cream for this recipe.

NUTRITIONAL INFORMATION PER SERVING: 103.0 calories, 1.2g protein, 16.7g carbohydrates, 1.7g fiber, 7.5g sugar, 3.7g fat, 3.2g saturated fat, 0.0mg cholesterol, 83.0mg sodium

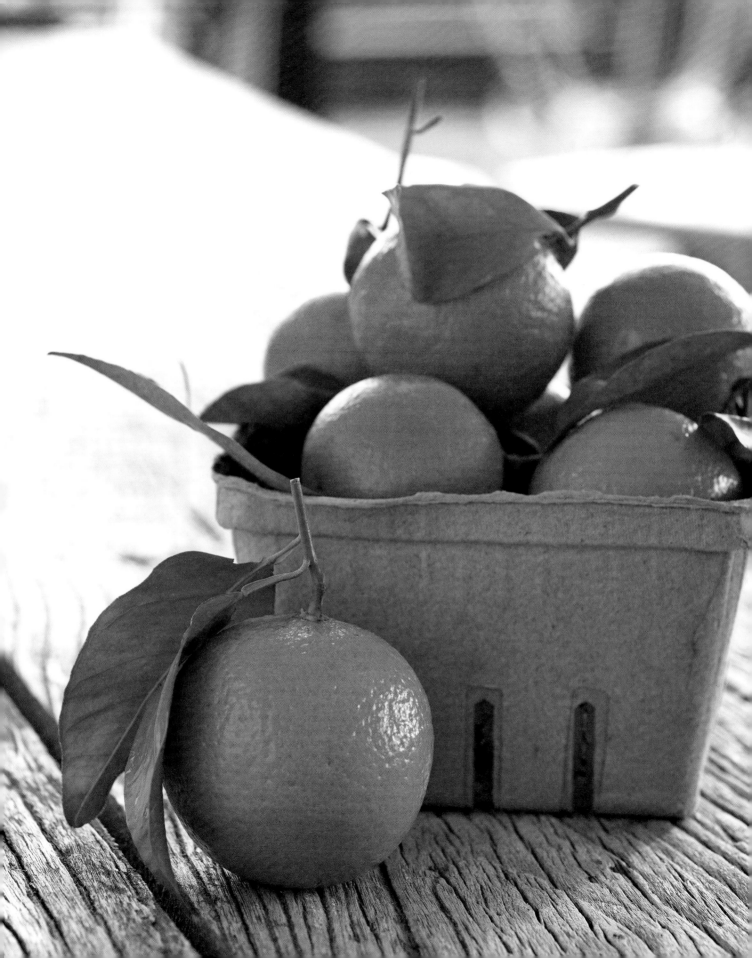

"If you're really busy, you don't have time NOT to eat healthy and exercise!"

Warriors keep an arsenal of healthy alternatives ready. One of the secrets of reigning victorious is to never feel deprived. Replace your favorite snacks with healthy alternatives.

SWAP THIS FOR THAT

As you wean yourself off unhealthy foods, use these super swap strategies:

- Drink green tea or herbal tea with a few drops of stevia instead of coffee.
- Have a decaf almond milk cappuccino as a comfort drink.
- Use coconut milk in your tea or coffee instead of half-and-half or soy creamer.
- Drink sparkling water sweetened with flavored stevia instead of diet soda.
- Squeeze lemon or lime or a few drops of stevia into seltzer to replace wine.
- Replace dairy and soy with almond or coconut milk.
- Replace candy with Brain on Joy or Brain in Love bars. They can be found on the website www.brainmdhealth.com.
- Replace ice cream with Coconut Avocado Protein Pudding (page 219), or just a handful of frozen grapes.
- Eat half an apple with almond butter instead of cookies and candy.
- Eat a pumpkin protein bar or ¼ cup raw, unsalted nuts and one piece of dark chocolate that's 70 percent cacao instead of muffins, candies, and cookies.
- Use avocado or hummus as a spread instead of butter.

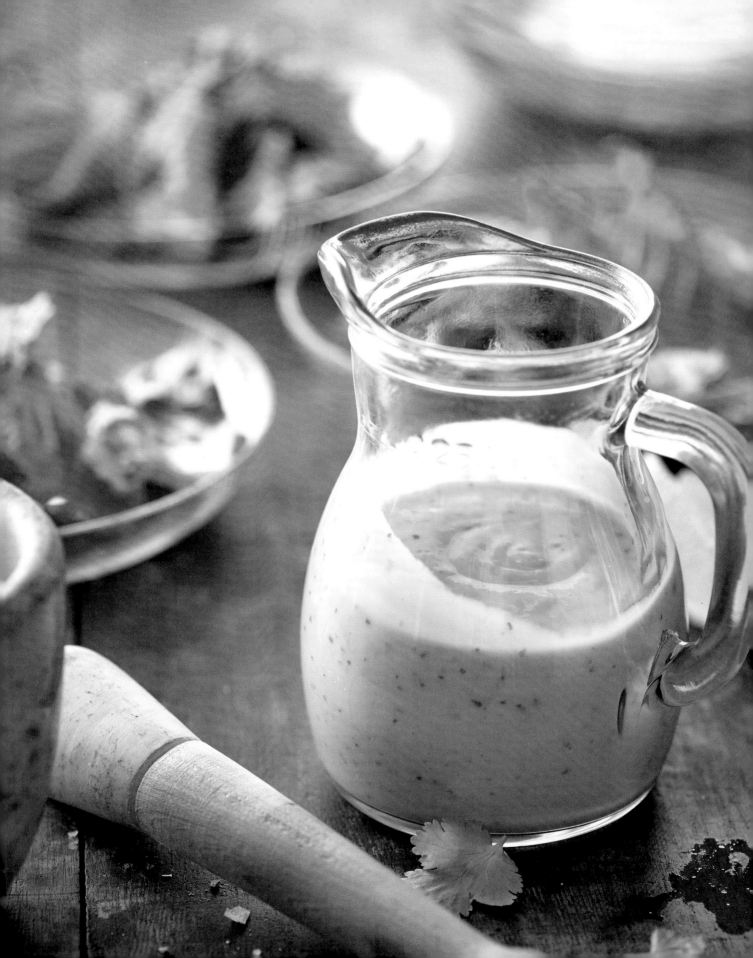

Sauces, Spreads, and Condiments

∎

Man is a moving being. If he does not move to what is good, he will surely move to what is not.

—ISSAI CHOZANSHI

S auces, spreads, and condiments can make or break any health program. No one wants to eat boring, dry food, and by making a few simple swaps, you don't have to. Great health is about abundance, not deprivation. We have no intention of eating a diet that makes us suffer, and we don't expect you to either. These recipes are party favorites and kid approved (including the big kid that sleeps next to you). With a little creativity, your family won't even realize you've hijacked their garbage food until they are healthy and vibrant. By then they will be happy about it.

Brain Warrior Food Refining

Remove extra calories, harmful chemicals, and food additives. At home, use the recipes in this section. When dining out, make these simple swaps:

1. Replace mayonnaise with hummus or Nayonnaise (page 257).

2. Replace ketchup with salsa.

3. Replace gluten-filled soy sauce with organic low-sodium tamari sauce.

4. Replace butter with avocado.

5. Replace commercial salad dressing with a little lemon and olive oil.

■

Tart and Tangy Barbecue Sauce

PREPARATION:

1. Heat oil in a saucepan over medium heat.

2. Add onion to cook until nearly caramelized. Add garlic and cook 1 more minute.

3. Add remaining ingredients, and bring to a simmer for 10 minutes.

4. Allow to cool, then puree the sauce with an immersion blender or regular blender till smooth.

5. Add salt and pepper and any other optional seasonings you like.

SERVES 16 (2 CUPS)

INGREDIENTS:

2 tablespoons avocado oil

1 onion, chopped

4 garlic cloves, minced

2 (6-ounce) cans tomato paste

½ cup erythritol

⅓ cup apple cider vinegar

1 tablespoon yellow mustard

OPTIONAL INGREDIENTS:

salt and pepper

seasonings, such as cumin, chipotle, paprika, coriander, or oregano, to taste

NUTRITIONAL INFORMATION
PER SERVING: 40.7 calories, 1.3g protein, 11.8g carbohydrates, 1.3g fiber, 3.0g sugar, 1.9g fat, 0.3g saturated fat, 0.0mg cholesterol, 205.0mg sodium

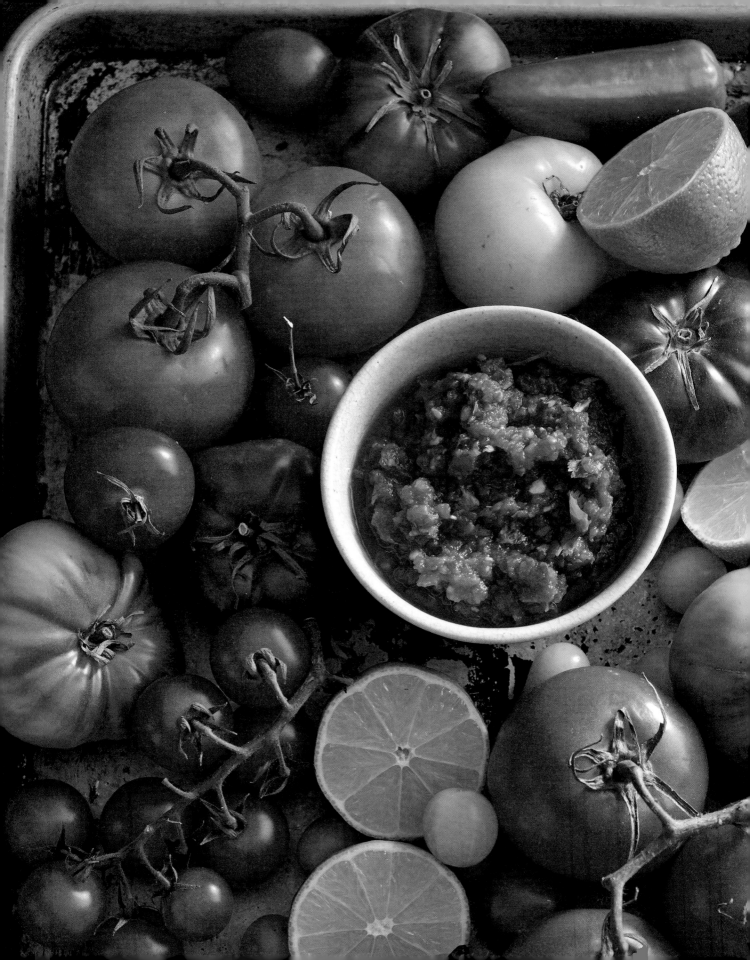

Restaurant-Style Salsa

PREPARATION:

1. In a food processor, chop the garlic cloves and jalapeño pepper, if more heat is desired.

2. Add the tomatoes, lime zest, lime juice, and the cilantro. Pulse till smooth.

3. Add the reserved tomato juice slowly until you reach the desired thickness.

INGREDIENTS:

2 garlic cloves

1 (28-ounce) can San Marzano whole tomatoes, juice separated and reserved, or 3 large fresh tomatoes

zest and juice of 1 lime

¼ cup cilantro leaves

salt and pepper, to taste

OPTIONAL INGREDIENT:

1 jalapeño pepper—add the seeds and ribs if you prefer more heat

NUTRITIONAL INFORMATION
PER SERVING: 36.3 calories, 1.4g protein, 28.0g carbohydrates, 2.3g fiber, 4.6g sugar, 0.1g fat, 0.0g saturated fat, 0.0mg cholesterol, 21.0mg sodium

Wholesome Hummus

SERVES 10

INGREDIENTS:

¼ cup fresh lemon juice

¼ cup tahini

1 small garlic clove, minced

2 tablespoons olive oil, plus drizzle of olive oil for serving

salt to taste

1 (15-ounce) can garbanzo beans, drained and rinsed

2 to 3 tablespoons water

dash of ground paprika

OPTIONAL INGREDIENT:

½ teaspoon ground cumin

Hummus is a great snack and makes a perfect dip for veggies. Remember, it's not intended to be a meal; just use a couple tablespoons, just enough to get the flavor and a satisfactory snack. Make the veggies the staple.

PREPARATION:

1. In a food processor, combine lemon juice and tahini, and pulse for about a minute. Scrape sides and pulse again for a few minutes.

2. Add garlic, 2 tablespoons of the olive oil, the salt, and cumin if desired. Pulse for about a minute. Scrape sides of bowl and pulse again.

3. Add about half of the garbanzo beans and pulse until smooth. Check consistency and add a tablespoon of water as needed. Add more garbanzos and pulse again, stopping to add water as necessary. If the mixture is really thick, add a couple more teaspoons of olive oil.

4. Once all of the beans are blended and water has been added to make the desired consistency, scrape sides and pulse the mixture again in the processor for another 30 to 60 seconds to ensure a smooth and creamy hummus.

5. Transfer hummus to serving bowl. Circle a spoon around the top, creating a smooth, circular surface. Drizzle remaining olive oil (about 1 teaspoon) around the top. Sprinkle with paprika.

6. Store in an airtight container until you are ready to serve it.

NUTRITIONAL INFORMATION PER SERVING: 104.5 calories, 2.9g protein, 10.0g carbohydrates, 2.16g fiber, 0.0g sugar, 6.4g fat, 0.9g saturated fat, 0.0mg cholesterol, 130.2mg sodium

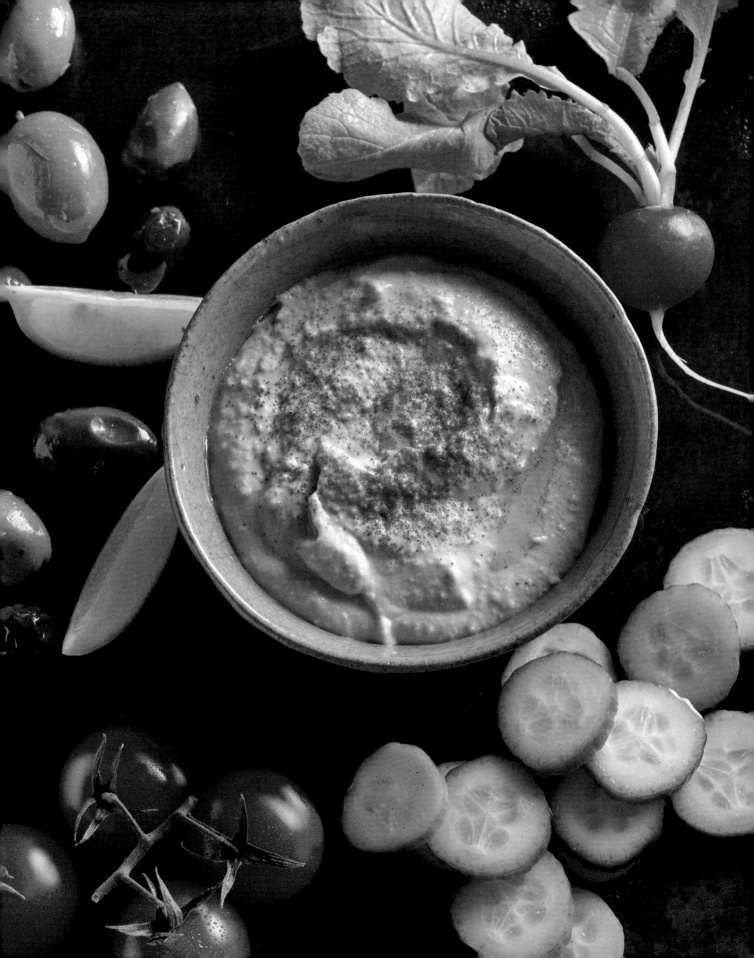

"God's Butter" Guacamole

SERVES 12

INGREDIENTS:
4 ripe avocados, peeled and pitted

garlic salt, to taste

OPTIONAL INGREDIENTS:
1 large tomato, finely diced

¼ cup cilantro, chopped

1 tablespoon lime juice

Guacamole is a go-to favorite spread for many things in our house. When our daughter was two years old, she called avocados "God's butter," and she has loved them ever since. We put them on eggs, coconut wraps, chopped veggies, soups . . . Just about anything tastes better with avocado! But remember, avocados are calorie dense, so make a little go a long way. Guacamole is intended to be a condiment.

My family tends to like things very simple, just avocados and a bit of garlic salt, but try experimenting with some of your favorite spices.

PREPARATION:

1. If you prefer chunky guacamole, mash avocados with a fork in large bowl. If you like your guacamole smoother, put the avocados in a food processor along with all other ingredients and pulse until smooth. Don't overprocess.

2. If you are hand mashing, add all other ingredients after avocados are thoroughly mashed. You may choose to keep cilantro out and add as a garnish.

3. Transfer to an airtight container until ready to serve. Guacamole doesn't last long, but the addition of lime or lemon juice will help keep it from turning brown quickly.

NUTRITIONAL INFORMATION PER SERVING: 96.3 calories, 1.1g protein, 5.0g carbohydrates, 3.9g fiber, 0.2g sugar, 8.9g fat, 1.2g saturated fat, 0.0mg cholesterol, 4.5mg sodium

Sour "Cream" Topping

This simple dairy-free recipe is the perfect sour cream alternative.

PREPARATION:

1. In a mixing bowl, blend coconut cream, vinegar, salt, and garlic, if desired. Whip all ingredients together until blended smoothly.
2. Place in refrigerator until ready to use.

> **NOTE:** Refrigerate a can of coconut milk and skim the thicker cream off the top to get the coconut cream for this recipe.

SERVES 8

INGREDIENTS:
1 cup coconut cream
2 tablespoons apple cider vinegar
¼ teaspoon salt

OPTIONAL INGREDIENT:
1 small garlic clove, minced

NUTRITIONAL INFORMATION PER SERVING: 60.0 calories, 0.0g protein, 1.0g carbohydrates, 0.0g fiber, 1.0g sugar, 6.0g fat, 6.0g saturated fat, 0.0mg cholesterol, 19.4mg sodium

Ranch-Style Dressing

This simple dressing is perfect for crudités, salad, chicken wings, and wraps.

PREPARATION:

Mix all ingredients together in a medium-sized bowl. Place in an air-tight container and refrigerate until ready to serve.

SERVES 16

INGREDIENTS:
1 cup vegan mayonnaise or Nayonnaise (page 257)
½ teaspoon garlic powder
2 teaspoons onion powder
1 teaspoon fresh chives, minced
1 teaspoon fresh dill, chopped
¼ teaspoon sea salt

OPTIONAL INGREDIENT:
1 tablespoon red wine vinegar

NUTRITIONAL INFORMATION PER SERVING: 37.0 calories, 0.1g protein, 1.3g carbohydrates, 0.0g fiber, 0.0g sugar, 3.5g fat, 0.0g saturated fat, 0.0mg cholesterol, 84.2mg sodium

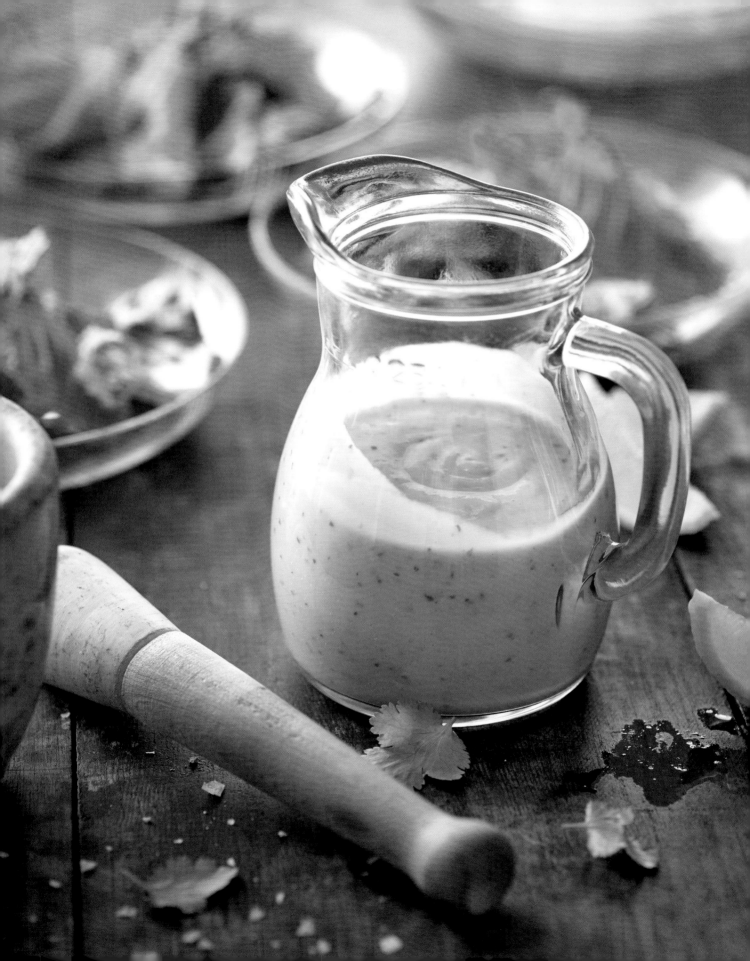

Avocado Cilantro Dressing

PREPARATION

1. In a blender or food processor, place avocado, garlic, lemon juice, cilantro, salt, and olive oil.

2. Pulse or mix on low setting for about 30 seconds or until well pureed.

3. Add water slowly, as necessary until mixture reaches a creamy consistency. Be careful not to make too thin.

4. Store in airtight container and refrigerate until ready to use.

SERVES 8

INGREDIENTS:

1 ripe avocado, peeled and pitted

1 garlic clove, halved

juice of 1 lemon

¼ cup cilantro leaves, cleaned and pulled from stem

¼ teaspoon salt

2 tablespoons olive oil

¼ cup water

NUTRITIONAL INFORMATION PER SERVING: 67.6 calories, 0.5g protein, 2.3g carbohydrates, 1.5g fiber, 0.2g sugar, 6.8g fat, 1.0g saturated fat, 0.0mg cholesterol, 21.2mg sodium

Zesty Aioli Dip

SERVES 8

INGREDIENTS:

¼ cup vegan mayonnaise

¼ cup tomato sauce or sugar-free ketchup

¼ teaspoon onion powder

¼ teaspoon garlic powder

¼ teaspoon salt

¼ to ½ teaspoon chili powder or ancho chile powder

PREPARATION:

1. Whisk all ingredients together in small bowl until smooth and creamy.

2. Divide mixture evenly into four small sauce cups, or store in an airtight container and refrigerate for future use. Sauce will last about 7 to 10 days.

**NUTRITIONAL INFORMATION
PER SERVING:** 91.4 calories, 1.9g protein, 9.9g carbohydrates, 2.3g fiber, 3.7g sugar, 5.3g fat, 0.4g saturated fat, 0.0mg cholesterol, 282.4mg sodium

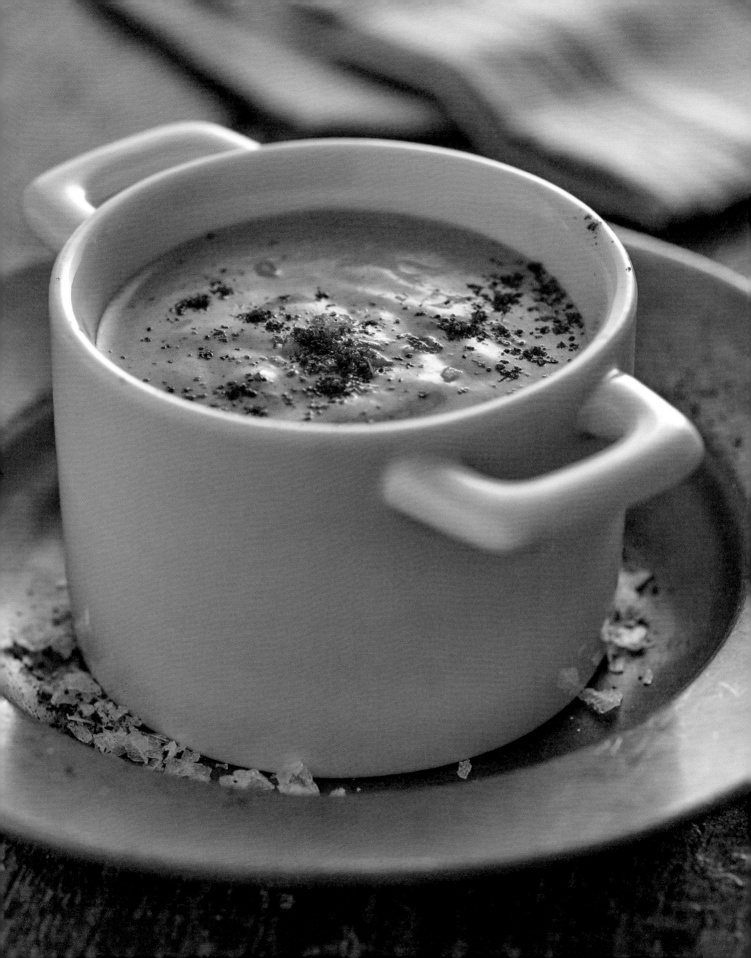

Guiltless Gravy

SERVES 8

INGREDIENTS:

2 tablespoons grass-fed butter or ghee

1 onion, chopped

2 to 4 garlic cloves

2 cups low-sodium chicken broth or bone broth (page 89)

1 to 2 tablespoons arrowroot, depending on desired thickness

salt and pepper, to taste

1 teaspoon dried rosemary or 1 tablespoon fresh, chopped

1 teaspoon dried thyme or 1 tablespoon fresh thyme, chopped

1 to 2 tablespoons coconut cream or full-fat coconut milk

OPTIONAL INGREDIENT:

¼ cup finely chopped precooked meat of your choice

PREPARATION:

1. In a medium-sized pot, melt butter over medium heat and add onions. Allow onions to caramelize, stirring occasionally for about 15 minutes or until onions are a light brown/translucent color. Be sure onions are not burning. Turn down heat if necessary.

2. After about 5 minutes, add garlic cloves to the onions. Add a bit more butter or ghee if necessary.

3. Add broth and turn up heat until mixture comes to a boil. Slowly add the arrowroot, stirring constantly to avoid clumping.

4. Add desired spices and herbs. Reduce the heat, add meat or poultry for flavor if desired, and simmer for 10 minutes.

5. Remove half of the mixture from the heat and transfer mixture to a high-powered blender.

6. Add coconut cream and blend on medium-high setting until the gravy is smooth. Stir the smooth gravy mixture back into the remaining chunky mixture with a spoon.

7. Serve over turkey or another favorite dish, such as Country-Style Biscuits (page 54) or Amen Holiday Stuffing (page 302).

> **NOTE:** In place of butter or ghee, feel free to use drippings from any meat or poultry you are cooking.

> **NOTE:** Uncured ham works well in this recipe as an optional meat, as it tastes like bacon when heated in a pan. Or use chicken, ground turkey, etc.

NUTRITIONAL INFORMATION PER SERVING: 55.0 calories, 1.0g protein, 2.8g carbohydrates, 0.4g fiber, 0.0g sugar, 4.5g fat, 4.0g saturated fat, 4.1mg cholesterol, 18.2mg sodium

Simple Fresh Tomato Sauce

PREPARATION:

Combine ingredients in a blender. Blend until smooth.

INGREDIENTS:

2 cups cherry tomatoes

2 garlic cloves, chopped

2 tablespoons fresh basil

1 tablespoon red wine vinegar

2 tablespoons extra-virgin olive oil

NUTRITION INFORMATION: 67.0 calories, 0.5g protein, 2.0g carbohydrates, 0.6g fiber, 1.2g fat, 0.5g saturated fat, 0.0mg cholesterol, 2.0mg sodium

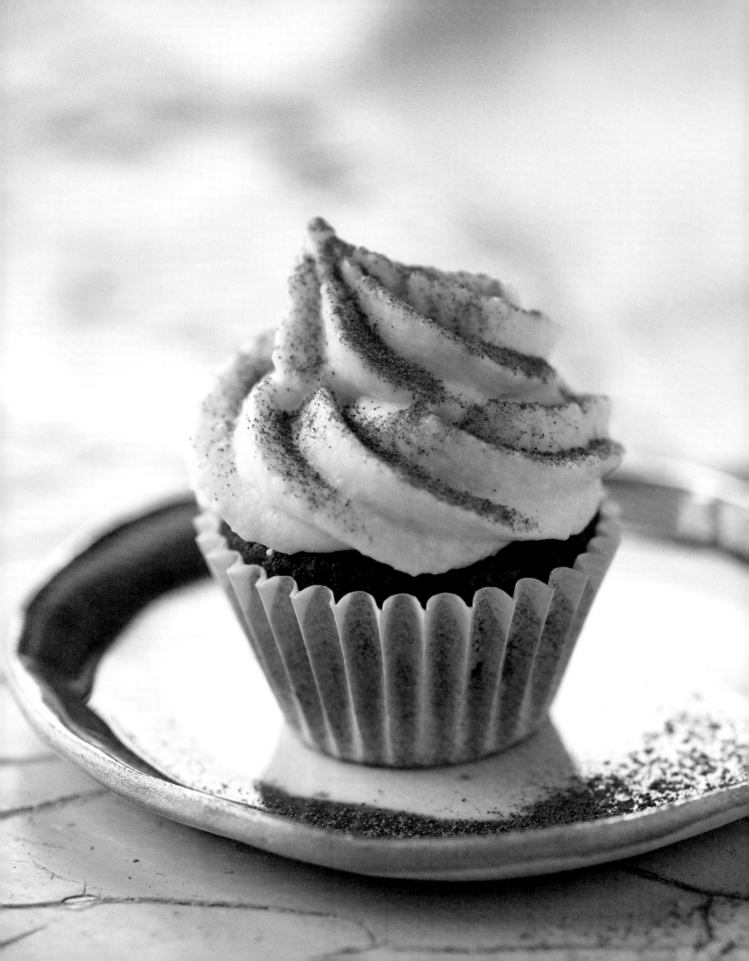

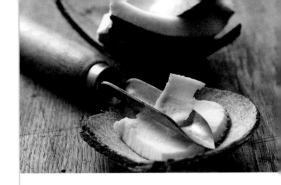

Heavenly Coconut Cream Frosting

This is a healthy, dairy-free version of processed cream cheese frosting. It's very tasty and it might be tempting to dig in and devour it, but it is high calorie and high fat, just as cream cheese frosting is. It is intended to be a spread or topping for a dessert, used in very small amounts.

This recipe calls for the meat from one or two young Thai coconuts. Some people are intimidated by the idea of opening coconuts to get the meat. It's easier than it sounds, and well worth the minimal effort! The fresh coconut water and delicious meat are amazing treats. The only thing you need is a meat cleaver or a heavy 10-inch kitchen knife to get started. Young Thai coconuts can be found at Asian markets or health food stores and come wrapped in plastic. You can use other types of coconut, but the meat is often not as soft. The meat from a young Thai coconut is usually similar to the consistency of tofu, very soft.

PREPARATION:

1. Open coconuts at top near the "soft" spot, using a large kitchen knife. Pour coconut water into an airtight container and refrigerate for future use. Using a spoon, scrape inside coconut, removing meat. Be careful not to leave behind any of the meat. Scoop and place in a bowl.

2. In a high-powered blender, place the coconut meat and honey or stevia. Add ¼ cup coconut cream.

3. Mix until creamy and smooth. Place in airtight container and refrigerate until ready to use.

4. Set out 15 minutes before spreading, to soften.

> **NOTE:** Refrigerate a can of coconut milk and skim the thicker cream off the top to get the coconut cream for this recipe.

> **NOTE:** To make Chocolate Coconut Cream Frosting, break up 2 ounces of dark chocolate (sugar free and dairy free) and put in microwave-safe bowl with about 1 tablespoon coconut milk. Microwave for 30 seconds. Stir and microwave for another 30 seconds if necessary, until chocolate is lightly melted. Add the chocolate to blender during step 2.

SERVES 16

INGREDIENTS:
1 cup fresh coconut meat from young Thai coconuts (about 2 coconuts, sizes vary)

2 to 3 tablespoons raw honey or 10 drops liquid stevia, vanilla-flavored

¼ to ½ cup full-fat coconut cream (depending on desired consistency)

OPTIONAL INGREDIENTS:
pinch of cinnamon

pinch of salt

1 teaspoon pure vanilla extract

NUTRITIONAL INFORMATION PER SERVING: 187.0 calories, 2.0g protein, 8.9g carbohydrates, 2.4g fiber, 4.8g sugar, 67.5g fat, 16.0g saturated fat, 0.0mg cholesterol, 18.1mg sodium

Stimulating Lemon Basil Dip

SERVES 16

INGREDIENTS:

1½ cup frozen peas, rinsed in warm water to defrost

½ cup yogurt

2 tablespoons basil, chopped

1 lemon, zest and juice

salt and pepper

This party favorite is a fresh, tangy dip for veggies. It's also a great alternative to hummus for those who prefer lighter flavors. It can be used as a dip for veggies, or spread on sliced turkey and cut into rolls for a snack.

PREPARATION:

1. Combine the peas, yogurt, basil, and lemon zest in a food processor or blender, and puree till smooth.

2. Season with lemon juice, salt, and pepper to taste.

NUTRITIONAL INFORMATION FOR 1 TABLESPOON LEMON BASIL DRESSING: 63.1 calories, 4.5g protein, 10.3g carbohydrates, 2.4g fiber, 5.3g sugar, 0.7g fat, 0.3g saturated fat, 1.9mg cholesterol, 82.1mg sodium

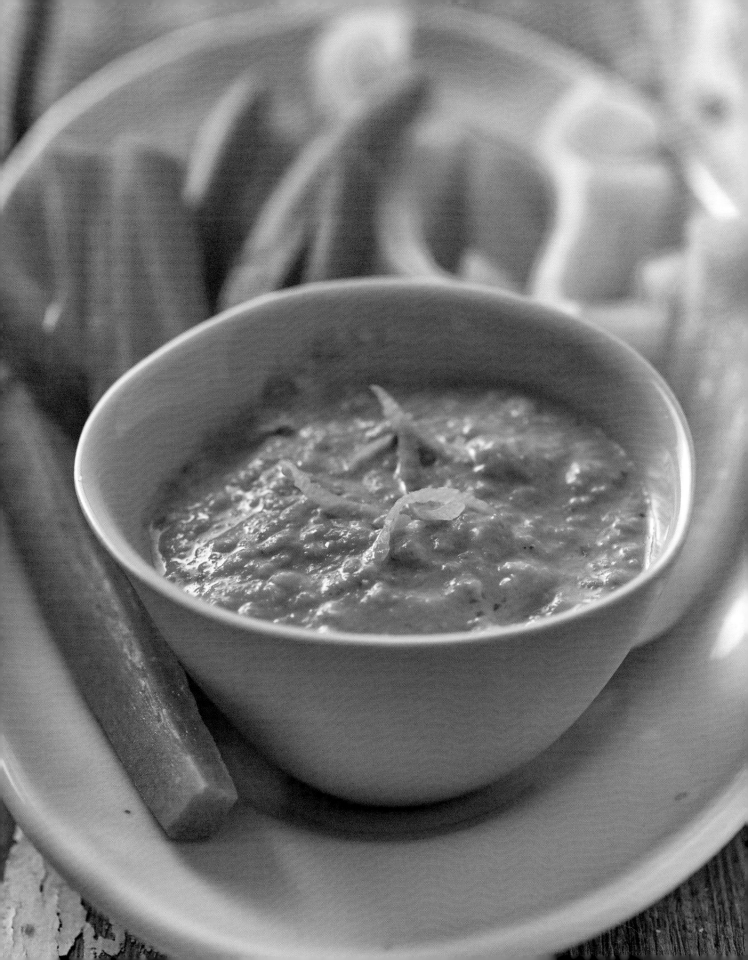

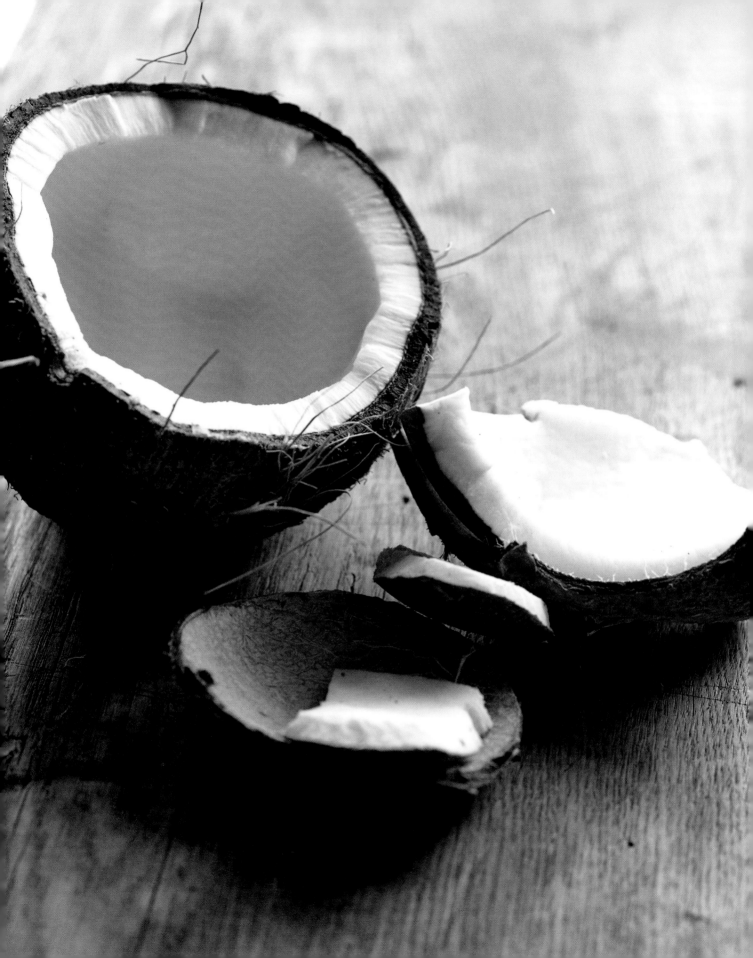

Silky Coconut Whipped Cream

This is one of my favorite toppings for berries, muffins, and other desserts. It's simple, fresh, and satisfying. In a pinch, you can skip the mixing process and simply use the coconut cream that has been separated from the fat in the can. It will hold together fairly well for a short time. Whipping the coconut cream gives you a fluffier end product that will store refrigerated for nearly a week without breaking down. It will also hold better if served over something warm.

PREPARATION:

1. Add coconut cream to a cold bowl, being careful not to get the coconut water in with the solids. Two cans of coconut milk should yield about 2 cups of coconut cream. Add erythritol or honey, if desired.

2. If you have a stand mixer, start on the low setting, increasing every few minutes until it's on the high setting. Mix coconut fat until it reaches whipped cream consistency, a process that can take 15 to 20 minutes.

3. Keep refrigerated until ready to serve.

> **NOTE:** If you don't have a stand mixer, you can use a handheld electric mixer, but it takes patience.

> **NOTE:** Refrigerate a can of coconut milk and skim the thicker cream off the top to get the coconut cream for this recipe.

SERVES 16

INGREDIENTS:

2 cups coconut cream (about 2 cans coconut milk)

2 to 3 tablespoons erythritol or 2 tablespoons raw honey

NUTRITIONAL INFORMATION PER SERVING: 69.0 calories, 0.7g protein, 1.7g carbohydrates, 0.0g fiber, 0.0g sugar, 7.2g fat, 6.3g saturated fat, 0.0mg cholesterol, 5.0mg sodium

Piquant Chimichurri Sauce

INGREDIENTS:

¼ cup fresh flat-leaf Italian parsley

1 cup packed fresh cilantro

2 tablespoons fresh oregano or
1 teaspoon dried

2 garlic cloves, peeled

2 tablespoons chopped shallot

3 tablespoons red wine vinegar

½ to ¾ cup extra-virgin olive oil

salt and white pepper

OPTIONAL INGREDIENT:
pinch of cumin

Use it as a marinade, serve it over meats, dip veggies in it, eat it on eggs, dollop it on top of a bowl of soup, or even use it as a condiment for just about anything—this chimichurri sauce is versatile!

PREPARATION:

1. Puree all ingredients, except oil, in a food processor.

2. Add the olive oil until the mixture reaches the consistency you would like. Adjust salt and pepper as desired.

> **NOTE:** Try this with the Omega Egg Burrito to Go (page 56) or Fajita-Style Roasted Veggies (page 147)

NUTRITIONAL INFORMATION
PER SERVING: 28.2 calories, 1.3g protein, 6.4g carbohydrates, 2.2g fiber, 0.4g sugar, 0.6g fat, 0.1g saturated fat, 0.0mg cholesterol, 6.6mg sodium

Mood-Boosting Chocolate Sauce

There's a reason that chocolate is the international food of love. Cacao contains phenethylamine (PEA), a plant compound that alerts your brain something fun is coming. This recipe includes the best of the cacao without the harmful effects of the sugar.

PREPARATION:

1. Place chocolate chips and coconut oil in a microwave-safe bowl.

2. Put bowl in microwave for 20 to 30 seconds. Remove from microwave and stir. Heat again for 20 to 30 seconds more, then remove and stir.

3. Continue heating, stirring until chocolate is melted and smooth. Be sure to heat in 20- to 30-second intervals to avoid burning the chocolate.

> **NOTE:** You can use sugar-free chocolate chips or chocolate bars broken into pieces for this recipe. See the Recommended Brand List (pages 338–39) for suggestions.

SERVES 16

INGREDIENTS:

8 ounces dark chocolate, sugar free and dairy free

2 tablespoons coconut oil

NUTRITIONAL INFORMATION PER 1-TABLESPOON SERVING:
58.5 calories, 0.9g protein, 7.1g carbohydrates, 3.75g fiber, 0.0g sugar, 5.9g fat, 3.4g saturated fat, 0.0mg cholesterol, 0.9mg sodium

Perfect Pesto

SERVES 16

INGREDIENTS:

2 packed cups basil or cilantro

4 garlic cloves

salt, to taste

white pepper, to taste

½ cup hemp seeds, walnuts, or pine nuts

juice of one lemon

½ cup extra-virgin olive oil

OPTIONAL INGREDIENT:

2 tablespoons nutritional yeast

Pesto can be tossed with quinoa, rice, gluten-free pasta, zucchini noodles, or roasted veggies. Also try pesto as a dip for fresh veggies, as a marinade for chicken or seafood, or as a dollop on top of soup.

PREPARATION:

1. In a food processor or blender, put the basil or cilantro, 1 garlic clove and a pinch of salt and pepper if desired, and pulse until the basil is finely chopped.

2. Add the hemp seeds, yeast if desired and 2 tablespoons lemon juice. Slowly drizzle in the oil while pulsing until you get to the consistency you'd like.

3. Taste, and adjust garlic, lemon, salt, and pepper to your preference.

NUTRITIONAL INFORMATION PER SERVING: 92.0 calories, 0.8g protein, 1.2g carbohydrates, 0.4g fiber, 0.2g sugar, 10.0g fat, 1.2g saturated fat, 0.0mg cholesterol, 0.4mg sodium

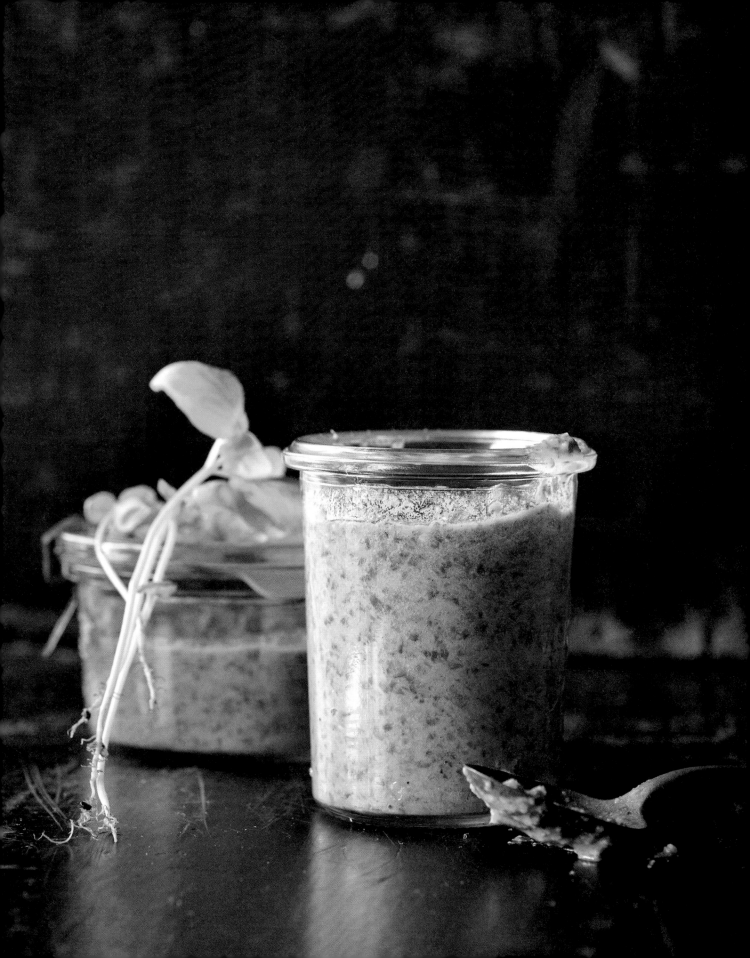

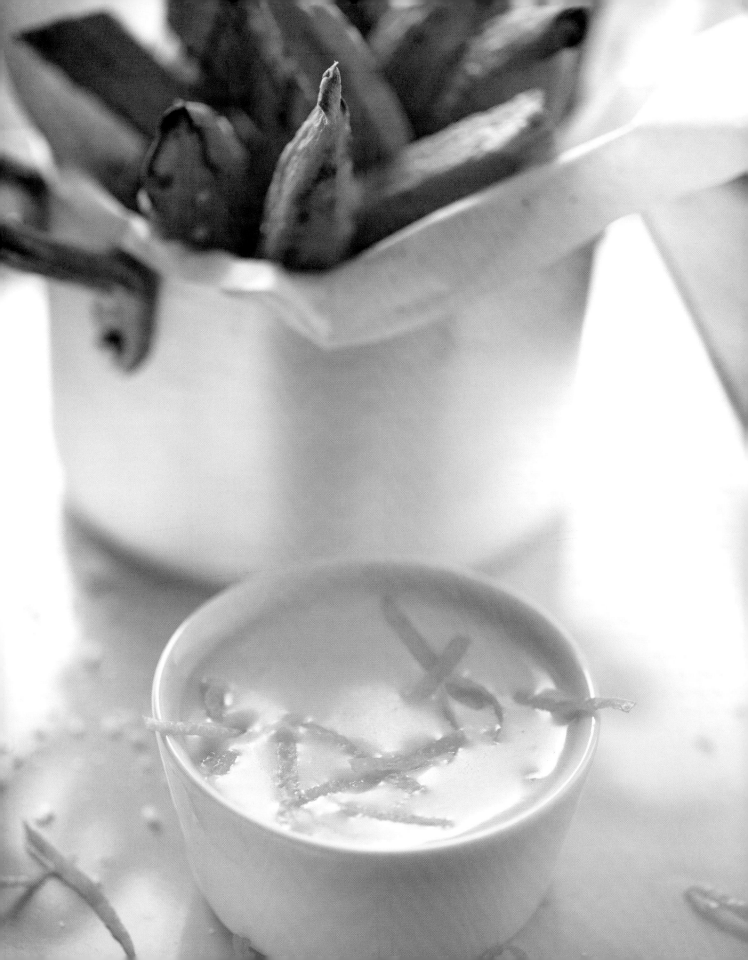

Nayonnaise

Making your own mayonnaise isn't hard, but it does require a bit of patience. If you add the oil too quickly and don't mix long enough, the mayonnaise will not thicken properly. It's very important to purchase high-quality pasteurized eggs when making any recipe containing uncooked eggs.

PREPARATION:

1. For traditional version: put egg, egg yolk, and mustard in a blender or food processor on the lowest setting. For vegan, add coconut milk to blender or food processor with mustard and run on lowest setting.

2. Drizzle ¼ cup of the olive oil or macadamia nut oil or avocado oil into the egg mixture as it is blending. Do this very, very slowly (over several minutes).

3. Add vinegar and salt as desired (I usually add about ½ teaspoon). Keep mixture blending the entire time. It should start to thicken.

4. Slowly drizzle the remaining ¼ cup of olive oil, macadamia nut oil or avocado oil into the mixture, as the mayonnaise is blending. Add coconut oil and allow mixture to blend for another minute or so. Mayonnaise should blend for a total of about 7 to 8 minutes from start to finish and be fairly thick at the end. It will thicken further when refrigerated. Put in airtight container and refrigerate for about 1 hour until mixture thickens. Discard any unused portion after a week.

NOTE: The vegan version will be looser without the egg, but it will set when refrigerated.

TRADITIONAL RECIPE:
SERVES 12 /
VEGAN: SERVES 16

INGREDIENTS:

TRADITIONAL:
1 whole egg plus one egg yolk

½ teaspoon Dijon mustard

½ cup olive oil, macadamia nut oil or avocado oil

¼ cup coconut oil

2 teaspoons fresh lemon juice or red wine vinegar

salt, to taste

VEGAN:
½ cup almond milk or coconut milk

½ teaspoon Dijon mustard

1 cup olive oil, macadamia nut oil, or avocado oil

1 to 2 teaspoons red wine vinegar or fresh lemon juice

pinch of salt

NUTRITIONAL INFORMATION PER SERVING FOR TRADITIONAL NAYONNAISE: 93.8 calories, 0.5g protein, 0.5g carbohydrates, 0.0g fiber, 0.1g sugar, 10g fat, 5.3g saturated fat, 0.0mg cholesterol, 1.4mg sodium

NUTRITIONAL INFORMATION PER SERVING FOR VEGAN NAYONNAISE: 44.21 calories, 0.0g protein, 0.1g carbohydrates, 0.0g fiber, 0.0g sugar, 9.4g fat, 1.3g saturated fat, 0.0mg cholesterol, 5.9mg sodium

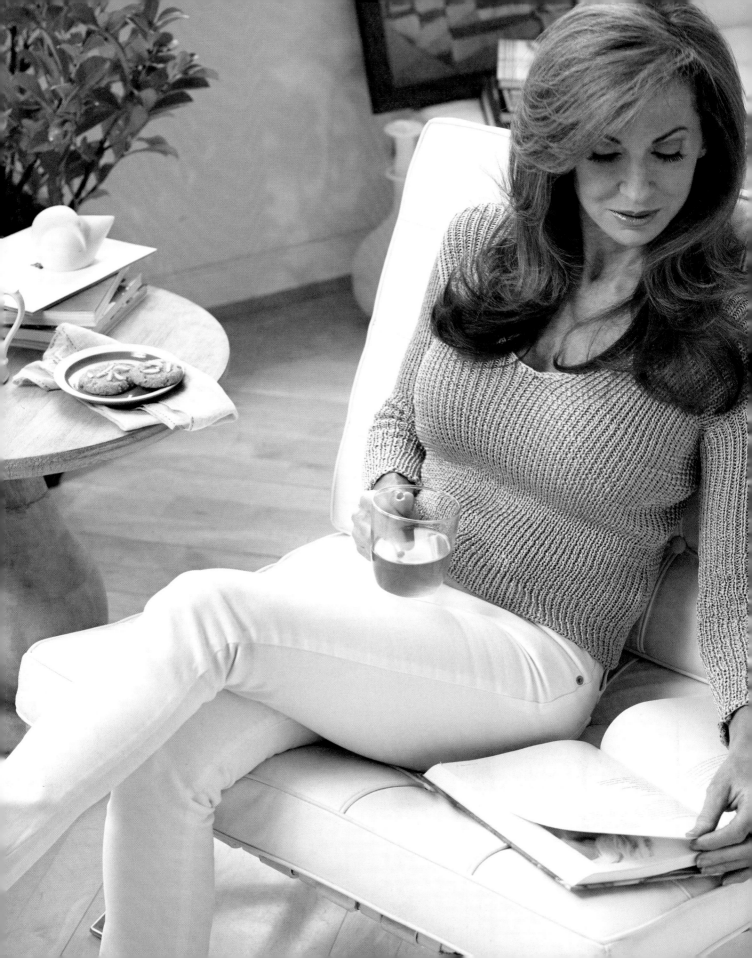

"Celebrate your victories. Rejuvenate your soul."

"Once you understand the mindset of a Brain Warrior, there is no suffering. Lose your story about being 'deprived' and you will have gratitude for food that serves you."

Bakery

Brain-Healthy Treats,
Breads, and Desserts

■

Accept challenges so that you may know the exhilaration of victory!

—GEORGE S. PATTON

There is no suffering required to be a Brain Warrior. People often say they don't want to get healthy because they don't want to be deprived. They love "treats." The real treat is being healthy and living your mission. But we understand that you want something tasty after a long day and a healthy meal. Frankly, there's no way I'd get anyone in my family to give up chocolate without a fight, and there's no reason to. Dozens of studies show the benefits of dark chocolate, minus the dairy and sugar. And there are plenty of other "treats" that are loaded with brain-healthy nutrients also.

These desserts are proof that being healthy doesn't mean suffering or deprivation. However, I don't recommend making a meal of them. Don't sacrifice the nutrient-dense meals in the book for dessert. Enjoy them as the treat they are intended to be.

Brain Warrior
Planning for Sweet Success

1. Keep some peeled bananas in the freezer. They can quickly be turned into tasty treats.

2. Freeze fresh fruit that goes uneaten and make sorbet.

3. Melted dark chocolate (sugar free and dairy free) makes even the healthiest snack taste decadent when lightly drizzled over the top.

4. Frozen desserts can be prepared ahead and kept on hand for surprise visitors.

■

One-Minute, Three-Ingredient Mug Cake

While microwave cooking isn't my first choice, there are times when it makes more sense to use the microwave than to eat fast food from unreliable sources. Sometimes we're just busy. I'd prefer our clients make this simple, wholesome treat for their kids, using a microwave, over processed, store-bought snacks loaded with sugar and chemicals. If you prefer the traditional route, prepare the ingredients the same way, but bake in a preheated oven (350 degrees F) for about 20 minutes, depending on the size of the oven-safe mugs.

PREPARATION:

1. Put chocolate in a microwave-safe bowl. Heat in 20- to 30-second increments, stopping to stir chocolate so it doesn't burn. As soon as chocolate is melted, remove the bowl from the microwave.

2. While chocolate is melting, put eggs in blender and blend on low speed (or use a handheld electric mixer, but the blender is faster). Let eggs whip until they stiffen and form peaks, about 90 seconds to 2 minutes.

3. Add baking powder and eggs to the chocolate. Stir in erythritol if desired. Gently stir until eggs and chocolate are completely blended. Be careful not to overmix or eggs will collapse. Mixture should look fluffy.

4. Divide evenly between two small microwave-safe dessert dishes or two regular-sized mugs. Put in the microwave for 1 minute each. Cook individually for best results.

5. Remove and allow to cool for 2 to 3 minutes. (They are really hot!)

6. If you wish to add the topping, place topping ingredients into a microwave-safe cup. Microwave all ingredients in 20-second increments, stopping to stir, until mixture is warm and creamy. Spread over cakes like a ganache.

7. For best results, serve warm so cake remains soft and moist inside.

NOTE: Refrigerate a can of coconut milk and skim the thicker cream off the top to get the coconut cream for this recipe.

SERVES 2

INGREDIENTS:

CAKE:
4 to 5 ounces dark chocolate, sugar free and dairy free

2 eggs

¼ teaspoon baking powder

OPTIONAL INGREDIENT:
1 tablespoon erythritol

TOPPING:
1 ounce dark chocolate, sugar free and dairy free

1 tablespoon cashew or almond butter

1 tablespoon coconut cream

NUTRITIONAL INFORMATION PER SERVING: 153.2 calories, 10.3g protein, 11.0g carbohydrates, 3.0g fiber, 1.2g sugar, 12.8g fat, 7.6g saturated fat, 186.0mg cholesterol, 354.6mg sodium

Two-Ingredient
Nutty Butter Cups

SERVES 12

INGREDIENTS:

8 ounces dark chocolate, sugar free and dairy free

¼ cup almond butter or seed butter (no stir)

OPTIONAL INGREDIENTS:

2 tablespoons coconut oil

Try serving these at a party. No one will believe they aren't peanut butter cups!

PREPARATION:

1. Line a mini muffin pan with candy paper or mini muffin liners. Standard muffin liners will be too large.

2. In a microwave-safe bowl, put about 2½ ounces of the chocolate and coconut oil if desired. If using chocolate bars, break into pieces. Coconut oil is not necessary, but it will give you a bit of grace, guaranteeing you don't burn your chocolate, and that you get smooth, creamy sauce every time. Heat chocolate in 20- to 30-second intervals, stirring each time. Heat until the chocolate is completely melted and smooth, being careful not to burn it. If you prefer heating chocolate over the stove, either heat over low heat using a double boiler, or use a small pot and stir constantly so the chocolate doesn't burn.

3. When chocolate is liquefied, spoon about ½ teaspoon of the chocolate mix into each candy paper, just enough to cover the bottom of the paper.

4. Put pan in the freezer for about 5 minutes so chocolate hardens.

5. While chocolate is cooling in the freezer, melt remaining chocolate (and coconut oil if desired).

6. Remove pan from freezer. Drop about ½-teaspoon–sized balls of nut butter in the middle of each cup, on top of the hardened chocolate base. Press lightly to flatten the ball so that the nut butter doesn't protrude over the top of the cup, but don't smash it down. The nut butter should remain in the center and not bleed out over the edges of the chocolate base.

7. Spoon remaining chocolate mixture into each cup, covering the nut butter completely. Be sure you get the sauce around the sides. If necessary, flatten the top and smooth over with chocolate. If chocolate doesn't surround the sides of the nut butter, the nut butter will show through, and the cups will fall apart.

8. Freeze for about 15 minutes before serving.

> **NOTE:** Be sure you use a firm "no-stir" brand of almond butter or seed butter. Most other nut butters are oily and separate. If it is too oily, it will bleed through the chocolate and cause the cups to fall apart. Also, keeping the cups small will make them easier to work with.

NUTRITIONAL INFORMATION
PER SERVING: 58.8 calories, 1.5g protein, 5.35g carbohydrates, 2.35g fiber, 0.0g sugar, 5.5g fat, 2.04g saturated fat, 0.0mg cholesterol, 1.1mg sodium

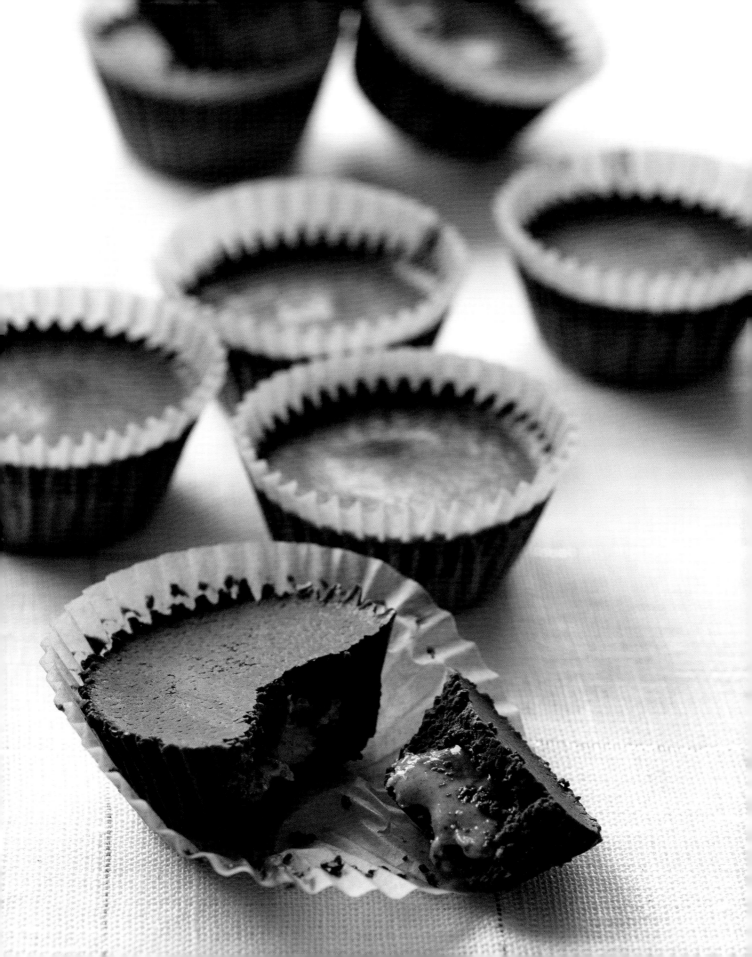

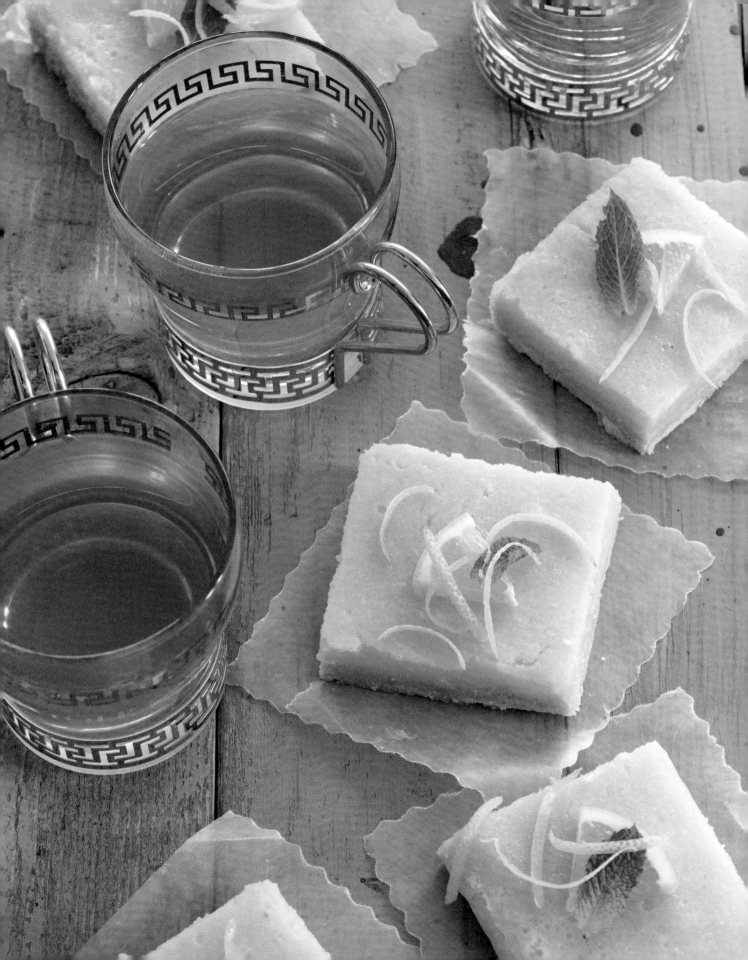

Luscious Lemon Squares

PREPARATION:

1. Preheat oven to 325 degrees F and generously rub an 8 x 8-inch baking pan with coconut oil, or line with parchment paper to ensure the lemon bars don't stick.

2. In a medium-sized bowl combine coconut oil, erythritol, flour, and salt, if you desire, to create the crust. Mix until a smooth dough forms.

3. Press dough evenly into the bottom of the prepared pan and place in oven for 10 to 12 minutes or until crust is a light golden brown. Once the crust is baked, let it cool for 15 to 20 minutes.

4. While crust is cooling, hand-whisk the remaining ingredients, adding the arrowroot last and slowly. Continually whisk while adding arrowroot to avoid clumping.

5. Pour lemon mixture over top of cooled crust and bake for about 25 to 30 minutes or until set. Let cool. For best results, place in refrigerator in an airtight container for at least 1 or 2 hours after cooling. This allows the crust to set.

6. Cut the bars into 16 squares.

> **NOTE:** Store bars in the refrigerator, and remember to remove from refrigerator 15 minutes prior to serving so they won't be hard. Coconut oil gets very firm in the refrigerator.

SERVES 16

INGREDIENTS:
½ cup coconut oil, at room temperature

⅓ cup erythritol

1 cup almond or coconut flour (or ½ cup of each for best results)

3 large eggs

½ cup erythritol

¼ cup raw honey

2 teaspoons arrowroot or ½ teaspoon baking powder

½ cup fresh lemon juice

OPTIONAL INGREDIENT:
½ teaspoon salt

NUTRITIONAL INFORMATION PER SERVING: 135.5 calories, 2.7g protein, 16.5g carbohydrates, 0.8g fiber, 4.5g sugar, 11.4g fat, 7g saturated fat, 34.9mg cholesterol, 28.6mg sodium

Double Chocolate
Mini Muffins

SERVES 12

INGREDIENTS:

⅓ cup coconut flour

¼ cup raw cacao powder

½ teaspoon baking powder

¼ teaspoon salt

4 eggs, beaten

1 teaspoon pure vanilla extract

2 tablespoons maple syrup

¼ cup erythritol

¼ cup coconut milk

¼ cup coconut butter, melted

¼ cup dark chocolate chips or dark chocolate bar, sugar free and dairy free

PREPARATION:

1. Preheat oven to 350 degrees F and line a muffin tin with 12 muffin papers.

2. If using a chocolate bar, chop chocolate into chip-sized pieces.

3. Whisk together the coconut flour, cacao, baking powder, and salt.

4. Make a well in the middle of the dry ingredients and add all the remaining ingredients except the chocolate chips. Whisk together.

5. Fold in the chocolate chips. Let the batter set and thicken for 5 minutes before baking.

6. Divide batter between 12 paper-lined mini muffin cups.

7. Bake for 12 to 15 minutes depending on desired moistness.

8. Serve warm.

NUTRITIONAL INFORMATION PER SERVING: 142.3 calories, 4.3g protein, 17.1g carbohydrates, 3.4g fiber, 2.7g sugar, 8.7g fat, 3.7g saturated fat, 62.0mg cholesterol, 63.5mg sodium

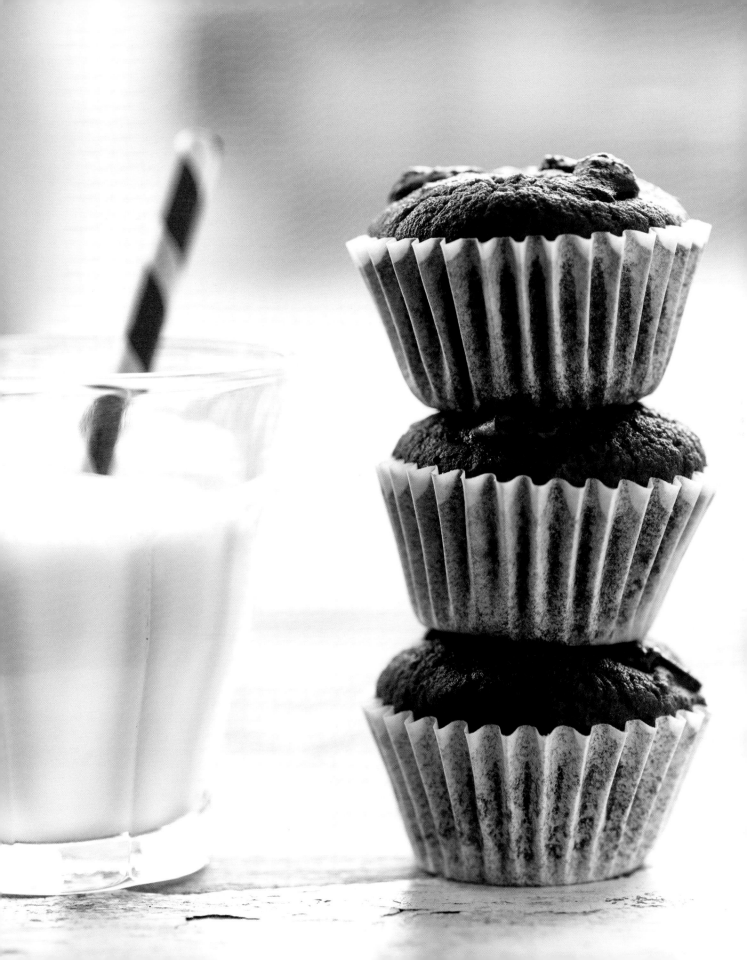

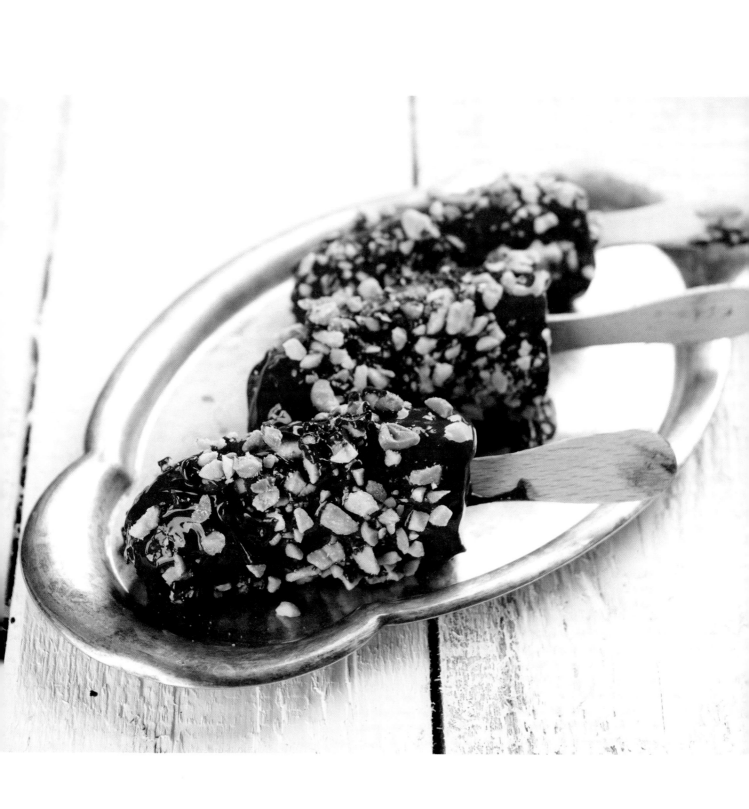

Whiz Kid Frozen Bananas

You will need four wooden ice pop sticks for the bananas.

PREPARATION:

1. Line a small cookie tray with parchment paper and set aside.

2. Place chocolate in a microwave-safe bowl. Add coconut oil. Melt in 15- to 20-second increments, stopping to stir after each increment. Chocolate should be melted within 60 to 75 seconds. Do not heat all at once or chocolate will burn. After chocolate is melted, add stevia if desired.

3. While chocolate is melting, push wooden sticks into the flat ends of the halved bananas.

4. Pour melted chocolate sauce into a wide saucer or small plate so it's easy to dip and roll the bananas.

5. Put nuts or coconut in another wide saucer or dinner plate next to chocolate.

6. Holding the stick, dip each banana into the chocolate sauce, rolling and coating the entire banana.

7. Immediately dip the bananas in the nuts or coconut, rolling to coat banana completely.

8. Lay coated bananas on waxed paper and place tray in freezer for at least 20 minutes to allow chocolate to set.

9. Refrigerate leftover sauce in airtight container for later use. Sauce will store for over a week.

NOTE: Leftover sauce makes a great dip for mixed berries.

SERVES 4

INGREDIENTS:
4 ounces dark chocolate, sugar-free and dairy-free bar broken into chunks or use chocolate chips

2 teaspoons coconut oil

2 slightly green bananas, peeled and halved

OPTIONAL INGREDIENTS:
5 to 10 drops liquid stevia, chocolate flavor

¼ cup finely chopped cashews or walnuts

¼ cup shredded coconut, unsweetened

NUTRITIONAL INFORMATION PER SERVING: 193.4 calories, 2.4g protein, 26.3g carbohydrates, 10.1g fiber, 5.0g sugar, 15.9g fat, 9.7g saturated fat, 0.0mg cholesterol, 2.5mg sodium

Revitalizing Lemon Almond Cookies

SERVES 12

INGREDIENTS:

¾ cup almond flour

¾ cup coconut flour

1 teaspoon baking soda

¼ teaspoon salt

1 egg

3 tablespoons raw honey

¼ cup coconut oil, melted

zest and juice of 1 lemon

½ teaspoon pure vanilla extract

¼ cup slivered almonds

PREPARATION:

1. Preheat oven to 350 degrees F.

2. Combine dry ingredients—the flours, baking soda, and salt—in a bowl, and whisk.

3. Combine wet ingredients—the egg, honey, coconut oil, lemon zest and juice, and vanilla extract—and stir until thoroughly combined. Add wet ingredients to dry ingredients and mix until a smooth dough forms. The dough will be very thick.

4. Form into 12 equal-sized cookies and place on a parchment-lined baking sheet. Press dough down to flatten with the back of a spoon dipped in water. Place several almond slivers on top of each cookie.

5. Bake about 8 to 10 minutes depending on desired crispness.

6. Allow to cool and set for a few minutes before serving.

NUTRITIONAL INFORMATION PER SERVING: 160.4 calories, 4.0g protein, 10.0g carbohydrates, 2.4g fiber, 4.8g sugar, 12.2g fat, 4.9g saturated fat, 15.5mg cholesterol, 124.0mg sodium

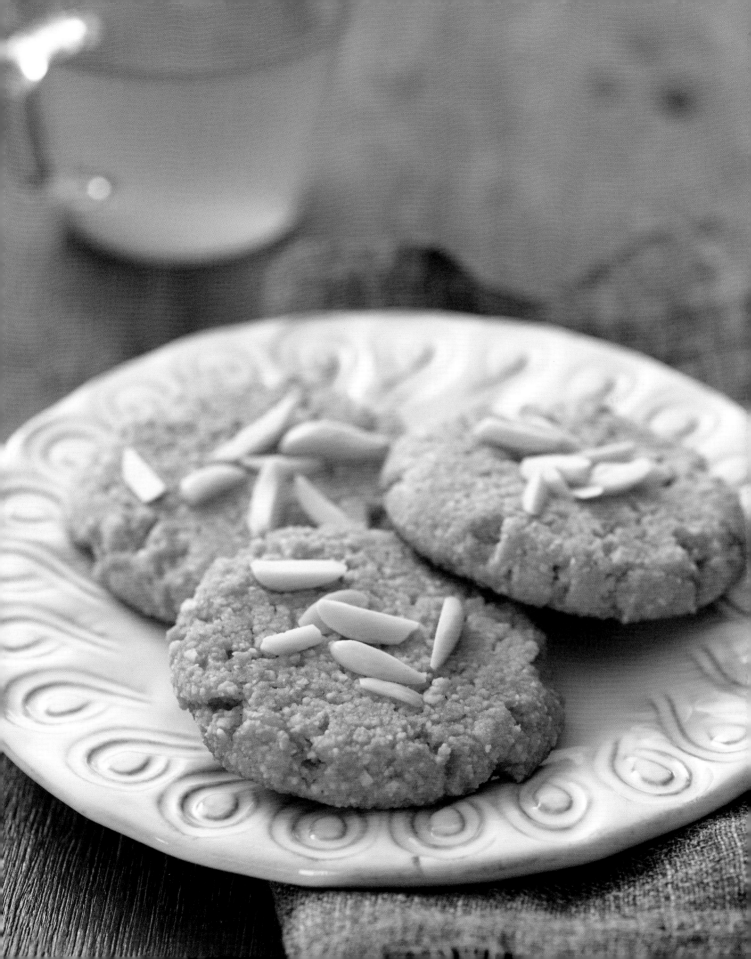

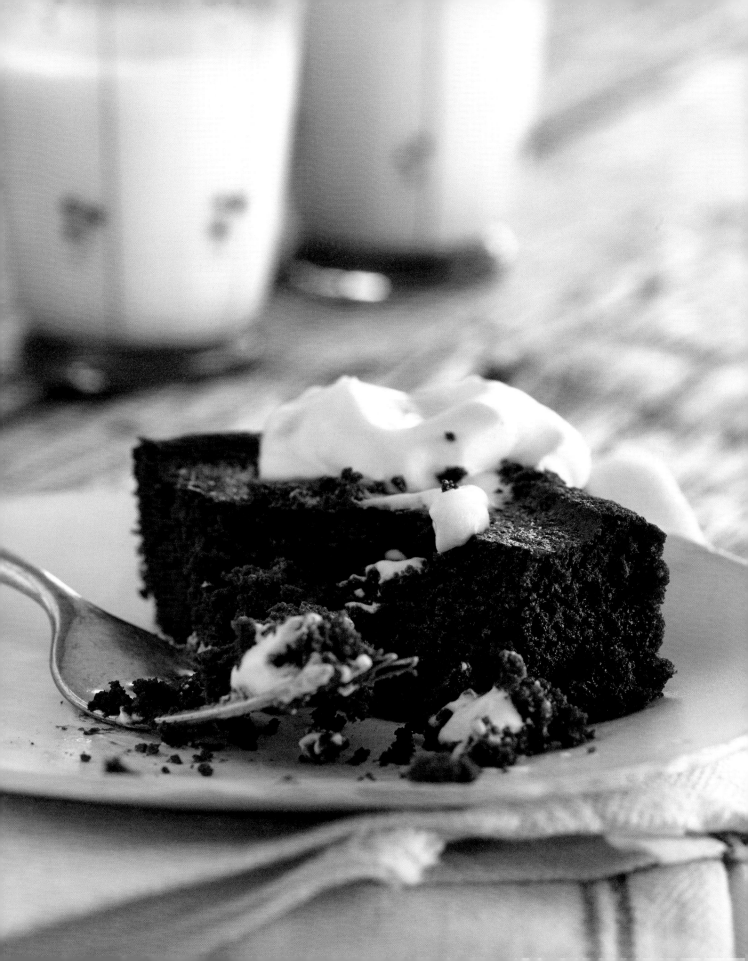

Fudgy Brownie Bites—
Two Ways

Fudgy Brownie Bites with Egg

Guests often look at us a little funny when I serve these delicious Brownie Bites, because they just don't taste healthy. The fudgy, rich chocolate and natural sweetness belie the fact that they are grainless and low glycemic. You can use either banana or canned organic pumpkin.

PREPARATION:

1. Preheat oven to 350 degrees F.

2. In a small saucepan over low heat, place coconut cream, chocolate (broken into pieces if it's a chocolate bar), cacao, and coconut oil. Stir frequently until ingredients are melted and thoroughly blended. Remove from heat.

3. In a medium-sized mixing bowl, place coconut flour, arrowroot, and baking soda. Blend together.

4. Add macadamia nut oil, eggs, and either mashed banana or canned pumpkin to dry ingredients.

5. Add chocolate mixture and erythritol or maple syrup to all other ingredients. Blend with a handheld electric mixer until wet and dry ingredients are thoroughly blended.

6. Spray a 9 x 11 baking dish with coconut oil or grease well. Pour brownie batter into pan evenly so there are no high spots.

7. Bake for 25 to 30 minutes depending on desired chewiness. Allow to cool before serving.

Serve warm or at room temperature. The longer they cool, the more "brownielike" they will be as the coconut oil sets. Store remaining brownies in an airtight container. Freeze leftovers within a couple of days.

> **NOTE:** Refrigerate a can of coconut milk and skim the thicker cream off the top to get the coconut cream for this recipe.

> **NOTE:** I often use erythritol in place of maple syrup to make these a very low-glycemic dessert. If you prefer a sweeter taste, or can't use erythritol, you may use maple syrup instead, or add a couple of tablespoons of maple syrup in addition to erythritol. They will still be much healthier than traditional brownies!

SERVES 20

INGREDIENTS:

¼ cup coconut cream

3 ounces dark chocolate, sugar free and dairy free

¼ cup raw cacao

¼ cup coconut oil

⅓ cup coconut flour (almond meal works but can be crumblier and contains more oil)

¼ cup arrowroot

½ teaspoon baking soda

¼ cup macadamia nut oil, almond oil, or avocado oil

3 eggs

2 bananas, mashed (about ¾ cup) or ¾ cup organic canned pumpkin

⅓ cup erythritol and/or 2 to 4 tablespoons maple syrup

OPTIONAL INGREDIENT:
1 teaspoon pure vanilla extract

NUTRITIONAL INFORMATION
PER SERVING: 90.0 calories, 1.3g protein, 3.6g carbohydrates, 0.8g fiber, 2.8g sugar, 8.1g fat, 4.3g saturated fat, 26mg cholesterol, 13mg sodium.

Adding 2 tablespoons of maple syrup increases the calories by 5.0 grams per serving and sugar by 1.2 grams per serving.

2 ounces dark chocolate, sugar free and dairy free

¼ cup coconut oil

¼ cup almond butter

¼ cup raw cocao

2 bananas, mashed

1 to 2 tablespoons arrowroot

1 teaspoon baking soda

¼ cup erythritol and/or 2 tablespoons pure maple syrup

OPTIONAL INGREDIENTS:

1 teaspoon cinnamon

1 teaspoon pure vanilla extract

pinch of salt

NUTRITIONAL INFORMATION PER SERVING: 89.0 calories, 1.5g protein, 7.2g carbohydrates, 1.3g fiber, 3.9g sugar, 6.8g fat, 4.0g saturated fat, 1.0mg cholesterol, 12.0mg sodium.

Adding 2 tablespoons of maple syrup increases the calories by 5 grams per serving and sugar by 1.2 grams per serving. Total calories will be 94 and total sugar will be 5.1 grams.

Grainless Brownie Bites—Vegan

This recipe is one of the simplest and lowest-glycemic dessert recipes I have created and is a wonderful option for anyone with egg allergies. The brownies will be a bit thinner than the version that contains eggs, but are delicious nonetheless. It takes about five minutes to prepare the ingredients for baking.

PREPARATION:

1. Preheat oven to 350 degrees F.

2. In a small saucepan over low heat, melt chocolate, coconut oil, almond butter, and cacao. Stir frequently until ingredients are melted and thoroughly blended. Remove from heat.

3. In medium mixing bowl, place mashed banana, arrowroot, baking soda, and erythritol and/or maple syrup if desired. Blend together.

4. Add chocolate sauce to banana mixture. Using a handheld electric mixer, start mixing on the low setting and increase speed until bananas are smooth and all ingredients are well blended.

5. Spray an 8 x 8 baking dish with coconut oil or grease well. Pour brownie content into pan evenly so there are no high spots.

6. Bake for 20 to 25 minutes depending on desired chewiness. Allow to cool before serving.

Serve warm or at room temperature. The longer they cool, the more "brownielike" they will be as the coconut oil sets. Store remaining brownies in an airtight container. Freeze leftovers within a couple of days.

Chocolate Protein Sorbet

1. Blend frozen bananas, chocolate protein powder or cacao powder, coconut cream, ice, and stevia if desired in a high-powered blender. Mixture should be very thick.

2. Pour into small serving dishes and top each dish with equal amounts of chocolate chips if desired.

3. Freeze in dessert bowls for 30 minutes before serving.

> **NOTE:** Refrigerate a can of coconut milk and skim the thicker cream off the top to get the coconut cream for this recipe.

SERVES 4

INGREDIENTS:

2 bananas, frozen (peel, halve, and freeze in advance)

2 scoops chocolate protein powder (plant based, sugar free) or 2 tablespoons cacao powder

¼ cup coconut cream, or a bit more for desired thickness

1 cup ice, approximately

OPTIONAL INGREDIENTS:

5 to 10 drops liquid stevia, chocolate flavor

2 tablespoons chocolate chips, sugar free and dairy free

NUTRITIONAL INFORMATION PER SERVING: 145.2 calories, 11.4g protein, 13.8g carbohydrates, 2.9g fiber, 5.0g sugar, 6.35g fat, 4.6g saturated fat, 0.0mg cholesterol, 1.5mg sodium

Chilled Mocha Melts

SERVES 16

INGREDIENTS:

1 ounce dark chocolate, sugar free and dairy free

1 cup coconut oil, softened

¼ cup almond butter, or other nut or seed butter

2 teaspoons organic ground coffee, regular or decaf

1 to 2 tablespoons pure maple syrup (it tastes great without much sweetener)

½ teaspoon pure vanilla extract

5 to 10 drops liquid stevia, chocolate flavored

pinch of salt

When I'm in a hurry, I make this dessert as a bark by freezing it in one large tray and breaking it into pieces when it's ready. If you prefer a more elegant look, you can mold it into candy paper. Just be sure to have 16 candy papers on hand before you get started.

PREPARATION:

1. Line a 9 x 9 baking sheet with parchment paper for bark. Or if you prefer individual candies, line a mini muffin pan with 16 candy papers.

2. Shave or finely chop the chocolate and set aside.

3. Place all ingredients except shaved chocolate in a blender. Blend until smooth and creamy. You may mix ingredients in a bowl with a rubber spatula, but the blender gets the lumps out of the coconut oil and almond butter. Transfer mixture to a medium-sized bowl.

4. If you are making a single sheet of bark, pour the mixture onto the parchment-lined baking sheet. For candies, spoon the mixture evenly between the candy cups.

5. Using a teaspoon, sprinkle the top with shaved chocolate.

6. Place the baking sheet in the freezer for at least 30 minutes or until the pieces solidify.

7. Break up the sheet into 16 pieces bark of similar size, or serve in individual candy cups.

NUTRITIONAL INFORMATION PER SERVING: 156.5 calories, 0.8g protein, 1.9g carbohydrates, 0.4g fiber, 1.2g sugar, 15.9g fat, 12.2g saturated fat, 0.0mg cholesterol, 12.6mg sodium

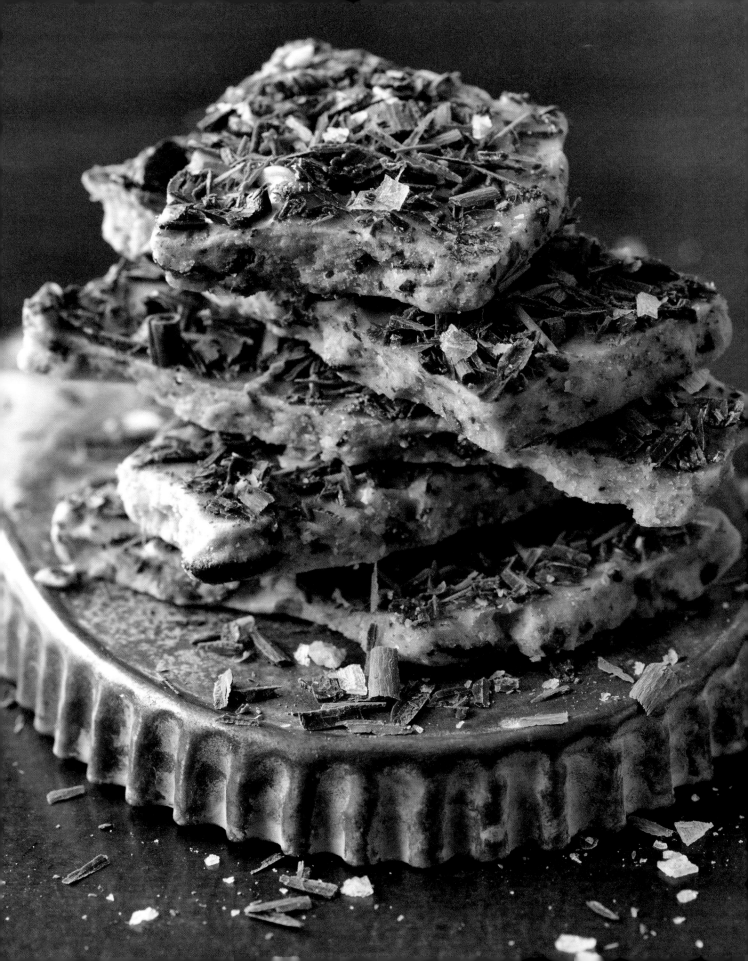

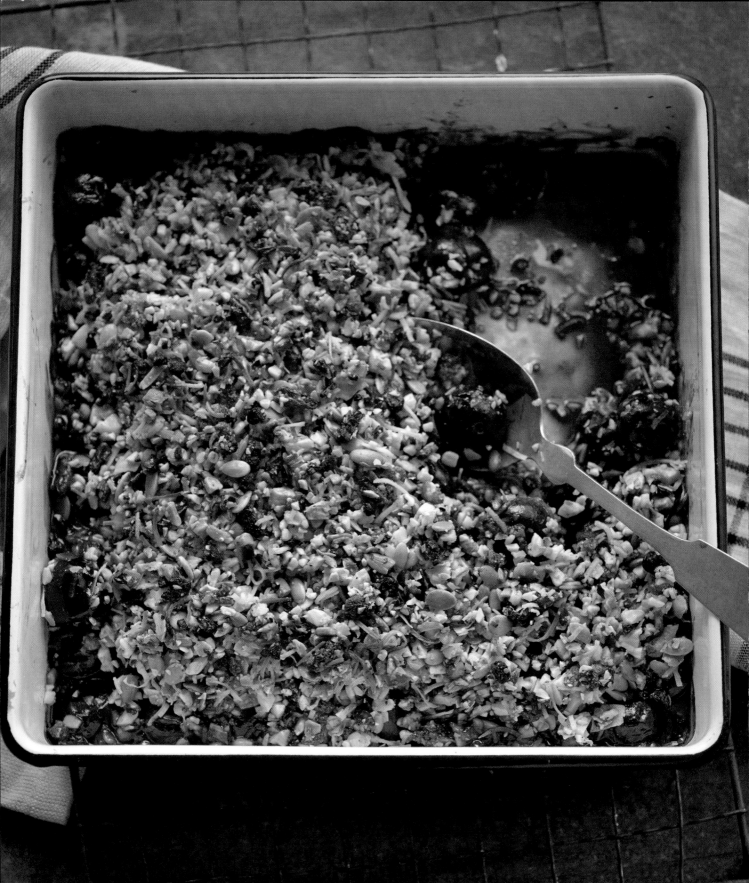

Cherry Crisp in a Jiff

If your house is anything like mine, there are lots of kids in and out, and I like it that way. My best chance of having influence over my daughter and her friends is by creating a fun environment for them. So I have to have food they will eat and a lot of it.

This recipe can be thrown together in a moment's notice. The cherries give it a higher sugar content than most of the other dessert recipes, but it's still healthier than any commercial dessert I know of, and a small amount is quite satisfying.

If you don't have premade Sunrise Grainless Granola on hand, you can use Steve's PaleoKrunch granola and skip adding the ghee or coconut oil.

PREPARATION:

1. Preheat oven to 350 degrees F.

2. Grease a baking pan, approximately 9 x 9 inches. Put cherries in pan.

3. In a medium-sized bowl mix granola and ghee or coconut oil by hand. Blend until well mixed but formed into small clumps. If you're using Steve's PaleoKrunch, you may need to break it up, as it tends to be very chunky.

4. Sprinkle a thin layer of the granola over the cherries, making sure to spread evenly and cover entire pan.

5. Bake for approximately 20 minutes or until you see it beginning to bubble. Remove and allow to cool for about 10 minutes before serving.

NOTE: Goes wonderfully topped with Silky Coconut Whipped Cream (page 251).

SERVES 8

INGREDIENTS:

20 ounces frozen, pitted cherries, thawed and juice drained

1 cup Sunrise Grainless Granola (page 53)

2 tablespoons coconut oil or ghee, or you can use grass-fed butter, melted

OPTIONAL INGREDIENTS:

⅓ cup erythritol or ¼ cup raw honey (it's often sweet enough without)

1 tablespoon arrowroot (thickens the juice from cherries as they bake)

NUTRITIONAL INFORMATION PER SERVING: 161.5 calories, 5.3g protein, 17.8g carbohydrates, 3.1g fiber, 10.2g sugar, 13.1g fat, 7.3g saturated fat, 0.0 mg cholesterol, 69.0 mg sodium

Apple Cinnamon Crisp

SERVES 8

INGREDIENTS:
coconut oil nonstick cooking spray

7 apples, peeled, cored and chopped

1 teaspoon cinnamon

½ teaspoon nutmeg

¼ teaspoon ginger

¼ cup pecans or walnuts

¼ cup almond flour

2 tablespoons unsweetened almond butter

6 dates

OPTIONAL INGREDIENT:
½ cup erythritol

PREPARATION:

1. Preheat oven to 350 degrees F and spray a 9 x 9-inch baking dish with coconut oil nonstick cooking spray.

2. Heat apples in a large sauté pan over medium heat. Apples will release fluid and begin to dehydrate after a couple of minutes. Add cinnamon, nutmeg, ginger, and erythritol, if desired. Cook until apples are hot and soft, about 15 minutes. Don't allow apples to dry out and burn.

3. Remove apples from heat and pour into the baking dish.

4. Mix nuts, flour, almond butter, and dates in food processor until well blended and chunky.

5. Remove crumble topping from food processor and sprinkle on top of the apples in baking dish. Bake the apple crisp for 15 minutes.

6. Use an ice cream scoop to spoon small portions into dessert bowls. Serve warm or cold.

> **NOTE:** Try using the slicer attachment on a food processor as a shortcut when cutting up the apples.

NUTRITIONAL INFORMATION PER SERVING: 84.5 calories, 1.9g protein, 6.8g carbohydrates, 1.7g fiber, 4.5g sugar, 6.3g fat, 0.5g saturated fat, 0.0mg cholesterol, 0.1mg sodium

Three-Ingredient Banana Nut Cookies

These amazing cookies are about as wholesome a snack as you'll find. Kids absolutely love them. I love having something I can throw together in a jiffy. On rare occasions you can even make these for breakfast so kids think you're really cool. This is a fun recipe for treating your kids to "cookies for breakfast," especially at sleepovers where there are sure to be a few picky eaters in the group. If you don't have grainless granola on hand, you can substitute quick oats.

PREPARATION:

1. Preheat oven to 350 degrees F. Spray baking sheet with coconut oil or line with parchment paper.

2. In a medium-sized bowl combine mashed banana, granola, and add-in ingredient of your choice (nuts, chocolate chips, or berries). Mix until thoroughly blended.

3. Evenly place tablespoon-sized balls onto the baking sheet and bake for 12 to 15 minutes depending on desired crispiness.

SERVES 16

INGREDIENTS:

Coconut oil nonstick cooking spray

2 bananas, mashed

1 cup Sunrise Grainless Granola (page 53) or Steve's PaleoKrunch Granola, crumbled fine

¼ cup of your favorite cookie add-ins (chopped walnuts; sugar-free, dairy-free chocolate chips; or goji berries)

NUTRITIONAL INFORMATION PER SERVING: 36.3 calories, 0.9g protein, 7.8g carbohydrates, 0.85g fiber, 2.9g sugar, 0.4g fat, 0.1g saturated fat, 0.0mg cholesterol, 0.2mg sodium

Scrumptious Pumpkin Muffins

SERVES 10

INGREDIENTS:

1 cup organic canned pumpkin or fresh pumpkin puree

¼ cup coconut cream

2 tablespoons maple syrup

6 eggs

⅔ cup coconut flour

½ cup erythritol

¼ teaspoon salt

1 teaspoon baking powder

2½ teaspoons pumpkin pie spice

OPTIONAL INGREDIENT:

¼ cup pumpkin seeds, crushed

PREPARATION:

1. Preheat oven to 350 degrees F and line a muffin tin with 10 standard-sized muffin papers.

2. Whisk together the pumpkin, coconut cream, maple syrup, and eggs in a bowl.

3. In a separate bowl whisk the dry ingredients, except pumpkin seeds if using.

4. Add wet into dry and blend well.

5. Divide the batter equally between muffin papers. Top with pumpkin seeds.

6. Bake 30 to 35 minutes.

> **NOTE:** Frost with Heavenly Coconut Cream Frosting (page 247) or Silky Coconut Whipped Cream (page 251), if desired.

> **NOTE:** Refrigerate a can of coconut milk and skim the thicker cream off the top to get the coconut cream for this recipe.

NUTRITIONAL INFORMATION PER SERVING: 174.0 calories, 6.7g protein, 12.2g carbohydrates, 4.4g fiber, 3.3g sugar, 10.0g fat, 5.6g saturated fat, 111.6mg cholesterol, 109.4mg sodium

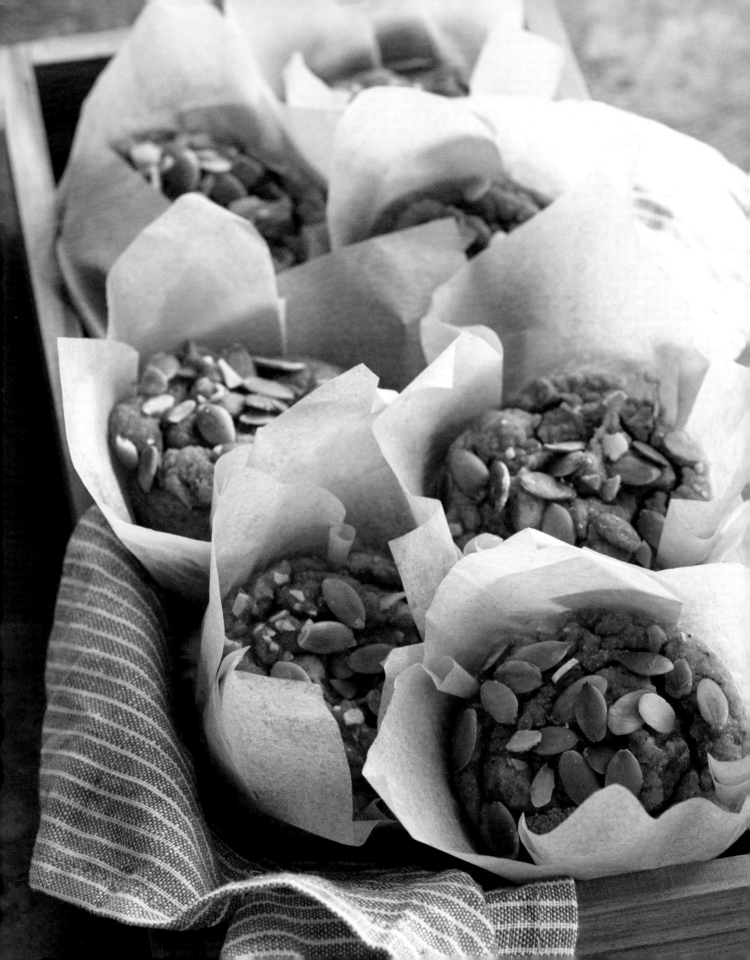

Chocolate Pumpkin Protein Bars

SERVES 16

INGREDIENTS:

coconut oil nonstick cooking spray

1 cup organic pumpkin

½ cup almond butter

½ cup chocolate or vanilla protein powder (plant based, sugar free)

½ cup erythritol

1 teaspoon baking soda

1 tablespoon pumpkin pie spice

1 cup coconut flour or almond flour

1 cup rolled oats or grainless granola

3 eggs

OPTIONAL INGREDIENTS:

2 tablespoons raw honey

1 teaspoon pure vanilla extract

1 ounce dark chocolate, sugar free and dairy free, melted or chopped (can be used as a drizzle or as chunks)

PREPARATION:

1. Preheat oven to 350 degrees F. Spray a 9 x 11-inch pan with coconut oil nonstick cooking spray, or line with parchment paper.

2. In a large mixing bowl, use a handheld electric mixer to combine pumpkin, almond butter, protein powder, erythritol, baking soda, spices, and honey and vanilla, if desired.

3. Add flour, oats, and eggs. Mix well, until thoroughly blended. Dough will be very thick.

4. Press dough into pan, spreading until it covers the entire pan evenly. Make sure the center isn't thicker than the corners.

5. Spread batter evenly into prepared pan. Sprinkle with chocolate chunks if desired, or wait to drizzle chocolate sauce.

6. Bake for 12 to 15 minutes or until a toothpick inserted comes out clean.

7. While bars are baking, place chocolate in a microwave-safe bowl if you wish to make a drizzle. Microwave for 15 to 20 seconds at a time, stopping to stir before microwaving for another 15 to 20 seconds. Chocolate should be thoroughly melted after 45 to 50 seconds. If a thinner sauce is desired, add a teaspoon of coconut oil while microwaving.

8. After pumpkin bars have cooled completely, use a small spoon to drizzle melted chocolate in zigzag lines across the pan. Refrigerate for 10 minutes to allow chocolate to set. Cut into 16 equal-sized bars. Freeze leftovers within a couple days.

NUTRITIONAL INFORMATION PER SERVING: 187.0 calories, 15.2g protein, 11.0g carbohydrates, 2.6g fiber, 1.3g sugar, 10.8g fat, 0.9g saturated fat, 34.9mg cholesterol, 45.5mg sodium

Sweet Potato Coconut Flan

PREPARATION:

1. Preheat the oven to 350 degrees F.

2. In a large saucepan, place the yam and just enough water to cover, and add salt. Bring to a boil, then turn down to simmer and cook till the yam is tender, about 20 minutes. Drain and cool.

3. When yam is cool, combine the yam and all ingredients except for coconut whipped cream in a food processor or blender and mix until smooth.

4. Divide the yam mixture among four small oven-safe soufflé dishes. Place the soufflé dishes in a towel-lined 8 x 8–inch pan. Fill the pan with very hot water, about 165 degrees F, until about halfway up the soufflé dishes. Place in the oven and cook for 30 minutes till the pudding is set.

5. Remove the pan from the oven, but allow the soufflé dishes to stay in the hot water for another 15 minutes to finish the cooking. Remove from the water and chill thoroughly, about 1 to 2 hours.

6. Garnish with Silky Coconut Whipped Cream and a pinch of ground cinnamon.

SERVES 4

INGREDIENTS:

1 large sweet potato or yam, peeled and diced

½ teaspoon salt

¾ cup coconut milk

2 eggs

1 tablespoon erythritol

1 tablespoon maple syrup

½ teaspoon ground ginger

½ teaspoon ground cinnamon

¼ teaspoon ground nutmeg

Silky Coconut Whipped Cream (page 251)

NUTRITIONAL INFORMATION PER SERVING: 93.8 calories, 3.9g protein, 12.2g carbohydrates, 1.4g fiber, 3.3g sugar, 3.2g fat, 1.1g saturated fat, 93.0mg cholesterol, 94.8mg sodium

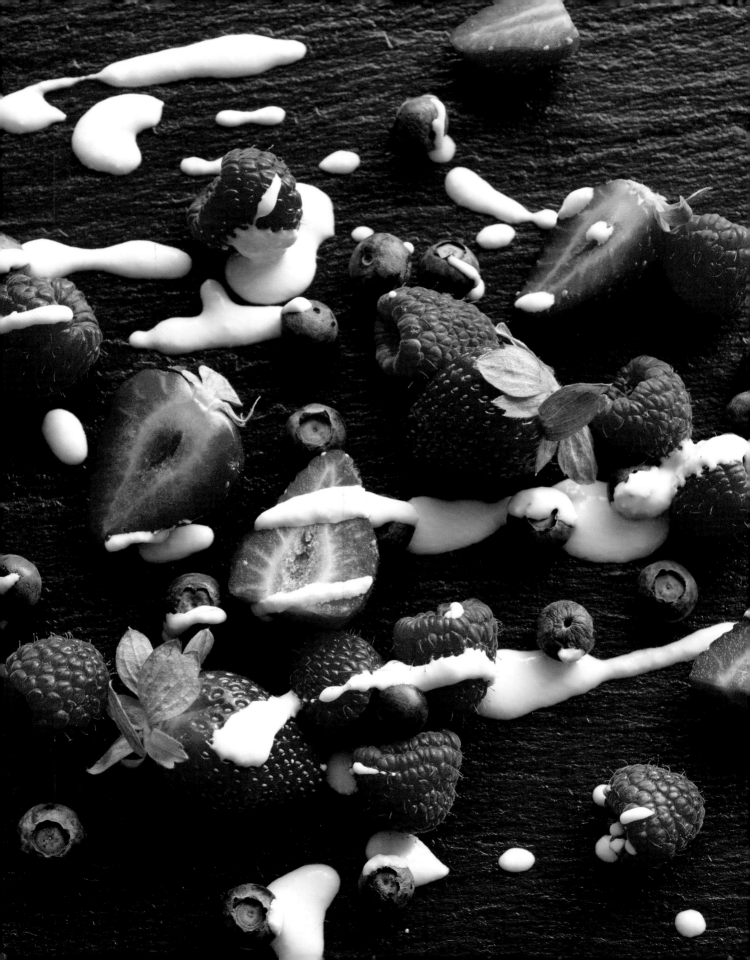

Fresh Berries with Macadamia Cream Sauce

This dessert is a favorite at parties. It's fresh and elegant. I like giving guests two options to choose from: Macadamia Cream Sauce or Simple Chocolate Sauce. Many people choose to drizzle both.

PREPARATION:

1. Mix berries and divide among four dessert bowls.

2. Add all Macadamia Cream Sauce ingredients to a high-powered blender. Blend until smooth and creamy. If sauce is too thick, add 2 to 4 tablespoons unsweetened almond or coconut milk until sauce reaches desired consistency. Transfer to serving bowl.

3. Drizzle sauce over berries and serve.

> **NOTE:** Instead of the Macadamia Cream Sauce, substitute with the Mood-Boosting Chocolate Sauce (page 253) for a chocolaty variation.

SERVES 4

INGREDIENTS:

FRESH BERRIES:
1 cup fresh blueberries

1 cup sliced fresh strawberries

1 cup fresh raspberries

MACADAMIA CREAM SAUCE:
½ cup macadamia nuts

2 tablespoons coconut, fine shredded, unsweetened

½ cup full-fat coconut milk

5 to 10 drops vanilla crème–flavored liquid stevia

OPTIONAL INGREDIENTS:
1 tablespoon raw honey

pinch of salt

NUTRITIONAL INFORMATION PER SERVING FOR BERRIES (AVERAGE):
46.8 calories, 0.8g protein, 11.4g carbohydrates, 3.9g fiber, 5.8g sugar, 0.3g fat, 0.0g saturated fat, 0.0mg cholesterol, 2.6mg sodium

NUTRITIONAL INFORMATION PER 1-TABLESPOON SERVING FOR MACADAMIA CREAM SAUCE:
70.6 calories, 1.1g protein, 3.4g carbohydrates, 0.4g fiber, 1.3g sugar, 6.2g fat, 0.1g saturated fat, 0.0mg cholesterol, 15.6mg sodium

Grainless Mini Maple Loaves

SERVES 12

INGREDIENTS:

½ cup almond flour

½ cup coconut flour

¼ cup flaxseed meal

½ teaspoon baking soda

½ teaspoon salt

5 eggs

¼ cup pure maple syrup

¼ cup macadamia nut oil, avocado oil, or almond oil

1 tablespoon pure vanilla extract

This delicious alternative to wheat-based bread makes a wonderful breakfast when combined with a bit of protein. It also makes a great afternoon snack.

PREPARATION:

1. Preheat oven to 350 degrees F and grease two mini loaf pans. You may line the pans with parchment paper if you wish to save cleanup time and avoid sticking.

2. In a medium-sized bowl mix dry ingredients: almond flour, coconut flour, flaxseed meal, baking soda, and salt.

3. In large bowl, whisk eggs, maple syrup, oil, and vanilla.

4. Add wet ingredients to dry ingredients. Mix thoroughly.

5. Pour mixture into two greased mini loaf pans. (Grainless breads often bake better in mini loaf pans.)

6. Place loaf pans in oven and bake for 25 to 30 minutes, until toothpick inserted into center of loaf comes out clean.

7. Cool and serve.

NUTRITIONAL INFORMATION PER SERVING: 170.2 calories, 5.5g protein, 1.5g carbohydrates, 3.2g fiber, 4.3g sugar, 11.0g fat, 1.6g saturated fat, 77.5mg cholesterol, 95.7mg sodium

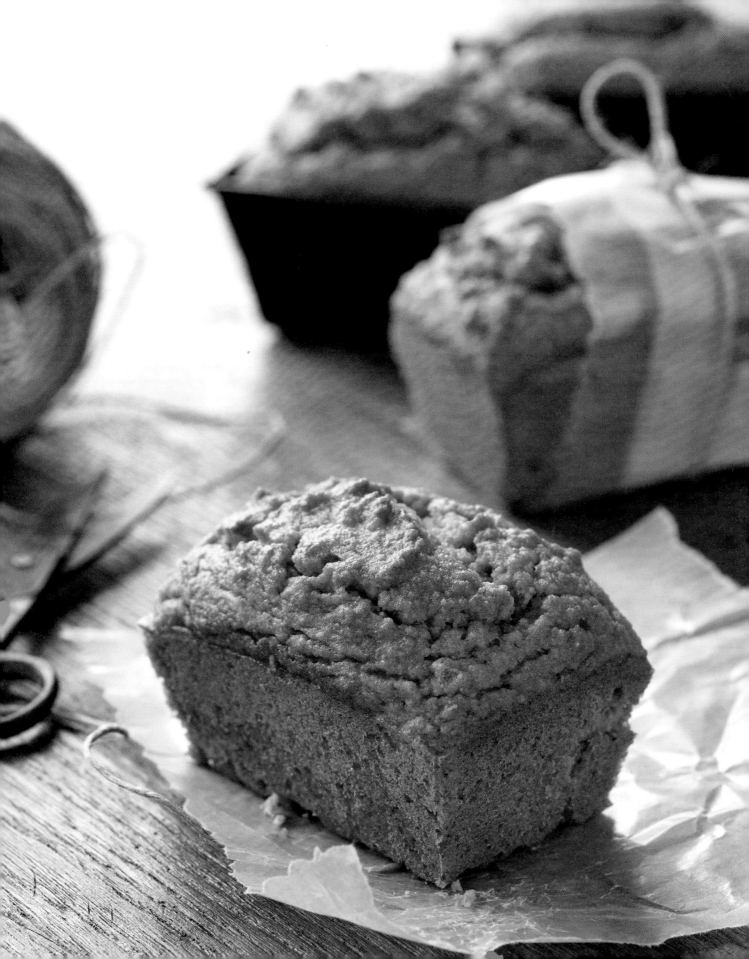

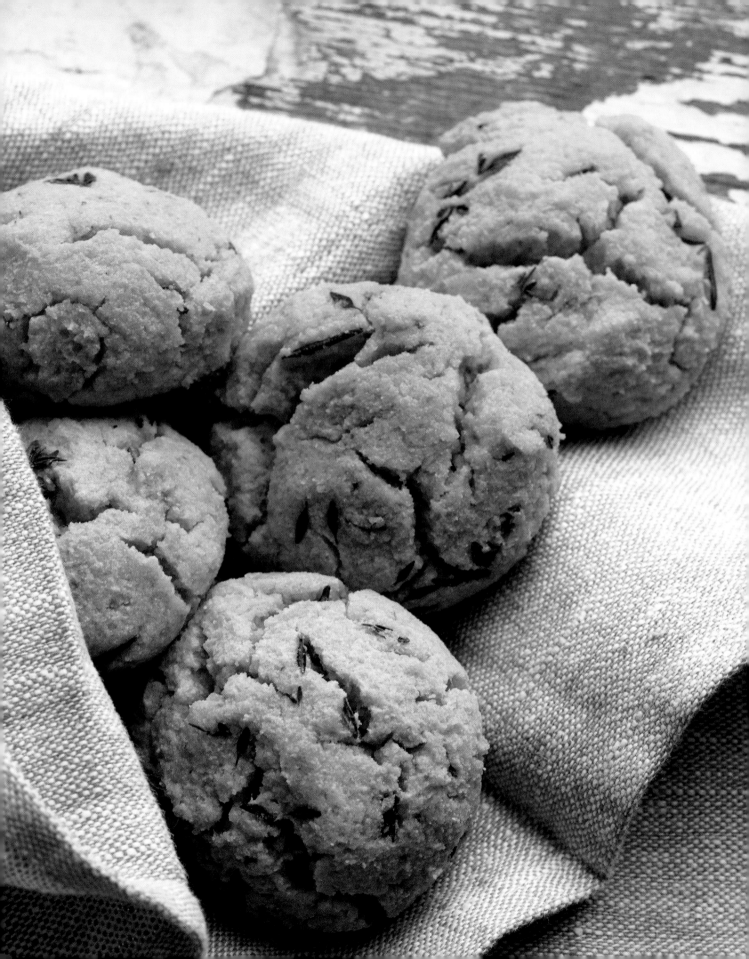

Savory Pumpkin Herb Biscuits

PREPARATION:

1. Preheat oven to 350 degrees F. In a medium-sized bowl, combine pumpkin, coconut milk, honey, eggs, coconut oil, and herbs. Mix thoroughly.

2. In separate small bowl, combine almond flour, salt, and baking powder. Mix thoroughly.

3. Add dry ingredients to the bowl of wet ingredients and stir until mixed.

4. Line a baking sheet with parchment paper. Portion the dough with an ice cream scoop for 8 equal-sized biscuits and place onto baking sheet.

5. Bake for 20 to 30 minutes until lightly browned and firm.

6. Serve warm.

SERVES 8

INGREDIENTS:

½ cup organic cooked pumpkin (canned is fine)

2 tablespoons light coconut milk

3 eggs

¼ cup coconut oil, melted

½ teaspoon fresh rosemary, chopped

½ teaspoon fresh thyme, chopped

1 cup almond flour or coconut flour

1 teaspoon baking powder

OPTIONAL INGREDIENTS:

2 tablespoons raw honey

¼ teaspoon salt

NUTRITIONAL INFORMATION PER SERVING: 196.4 calories, 5.5g protein, 7.5g carbohydrates, 1.7g fiber, 4.2g sugar, 16.3g fat, 8.0g saturated fat, 69.8mg cholesterol, 124.1mg sodium

Holiday Sugarless Cookies

SERVES 16

INGREDIENTS:

1 cup almond flour

¼ cup coconut flour

¼ cup erythritol

½ teaspoon baking soda

⅛ teaspoon salt

1 egg

2 teaspoons pure vanilla extract

¼ cup maple syrup or raw honey

2 tablespoons coconut oil, melted

OPTIONAL INGREDIENTS:

xylitol crystals or coconut sugar

2 tablespoons arrowroot for dusting if you are doing cutouts

PREPARATION:

1. Preheat oven to 350 degrees F.

2. Place dry ingredients in a large bowl and whisk together.

3. Add wet ingredients except coconut oil to dry ingredients and mix with a handheld electric mixer.

4. Turn mixer to low setting and slowly add coconut oil.

FOR SIMPLE ROUND COOKIES:

1. Drop rounded tablespoons of dough onto two parchment-lined baking sheets.

2. Sprinkle with xylitol crystals or coconut sugar and bake for 11 to 13 minutes, or a couple of minutes longer for crisper cookies.

FOR MAKING COOKIE-CUTTER CUTOUTS:

1. Refrigerate dough for several hours.

2. Using a fine dusting of arrowroot starch, dust two sheets of parchment paper and the surface of the dough.

3. Place the dough between the two sheets of paper and roll out into ¼-inch thickness. Remove the top sheet and press desired cookie cutters into the dough. Remove excess dough from around the cookie, but leave cookie undisturbed on parchment paper.

4. Place parchment paper with cookies (after filling the sheet with cutouts) on a baking sheet. Sprinkle with xylitol crystals or coconut sugar.

5. Bake for 12 to 15 minutes or until edges are browned.

6. Cool for five minutes before serving.

> **NOTE:** For holiday decorating, try adding a couple of drops of beet juice extract to the xylitol crystals or coconut sugar and mix well to turn the crystals red. Allow them to dry before decorating.

NUTRITIONAL INFORMATION PER SERVING: 90.8 calories, 2.4g protein, 9.9g carbohydrates, 1.5g fiber, 3.3g sugar, 6.1g fat, 2.0g saturated fat, 11.6mg cholesterol, 54.0mg sodium

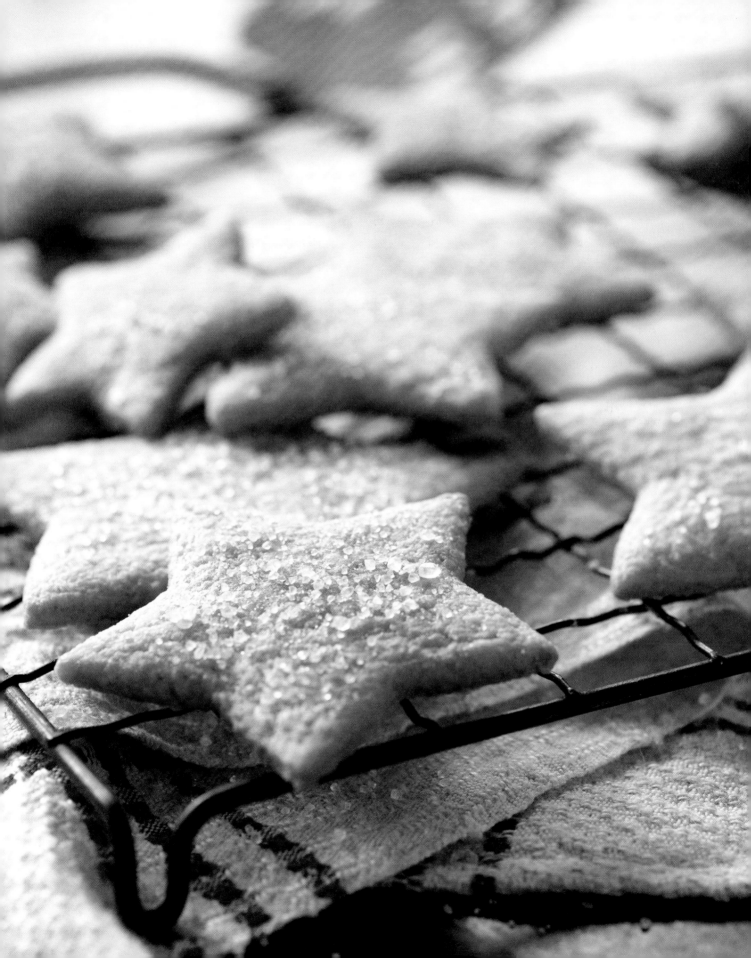

"Focus on love, service and giving thanks for the holidays."

—Daniel and Tana

SECTION 13

Brain Warrior
Holiday Meal Plan

Warriors Don't Wait Until January 1 to Start Training, They Train All Year!

■

The more you sweat in training, the less you bleed in combat.

—NAVY SEALS

Did you know that more heart attacks occur on December 25 than any other day of the year? Experts believe it's because of a combination of stress, overindulging in inflammatory foods and alcohol over the holidays, and lack of sleep. Travel and the decision to postpone seeking medical attention for serious symptoms also factor in.

Let's back up. It all starts with Halloween. Your bliss point, akin to a cocaine high, is triggered when you overwhelm the brain with excessive sugar. This sets sugar addiction, inflammation, and brain fog in motion. It's the start of lots of bad decisions. From there, the season of parties is just getting under way.

Thanksgiving, Christmas, and Chanukah have become less focused on giving and more focused on gluttony and self-indulgence. This isn't our opinion: this is a statistic. According to many experts, the average American easily consumes close to 3,000 calories in one meal. With lengthy family gatherings and second portions, that number has been estimated to be as high as 4,500 calories in a day. That's about how many calories an average man should eat in two days! And then the parties continue all the way through the New Year. It's a perfect storm for anyone to become vulnerable to illness. Then again, it's usually those vulnerable to illness who engage in this kind of activity. Yes, we're picking on you (out of love).

Daniel and I simply refuse to think of ourselves as "deprived" because we make the choice to feel energetic instead of overweight and foggy during the holidays when the focus is supposed to be on gratitude and helping others. We feel blessed and we want you to join us. You can enjoy the holidays more than ever with these simple recipe swaps.

Amen
Thanksgiving Menu

■

Tana's Marinated Turkey

If you're serious about having the most moist turkey anyone has ever tasted, try soaking the bird in a wet brine for 18 hours before starting on day-of prep. But beware: you will become the designated turkey maker in the family forever! This recipe requires marinating the turkey for a full 6 to 24 hours prior to cooking.

The turkey recipe can be adapted to roasted chicken. Cut ingredients in half and marinate according to same instructions. Preheat oven to 425 degrees F and roast for 1½ hours. Keep chicken breast side down for the first hour and turn over for the final 30 minutes.

You will need cheesecloth for baking the turkey.

PREPARATION TO BE DONE THE DAY BEFORE COOKING:

1. Start with a fully thawed turkey. Remove innards from cavity (set aside for stuffing if you choose) and rinse turkey well. Pat dry with paper towels.

2. Loosen the skin from the turkey, being careful not to remove the skin completely from the turkey. You just want to separate the skin from the meat. Try not to puncture the skin. The skin will remain attached at the legs' attachment points.

3. Mix all ingredients in the marinade with a whisk prior to marinating the turkey.

4. Evenly apply the marinade around the turkey meat, under the skin, with clean hands (always being careful to handle *all* meat with clean hands and not touch anything else prior to washing). Be sure to apply a thick coat of marinade.

5. Apply a final, thin coat of marinade to the inside cavity of the turkey and the outer skin. If you don't have enough left, you may choose to use salt with a little olive oil.

6. Cover turkey and refrigerate overnight.

PREPARATION TO BE DONE THE DAY OF COOKING:

1. Preheat oven to 400 degrees F. If desired, wrap turkey in cheesecloth to hold juices in during basting phase.

2. Place turkey breast down (for the most moist breast meat) in a roasting pan or directly on the lower rack above a roasting pan.

SERVES 16

INGREDIENTS:

1 (12-pound) turkey

1½ cups macadamia nut oil or avocado oil

¼ cup fresh squeezed lemon juice

2 tablespoons minced garlic

2 tablespoons fresh rosemary, finely chopped

2 tablespoons fresh thyme, finely chopped

salt and pepper, to taste

OPTIONAL INGREDIENTS:

½ cup ghee or grass-fed butter, for basting

½ to 1 cup chicken broth, as needed

(RECIPE CONTINUES)

3. Cooking time varies, but a general rule is about 15 minutes for every pound.

4. After 30 minutes, reduce the cooking temperature to 350 degrees F for the next two hours, and then reduce it again to 250 degrees F for the remaining time.

5. Use a baster to retrieve juices from the bottom of the pan and baste the turkey every 30 minutes or so. Add ghee to the roasting pan and add a bit of chicken broth if desired.

6. Use a meat thermometer to ensure the meat is fully cooked. The white meat should have an internal temperature of about 165 degrees F.

7. For the last 20 minutes of cooking time, turn the turkey over and increase the oven temperature to 300 degrees F. This will brown the skin of the breast.

NUTRITIONAL INFORMATION PER SERVING FOR 4 OUNCES TURKEY BREAST MEAT, NO SKIN: 232.0 calories, 34.0g protein, 0.0g carbohydrates, 0.0g fiber, 0.0g sugar, 10.0g fat, 1.3g saturated fat, 94.0mg cholesterol, 582.0mg sodium

NUTRITIONAL INFORMATION PER SERVING FOR 4 OUNCES DARK MEAT, NO SKIN: 262.0 calories, 32.6g protein, 0.0g carbohydrates, 0.0g fiber, 0.0g sugar, 14.1g fat, 2.9g saturated fat, 127.0mg cholesterol, 582.0mg sodium

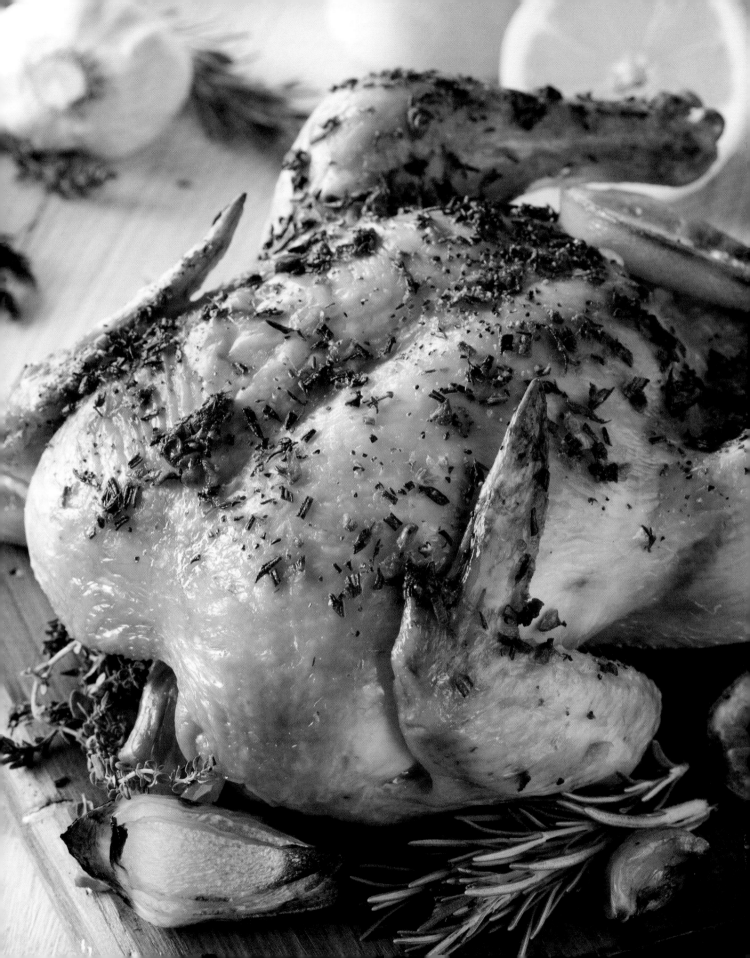

Amen Holiday Stuffing

SERVES 16

INGREDIENTS:

1 tablespoon ghee or grass-fed butter

4 cups butternut squash, peeled and cubed

1 medium onion, diced

1 apple, diced

4 stalks celery, diced

2 to 3 garlic cloves, minced

salt and pepper to taste

1 pound extra-lean ground turkey or bison

1 tablespoon fresh rosemary, finely chopped

1 tablespoon fresh thyme, finely chopped

1 tablespoon fresh sage, finely chopped

2 cups walnuts, finely chopped

salt and freshly ground pepper to taste (about ½ to 1 teaspoon each)

OPTIONAL INGREDIENTS:

1 cup pomegranate seeds

FOR RICHER STUFFING, ADD:

2 eggs, beaten

1 cup almond flour

½ cup chicken broth

This delicious, healthier version of traditional stuffing is a favorite in our house. It's so complete that we often eat it as a main course, topped with a bit of gravy and a big salad. The recipe is designed to feed a large group for the holidays. For smaller gatherings, simply cut the recipe in half. Make this a vegan stuffing by increasing the amount of squash, apple, and nuts and eliminating the meat.

PREPARATION:

1. Preheat oven to 375 degrees F.

2. Melt the ghee or butter in a large skillet placed over medium-high heat. Sauté the butternut squash, onion, apple, celery, and garlic for about 10 minutes, and season to taste with salt and pepper. Remove from pan and set aside.

3. Add turkey to the pan and sauté for about 2 minutes. Add a bit more ghee if necessary.

4. Add herbs and walnuts, and season with salt and pepper. Mix well.

5. Remove meat from heat. The meat should still be somewhat pink. The meat will finish cooking in the oven.

6. In a large bowl, combine squash mixture and meat mixture. Add optional ingredients (pomegranate seeds, eggs, almond flour and chicken broth) as desired. Mix thoroughly.

7. Put the mixture in a baking dish and bake uncovered for 30 to 45 minutes or until squash is tender.

8. Serve with Guiltless Gravy (page 244).

NUTRITIONAL INFORMATION PER SERVING: 186.0 calories, 12.1g protein, 8.4g carbohydrates, 3.5g fiber, 1.5g sugar, 13.2g fat, 1.6g saturated fat, 31.0mg cholesterol, 41.0mg sodium

Clever Kale Slaw

1. Combine kale, cabbage, carrot, and cashews.

2. In a small mixing bowl, combine Nayonnaise or vegan mayonnaise, vinegar, spices, herbs, sunflower seeds, cranberries, and stevia, if desired. Whisk until mixture is blended well. Toss with kale mixture.

3. Allow salad to refrigerate for 30 minutes prior to serving if possible so flavors can marry.

> **NOTE:** You can use 1 cup prepackaged coleslaw mix instead of cabbage if you prefer.

SERVES 8

INGREDIENTS:

2 cups finely shredded kale, thick stems removed

½ cup shredded green cabbage

½ cup shredded purple cabbage

¼ cup shredded carrot

½ cup chopped raw cashews

½ cup Nayonnaise (page 257) or vegan mayonnaise

1 tablespoon apple cider vinegar

½ teaspoon allspice

⅛ teaspoon cinnamon

⅛ teaspoon nutmeg

¼ teaspoon salt

¼ teaspoon pepper

1 teaspoon fresh oregano, finely chopped, or ½ teaspoon dried

1 teaspoon fresh thyme, chopped, or ½ teaspoon dried

⅓ teaspoon curry powder

¼ cup raw sunflower seeds

½ cup dried cranberries

OPTIONAL INGREDIENT:
½ packet stevia

NUTRITIONAL INFORMATION PER SERVING: 164.6 calories, 3.1g protein, 13.8g carbohydrates, 2.7g fiber, 7.2g sugar, 11.4g fat, 1.2g saturated fat, 0.0mg cholesterol, 62.4mg sodium

Cauliflower Mashed Potatoes

INGREDIENTS:

2 cups vegetable broth, bone broth (page 89) or water

1 head cauliflower, cut into large florets

¼ cup unsweetened almond milk

1 tablespoon ghee or grass-fed butter

2 garlic cloves, minced

½ teaspoon Italian seasoning

1 teaspoon fresh rosemary, chopped

2 teaspoons arrowroot mixed with 2 tablespoons water

salt and pepper, to taste

OPTIONAL INGREDIENT:

2 tablespoons finely chopped chives

PREPARATION:

1. Pour broth into a medium pot. Put cauliflower florets in pot and bring to a boil over medium-high heat. Cover, reduce heat to low, and simmer for 10 minutes. If you prefer using water, then steam cauliflower in a steamer basket, being sure not to allow the water to touch the cauliflower. If steaming, cook until fork tender, about 8 minutes.

2. While cauliflower is cooking, combine almond milk, ghee, garlic, Italian seasoning, and rosemary in a small saucepan over medium heat. When it reaches a boil, add the arrowroot mixture, stirring constantly until it is thickened and smooth. Remove from heat and set aside.

3. Drain as much liquid from cauliflower as possible and place florets in a food processor or blender, blending on high for about 1 minute. Add sauce and blend until smooth and creamy.

4. Season with salt and pepper to taste and garnish with chives if desired.

NOTE: Try serving Cauliflower Mashed Potatoes warm over a bed of baby spinach.

NUTRITIONAL INFORMATION PER SERVING: 110.0 calories, 4.9g protein, 7.5g carbohydrates, 3.0g fiber, 3.3g sugar, 7.5g fat, 5.2g saturated fat, 8.0mg cholesterol, 128.0mg sodium

"Never let the holidays be an excuse to hurt yourself."

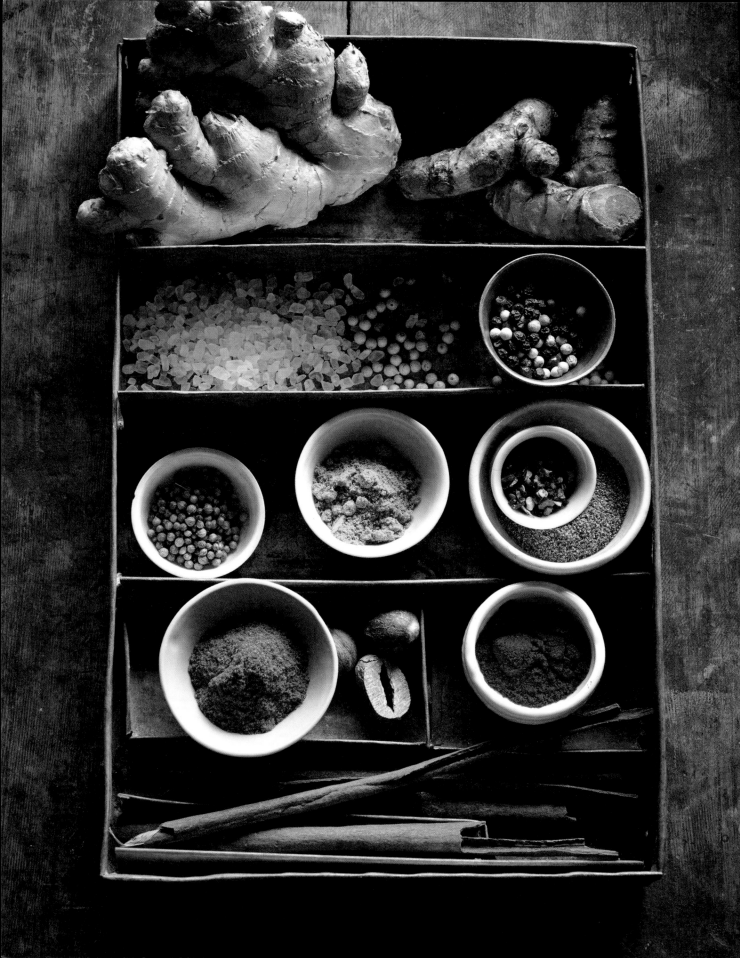

Brain Warrior Herbs and Spices

Get the Delicious Mental Edge

■

He who takes medicine and neglects his diet wastes the skill of his doctors.

—CHINESE PROVERB

I t is said that ninjas had an inseparable relationship with medicinal plants and herbs. They believed that a person couldn't be healthy unless they ate healthily *every day*, and that food was either medicine or poison. They used the plants and herbs that grew around them to treat people, and they also used them as weapons to destroy their enemies! Ninjas prided themselves on being as knowledgeable as most doctors (and often disguised themselves as such) due to their deep understanding of the healing power of herbs, spices, and healing arts.

What did your grandma have in common with ninjas? Hopefully she wasn't a spy, but she did use herbs and spices that boosted brain function and prevented illness. You may have thought Grandma's oregano marinara sauce, loaded with garlic and basil, was a culinary delight, but it was so much more! Grandma's food has the healing power that most people have lost with the introduction of convenient, processed, ready-made food.

Worth Going to War

See that spice rack in the corner of your kitchen collecting dust? Nations have gone to war over herbs and spices for thousands of years for their medicinal powers. You can literally spice up your brain, balance your blood sugar, improve your mood, *and* make your food taste better using those mysterious little "farm"-aceutical bottles in your kitchen. Fortunately the only war you'll have to fight to get them is the line at the grocery store.

SPICE UP YOUR BRAIN WITH A DAILY DOSE OF FARM-ACEUTICALS

- Add cinnamon, nutmeg, cacao, pure vanilla extract, cardamom, or mint to smoothies.
- Toss chopped fresh herbs, such as basil, chives, and cilantro, into salads.
- Blend garlic, fresh herbs, nuts, and olive oil to make delicious pesto sauce.
- Simmer herbs and spices into soups, stews, and chili.
- Sprinkle chopped fresh herbs over grilled meat and fish.
- Mix several kinds of spices to make a rub for grilled vegetables.
- Blend multiple herbs and spices with a little oil and lemon juice to make marinades for all types of meat.
- Add fresh mint to smoothies or fruit salad for a surprisingly bright taste twist.
- Add fresh ginger and berries to sparkling water for a refreshing summer drink.
- Cook with fresh herbs when possible, but for convenience, keep dried herbs and spices on hand.

Here are some specific herbs and spices with their intrinsic medicinal properties for your reference:

Basil   A potent antioxidant that has been used for medicinal purposes for thousands of years, basil improves blood flow to the brain and enhances overall brain function. Its anti-inflammatory properties also help improve cognitive function and prevent strokes and cancer. Basil also contains generous amounts of vitamin K and calcium, and preserves the integrity of DNA. A healthy way to dish it up: Chop and add to any salad, dressing, or sauce with an Italian flair.

Black Pepper   One of the most widely used and traded spices since ancient times, black pepper was used to prevent the growth of bacteria and to preserve meat in hot climates. It enhances the absorption of numerous compounds, including curcumin (a powerful antioxidant), and increases hydrochloric acid (stomach acid), which aids in digestion. Remember, you need a healthy gut to have a healthy brain. A healthy way to dish it up: Jazz up morning eggs with just a pinch.

Cayenne   The bold taste in cayenne is created by the capsaicin, which is well known for its many health benefits, including preventing ulcers and certain cancers, and relieving pain. It also increases hydrochloric acid (stomach acid), which aids in digestion. Cayenne pepper is loaded with vitamin A carotenoids. It helps fight inflammation, boost immunity, and stimulate metabolism to promote weight loss. Precautions should be taken not to overindulge if you suffer from hypertension. A healthy way to dish it up: Add a pinch to chili, soups or even smoothies for a unique twist.

Chili Powder   Made with ground chili peppers, chili powder contains the compound capsaicin, which inhibits inflammation and damage from oxidation. It also may reduce cholesterol and triglycerides, prevent blood clots, lower heart attack risk, boost immunity, lower the risk of prostate cancer, help with the regulation of insulin and blood sugar, reduce nasal congestion, and prevent certain types of cancer. A healthy way to dish it up: Transform a bland spread into a wonderful aioli sauce with just a pinch.

Cinnamon   Shown to improve working memory and ability to pay attention. A 2005 study in the *North American Journal of Psychology* found that chewing cinnamon gum speeds up the rate at which your brain processes visual cues so you can react to them more quickly. Cinnamon regulates blood sugar levels, which helps you maintain attention and improves cognitive performance. Research shows that the scent of cinnamon is enough to enhance these functions. Cinnamon also works as an aphrodisiac in men. A healthy way to dish it up: Sprinkle one teaspoon of cinnamon in your morning shake for a brain-healthy way to start your day.

Coriander   The phytonutrients in coriander may help control blood sugar and lower cholesterol levels. This concentrated form of cilantro contains substantial amounts of manganese, vitamin C, and vitamin K. A healthy way to dish it up: Add to marinades, or chew coriander seeds to combat bad breath.

Curry and Turmeric   These popular Indian spices contain a chemical called curcumin. A potent antioxidant, curcumin reduces inflammation and helps to prevent and break up the plaques thought to be responsible for Alzheimer's disease. There is also evidence that it offers protection from cancer and supports healthy liver function. There are

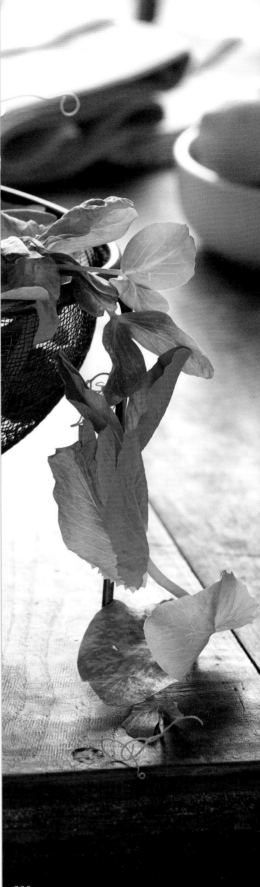

currently twenty-four published studies listed with the National Institutes of Health reporting the benefits of turmeric and curry related to the anti-inflammatory action of this natural chemical. For example, in a 2009 study in the *Journal of Alzheimer's Disease*, UCLA scientists mixed curcumin and vitamin D_3 in the blood of Alzheimer's patients in test tubes and found that they prevented the buildup of amyloid beta, an abnormal protein that is thought to be one of the causes of Alzheimer's disease.

Garlic

Although it is technically a vegetable, we think of garlic as herblike because of its potent flavor. Garlic has been used for medicinal purposes for over 5,000 years. Louis Pasteur confirmed the antibacterial effects of garlic in 1858. Compounds in garlic cause blood vessels to relax and dilate, increasing blood flow to the brain and improving brain function. Eating garlic regularly can help lower the risk of strokes, improve heart health, and boost the immune system's ability to fight off colds and flu. Allicin is the compound in garlic that performs this antioxidant action. Many researchers consider allicin in garlic to be the most potent antioxidant on the planet. Garlic also has insulin-sparing properties, which help to stabilize blood sugar. And it has been shown to decrease LDL ("bad") cholesterol and increase HDL ("good") cholesterol. A healthy way to dish it up: Combine garlic with tomatoes and basil for a brain-boosting marinara. To get the best effects, cut and peel the garlic and let the garlic stand for fifteen minutes before cooking.

Ginger

An anti-inflammatory agent, ginger may protect against neurodegenerative diseases and reduce the oxidative stress that causes brain cells to age and die. Ginger contains natural antiemetic agents to help decrease nausea and vomiting. It is also believed to help lower cholesterol. The antifungal and antibacterial nature of ginger makes it a great treatment for wounds. The next time you feel a migraine coming on, reach for the ginger before you take your usual migraine medication. "Ginger helps reduce the nausea that often comes with migraines, which may help with the absorption of other migraine medications so they can work better," says Roger Cady, MD, director of the Headache Care Center in Springfield, Missouri, and lead author of a 2005 study on a combination of ginger and feverfew for migraine relief. For the study, Cady's team of researchers treated people with sublingual ginger and feverfew when their headache was still in the mild stage. After two hours, 48 percent of the participants were pain free. In 34 percent, the pain remained mild and didn't become more severe. According to Cady, "If a headache doesn't go to full-blown migraine, that is considered a success." A healthy way to dish it up: For a fragrant ginger tea that settles your stomach, grate three teaspoons of fresh gingerroot, place it in one cup of boiled water, cover and steep for ten to fifteen minutes. Strain before drinking.

Note: Ginger has natural anticoagulant properties, so if you are taking an anticoagulant medication, check with your health care provider before using ginger supplements.

Marjoram   This culinary favorite promotes healthy digestion and can soothe minor digestive upsets. Marjoram has historically been a favorite herbal remedy in women's health because of how well it is believed to relieve muscle cramps. A great source of vitamin K, marjoram has been associated with preventing Alzheimer's disease by decreasing neuronal damage. Besides having anti-inflammatory and antibacterial properties, this sweet-tasting herb is loaded with vitamin C, beta-carotene, vitamin A, cryptoxanthin, lutein, and zeaxanthin, which is known to protect against age-related degenerative diseases and cataracts in the eyes. A healthy way to dish it up: Add a few leaves to a pot of water and bring to a boil. Reduce heat and steep for ten minutes to create a soothing tea.

Mint   One of the most versatile herbs in the kitchen has turned out to be nearly as versatile for boosting health. According to a study published in the *International Journal of Neuroscience*, the scent of peppermint improves memory and focus. Mint has been used for medical reasons by healers for hundreds of years for ailments such as digestive disturbance, diarrhea (irritable bowel syndrome), and bad breath, and for teeth whitening, and general tooth care. Mint is generally considered delicious by people of all ages and from most cultures. A healthy way to dish it up: Add mint leaves to water or smoothies, or chop and add to any salad to give a fresh summery twist.

Oregano   One of the strongest antioxidants known, oregano protects cells in the body and brain from free radicals that cause premature aging. Oregano is also a source of omega-3 fatty acids, which enhance brain function and offer protection from depression and premenstrual syndrome symptoms. It may also reduce insomnia and relieve migraine headaches. Oil of oregano is a potent antibacterial agent. A healthy way to dish it up: Chop several leaves and add to fresh marinara sauce.

Nutmeg   Like cloves, this aromatic spice contains eugenol, a compound thought to be cardioprotective. It also contains myristicin, which helps to prevent the formation of plaques in the brain believed to be responsible for Alzheimer's disease. Chinese medicine recommends nutmeg for the treatment of liver disease. Herbal medicine practitioners often use nutmeg to treat depression and anxiety. A healthy way to dish it up: Though commonly used for baking, nutmeg adds a delicious twist to lamb stew.

Rosemary   The caffeic and rosmarinic acids found in rosemary contribute to its legendary antioxidant and anti-inflammatory properties.

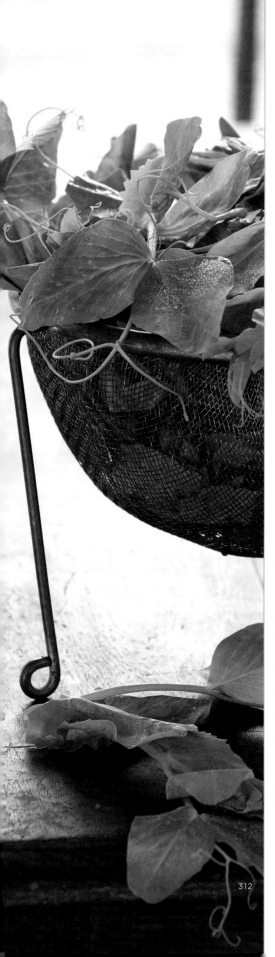

Improved circulation and digestion are but a couple of benefits you may enjoy along with the wonderful flavor of this herb. Rosemary also offers protection from cognitive decline associated with dementia and may provide new hope in the treatment of Parkinson's disease. Rosemary has been reported to help memory. A healthy way to dish it up: Probably one of the most versatile herbs for creating marinades and salad dressings, rosemary adds great flavor to salads, poultry, and meat.

Saffron   Got a case of the blues? Before you ask your doctor for antidepressants, try eating more saffron. In five studies conducted from 2004 through 2007, researchers at the University of Tehran, Iran, showed that saffron works as well as antidepressant medication in treating mild to moderate depression. The 2007 study involved giving forty depressed patients either saffron capsules or Prozac twice a day for eight weeks. At the end of the trial, the saffron proved to be as effective as the prescription medicine. Depression is associated with low levels of the neurotransmitter serotonin, and saffron seems to boost serotonin levels in the brain. In addition to adding a wonderful flavor to soups and other dishes, saffron can also improve memory and the ability to learn. This prized herb contains carotenoid compounds that boost immune function. A healthy way to dish it up: Add about one half teaspoon of saffron while cooking to two cups of rice or quinoa for a mood-boosting side dish.

Sage   When you keep losing your car keys, it's time for some sage. In a 2006 study, British researchers reported that this aptly named spice revs up memory in both the younger and the older generations, and it also minimizes the cognitive decline associated with Alzheimer's disease. Sage works because it inhibits an enzyme that breaks down the neurotransmitter acetylcholine, and you need to keep acetylcholine high in order to boost memory. The enzymes superoxide dismutase and peroxidase in sage have made it particularly popular with natural healers over the centuries for its effectiveness in fighting bacteria, preventing cancer, aiding digestion, and healing wounds. A healthy way to dish it up: Get smart and add two tablespoons of fresh chopped sage leaves to enhance the flavor of winter soups.

Thyme   Sixty percent of the solid weight of your brain is fat, and the highest percentage is a type of fat known as docosahexaenoic acid (DHA). DHA is important for rebuilding brain cells and protecting them against age-related degeneration. People who have low levels of DHA are more susceptible to Alzheimer's disease. Luckily, thyme is on your side. A 2000 study in the *British Journal of Nutrition* showed that it increases the amount of DHA in the brain. This flavorful spice helps to protect neurons in the brain from premature aging. It is also very high in pyridoxine, which helps keep the neurotransmitter gamma-aminobutyric acid (GABA) elevated, aiding in stress reduction. Thyme contains thymol, an essential oil known for its antifungal and antimicrobial properties. Thyme is so densely packed with polyphenols, vitamins, and minerals that it has one of the highest ORAC values of all herbs. (ORAC stands for *oxygen radical absorbance capacity*, and is a way of measuring the amount of antioxidant capacity in various foods.) A healthy way to dish it up: The next time you roast a turkey, rub it with two tablespoons of fresh chopped thyme leaves in addition to your other favorite spices before cooking.

If you begin to think of herbs and spices as natural medicine to boost your brain and body health, those exotic bottles may not seem so intimidating. There are no rules with herbs and spices. Be adventurous and try creating a new marinade, dressing, or infusion. The results may pleasantly surprise you.

THE WAR ON SALT

The importance of salt to human beings from the beginning of time is indisputable. Access to "the spice of life" has been a major contributor to the rise of many civilizations since the earliest recorded history, and it is responsible for the fall of just as many. Salt contributed to the rise of the Egyptian empire. The Romans built roads with the primary purpose of salt transportation during the early years of the Roman Republic. In fact, the word *salary* comes from the Latin word for salt because the Roman Legion paid soldiers with salt, which was "worth its weight in gold." Even the Bible has over forty metaphors referencing salt in positive terms.

Everything changed in 1904 when a group of French doctors made an anecdotal connection between a group of patients who had hypertension and who also happened to be salt fiends. Belief in this connection was solidified in the 1970s by a researcher who claimed to have indisputable evidence that salt causes hypertension. He fed rats *500 grams* of sodium each day (the average American *human* consumes between 3.5 and 8 grams of sodium per day). After studying population trends and making the connection between high sodium consumption and hypertension, it was decided that excessive salt consumption indeed contributes to hypertension. Unfortunately, no studies were done to account for genetics, other lifestyle factors, or possible environmental influences. Recommendations were made for Americans to cut their salt intake by up to 85 percent, and most people have accepted this as truth.

[CONTINUED]

On the other side of the salt war, many studies have shown opposite findings, that elevated sodium may have very little influence on hypertension, and may in fact have some health benefits. A massive study published by Intersalt in 1988 compared sodium intake with blood pressure in subjects from fifty-two international research centers. They not only discovered no relationship between hypertension and sodium intake, but there was an inverse relationship in some populations. Intersalt wasn't the only group to take up arms in this war. Studies published by the Cochrane Collaboration, *American Journal of Medicine* (2006), and *European Journal of Epidemiology* (2007), just to name a few, showed that there is little evidence that changing to a low-salt diet offers any benefits. In fact some studies showed the opposite, that consuming a low-sodium diet was detrimental, and that high-sodium diets lead to better health for many people.

For as much evidence that shows the benefits of decreasing sodium where hypertension is concerned, there is equal evidence showing the benefits of sodium. According to Dr. Michael Alderman from the Albert Einstein College of Medicine, this is because people respond individually as a result of how the kidneys function to compensate for sodium consumption. Alderman has suggested a large, controlled, government-sponsored study to obtain unbiased evidence. It's unlikely any such study will be done due to cost.

Now let's talk about the effect of salt on the brain. Let's face it, ultimately what's good for the brain is good for the heart. Salt makes food taste better. But when high amounts of salt are combined with excessive amounts of sugar and fat, especially cheap processed fat, it makes food taste *amazing!* In fact, it tastes so amazing, "I bet you can't eat just one!" Food companies know this and they capitalize on it. Processing food with high levels of salt, sugar, and fat overwhelms the brain so you don't register the feeling of fullness as easily. It also lights up the cells in the same part of your brain that heroin and cocaine trigger. This causes the neurotransmitter dopamine to be released. Dopamine is associated with pleasure. In other words, too much salt added to certain foods contributes to a "rush," followed by a similar comfort feeling of an opioid release, without the extreme cognitive disorientation. While you may not experience an acute cognitive disorientation from salt, sugar and fat, it does in fact contribute to long-term cognitive decline over time. According to a new study from the Baycrest Kunin-Lunenfeld Applied and Evaluative Research Unit in Toronto, people who consume more than 2,300 milligrams of sodium each day, *in combination with a sedentary lifestyle*, are at higher risk for Alzheimer's disease. The reason is not related to hypertension but rather, the supporting role salt may play in damaging blood vessels. The study also made the correlation. Many experts also made the connection that excessive salt intake is often associated with processed food consumption; therefore more studies may need to be done.

The Brain Warrior's Way is a program to get control of your health, conquer food addictions, and learn to see whole food as abundance. Salt is used in moderation in the recipes, often with options for low-sodium alternatives. Always consult your physician before making any drastic changes to your health program.

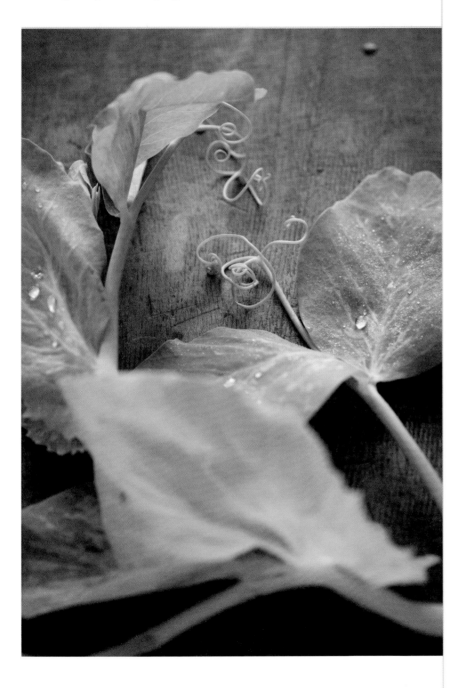

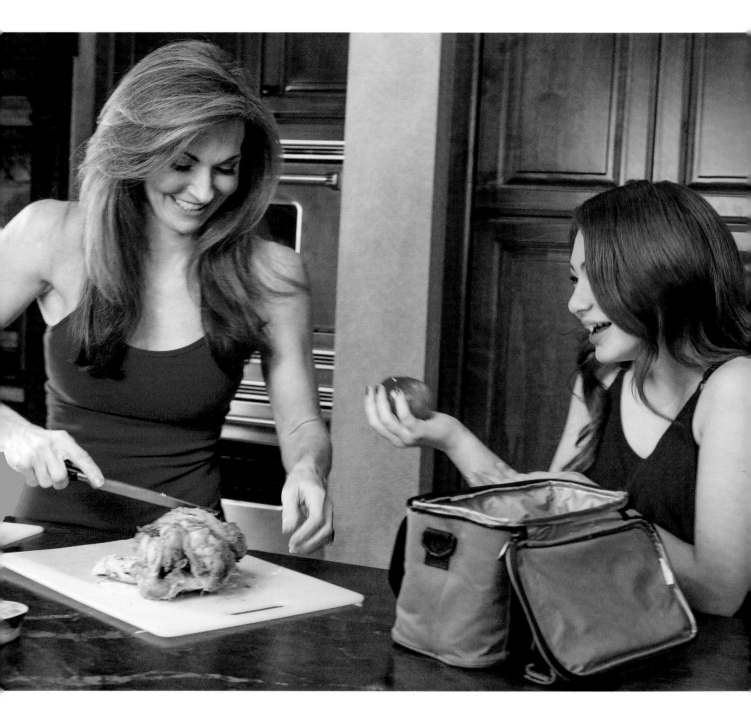

Rations for Brain Warriors on the Road

Surviving and Thriving on the Go

■

In preparing for battle I have always found that plans are useless, but planning is indispensable.

—DWIGHT D. EISENHOWER

Ancient warrior tribes all had one thing in common: they ate with purpose. Being a warrior was an honor that only the strongest and most elite could aspire to. Ancient warriors spent extensive time deployed away from home. Planning road rations was a critical part of warrior life. Food on the go was crucial for avoiding starvation in a time with no convenience stores, fast-food restaurants, or refrigeration. As a result, warrior tribes were acutely *conscious* of the food they ate. Having a mental and physical edge was the difference between life and death! Many warriors viewed food as medicine.

Modern-day Brain Warriors can glean tremendous wisdom from the ancient warriors, especially concerning food on the road. Always be prepared and ready. If you fail to plan, you plan to fail.

Lunches on the go, traveling, and at airports, parties, and restaurants are where Daniel and I both found it most challenging to stick to our lifestyle in the beginning. Our patients report the same challenges. When I began my journey in martial arts, all I was interested in was learning how to fight. But the early stages of training were very different from what I expected. I was taught the incredible value of preparation, awareness, avoidance, deflection . . . and exit strategies (including running really fast!). Eventually I learned how to fight, but my master explained that fighting should be reserved only for extreme situations because encounters with adversaries who outsize you are risky. So you have to fight smarter, not harder, and use effortless power.

This is the framework and metaphor Daniel and I both use, and that we teach patients.

▶ If mornings are rushed, pack your lunch and snacks the evening before.

▶ Have plenty of travel-sized storage containers on hand, and keep them in a convenient location in your kitchen.

▶ Premeasure portions into several containers and mark the containers with a permanent marker. For example: measure out 1 tablespoon into a small container and mark the spot. Do the same for ¼ cup, ½ cup, etc. You will never have to measure again; just fill the container up to the line. This is a tremendous time-saver.

▶ Immediately pack leftovers after dinner into lunch containers for the next day so you have a good supply of healthy, ready-to-eat foods.

▶ Always have an ice chest ready for on-the-go meals and snacks. Having a good supply of meals and snacks with you at all times helps keep you out of the drive-thru line.

▶ Always carry nuts and seeds in your pocket or purse so you can keep from getting too hungry if you're delayed.

▶ When traveling, make the grocery store your first stop upon arriving at a destination so that you don't have to go out to a restaurant for every meal or snack during your trip.

▶ Stock up on healthy items stored in snack-sized bags or containers that travel well and bring them on the road with you.

▶ Keep a list of dry foods prepacked in your travel bag (see our list below for suggestions).

▶ Call ahead and request a refrigerator in your room. Most hotels will accommodate you, so long as you give them notice. If not, ask them to clean out the minibar for your use. Don't move anything yourself or you may be charged.

AWARENESS

▶ Do an Internet search to find healthy restaurants and grocery stores before traveling.

▶ Many fast-food restaurants now serve wild-caught fish and steamed vegetables.

▶ Ask the hotel concierge for best recommendations for healthy stops.

- Look up menus for restaurants ahead of time so you can research menu items that you are not sure of and can plan out your options ahead of time.

- Call ahead to parties and find out what is being served so you can be prepared. Ask hostesses if they mind if you bring a dish (or two) to accommodate the way you eat. Most people appreciate the help, and this gives the hostess a heads-up that you don't eat a typical diet. You will set an example!

- Always keep on hand the list of alternatives for the things you most crave.

AVOIDANCE

- Do a pantry cleanse and get the toxic foodlike substances out of your house. You are kidding yourself if you believe you won't be tempted by them.

- If you can't find a healthy fast-food restaurant and you forgot your lunch, avoid the fast-food line. Instead stop at a grocery store and pick up a can of wild salmon or a hard-boiled egg and a salad. Don't let lack of preparation be an excuse to fail.

- Call ahead to alert restaurants that you have special dietary needs. Most will accommodate. Otherwise, find a different restaurant.

- When attending banquets and functions, eat in advance and then just pick at the veggies and salad. Ask if they are able to accommodate your dietary needs. Many venues now serve grilled fish or chicken with steamed vegetables available for people who have special dietary needs. In restaurants, ask the waiter not to leave bread on the table. Make one decision to avoid it, not thirty decisions to torture yourself and flirt with it!

- Take a wholesome, healthy dessert with you to parties so you won't be tempted by the cheesecake. If you don't want to make your own, find a "raw" food restaurant near you that serves outrageous desserts—but ask them to go easy on the sweetener. Raw desserts are usually made with unprocessed fruit and nuts that haven't had all of the nutrition and fiber cooked out of them.

- If you can't resist the sad faces of your kids when you decline the devious toys in fast-food restaurants, the ones designed to make you buy disease-promoting food, don't go there!

- ▶ Practice saying a polite and firm "No, thank you" or "I've already eaten" to well-meaning, but pushy family members who want to stuff your face with garbage that will make you regret it later.

- ▶ Steer clear of the samples that manufacturers hand out when you are shopping.

- ▶ Turn off the television or walk away when commercials appear with advertisements that are designed to lure you or your children into making poor eating choices.

- ▶ When restaurant servers try to supersize your order, sell you an additional item, or bring the dessert tray, hold up a hand and say, "I'm all set, thank you."

FIGHT BACK

Eventually there will come times that you need to take a firm stand for what you believe. If you have a plan, you'll feel less vulnerable. Also, it will be less awkward than if you just get frustrated.

There are many strategies for fighting back. When it comes to food fights, I'd like to suggest "firm, kind and polite." Gandhi transformed a nation employing similar strategies. The Italian proverb "You catch more flies with honey than vinegar" is apropos. People are more likely to listen to what you have to say if they are not confronted with hostility. Admittedly, this took a bit of practice for me, so I've listed some strategies that I've found work for me.

- ▶ Create your own "fun meal" and toys for your children when they eat healthy food. The fast-food industry doesn't own your children. If you find yourself infuriated by these schemes, fight back with an equally powerful tactic. Personally, I find well-placed bribery to be completely effective, as long as it buys me a teaching moment and ends with positive results.

- ▶ If family members or friends continue to be pushy after you've politely told them you aren't hungry, say to them, "I'm actually trying something new and eating more healthfully these days, and I just feel so much better when I stick to my plan. If you are interested, I can lend you this great cookbook I have . . ." Use this moment that could become uncomfortable and open the door to talk about what eating healthfully has done for your life and what it could do for their life as well. However, if you come from a family that is food centered like my very large, well-meaning Lebanese family, you may need to be a bit firmer. I will sometimes jestingly say with *love*, "It feels like you're loving me to death with food." Then I wink. I usually get the standard response, "You need more meat on your bones!" and we all laugh.

▶ When servers are pushy and insist that you should supersize or add another item because it's worth the extra dollar, tell them, "No, thank you—it's not about the money for me; it's about my health."

▶ When paying to attend events that don't allow you to bring in your own food, ask if they serve food that will accommodate your special dietary requirements. Usually they will allow you to bring your own food, but if not, calmly and politely ask to talk to the manager. Making your needs known is how changes are made, and as long as you are reasonable, the people you are talking to will be more understanding of your point of view. I've never had a manager refuse to allow me to bring a healthy snack in. In fact, there are three restaurants in our area that started carrying healthy snacks because of our loving persistence. Even the local movie theater now offers veggies with hummus and guacamole, and paninis (which I can eat minus the bread).

When changes like this do occur, be sure to acknowledge and celebrate them. I always comment, praise, and am sure to honor them by purchasing their food when I can.

▶ When your child's school asks you to go along with their attempt to teach "nutrition" to your child according to the food pyramid, and they ask you to tell your child that there are no "good" or "bad" foods, it's time to get involved. I wrote a document stating the reasons that I would not agree to such nonsense, and included scientific articles. I even offered to come teach a nutrition class, and that is something that you could do for your child. I still haven't received a response, but that doesn't stop me from modeling healthy eating at home and teaching our family a better way to eat. Where our classrooms fail us, we have to take up the responsibility at home while we continue to fight for changes in the way nutrition is taught. While the school has not officially acknowledged my tough-love stand, many of the individual teachers have. I have been asked for coaching by teachers for their families and for outside programs. Many of the teachers recommend my coaching to the parents of children with behavioral issues. And don't think this can't happen for you. We have many stories of our Brain Warriors starting mini-movements. These are not people with medical degrees. They are passionate people, caring about other people.

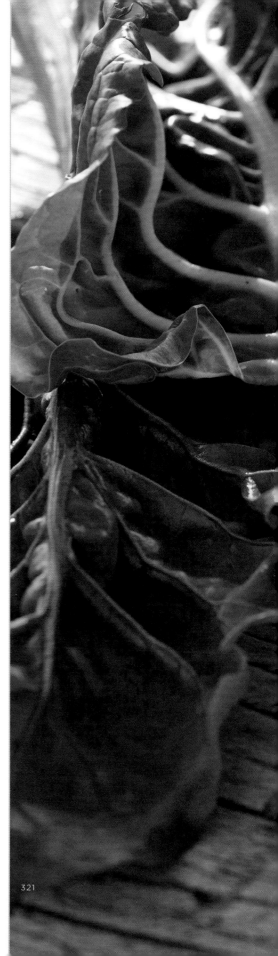

Improving the health of your brain is not only the goal; it is the only option! You must be willing to do what it takes to keep it healthy. We are your partners, but you must take the initiative. Don't be misled by food designers, or even well-meaning family members. Be the person who influences others to be healthy, and having respectful and open conversations with people when teachable moments present themselves is the best way to do that!

What to Pack and What to Order

Pack Ahead

DRY FOODS TO KEEP IN YOUR SUITCASE:

Here is a list of foods that I keep packed for my family. I simply rotate based on expiration dates. We are always prepared! I would also recommend keeping a list of safe foods to buy when you arrive at your destination.

- ▶ 3-ounce cans wild salmon (BPA free) with pop tops
- ▶ Coconut wraps
- ▶ Green tea
- ▶ Liquid stevia
- ▶ Dark chocolate (sugar free, dairy free)
- ▶ Plant-based protein powder (either premeasured into self-sealing bags or travel-sized pouches from the manufacturer)
- ▶ Grass-fed beef or turkey jerky
- ▶ Nut butter and coconut butter in travel-sized, single-serving packets

DAILY CHOICES FOR YOUR LUNCH BOX:

PROTEIN:
- ▶ Hard-boiled eggs
- ▶ Grilled chicken breast
- ▶ Canned wild salmon with pop-tops
- ▶ Smoked wild salmon
- ▶ Leftover entrée from last night's dinner
- ▶ Homemade Chocolate Pumpkin Protein Bars (page 286). Make a tray and freeze in advance.
- ▶ Deli meat (sugar free, nitrate free)
- ▶ Precooked wild shrimp
- ▶ Grass-fed jerky

CARBOHYDRATES:

▶ Chopped vegetables (broccoli, cauliflower, peppers, cucumbers, carrots, zucchini)
▶ Hummus
▶ Salsa for dipping
▶ Organic berries
▶ Organic apples
▶ Organic cherries
▶ Other low-glycemic fruit

HEALTHY FATS:

▶ ¼ to ½ cup nuts (depending on how long you will be gone)
▶ Olive oil for salad dressing
▶ Guacamole
▶ Sunflower or pumpkin seeds
▶ Coconut wraps (to replace bread)
▶ ½ ounce dark chocolate, sugar free, dairy free
▶ Nut butter in single-serving travel-sized packets
▶ Homemade trail mix
▶ Water: Always keep a nonplastic bottle of water on hand—when you think you are hungry you may just be thirsty! Use plastic bottles only in a pinch.

Ordering Out

THREE SIMPLE THINGS TO REMEMBER WHEN EATING OUT

1. Stick with 70/30: Focus your diet on 70 percent plants, 30 percent protein, with high-quality fat—*bread, rice, pasta, tortillas, and potatoes DO NOT count!*
2. Order items, not plates: instead of ordering chicken Parmesan with cream sauce, ask for chicken breast with marinara sauce and steamed vegetables or salad.
3. Make one decision, not thirty: Never let the waiter leave bread or fried appetizers. Make one decision to say, "No, thank you," instead of thirty decisions to resist once it's in front of you.

If you didn't have time to check out the menu online ahead of time, don't fret. When going to any restaurant, have one simple model in mind: stir-fry without rice. In other words, have lots of veggies, a little protein, and pile on the herbs and spices. However, you want to watch out for things like MSG, soy and gluten, so be sure to ask for the gluten-free options and ask if they use MSG. The stir-fry example is only a model to keep you on track. It can be transferred to any style of food.

Also, the simpler the recipe, the safer it generally is, but be sure to ask. Try to stick with basics. If they have a complicated recipe that includes chicken breast or broccoli, it likely means they have chicken breast and broccoli in its simple form. Since they likely want you as a customer, most restaurants will accommodate your requests, especially if you explain that they're for health reasons. I often explain, "It's not that I don't love it; it just doesn't love me back." That's usually enough to end the conversation.

If bread or appetizers are a trigger for you, make one decision not to have the waiter leave them on the table, instead of thirty decisions to use willpower to avoid them. Willpower rarely wins long term, especially when you're tired or hungry and brain function isn't at its strongest.

Here are a few examples of the adjustments we make and our recommendations when dining out:

CHINESE/JAPANESE FOOD SUGGESTIONS:
► Order stir-fry without rice and add extra veggies
► Have a seaweed salad or sashimi salad without ponzu sauce (which contains gluten)

- ▶ Ask for sushi rolls without rice (cucumber cut rolls)
- ▶ Order hand rolls on seaweed paper with no rice. Add your favorite fish and avocado
- ▶ Ask for gluten-free tamari sauce instead of soy sauce
- ▶ Ask if they serve grilled vegetable, shrimp and chicken skewers without breading
- ▶ Avoid restaurants that use MSG

Tamari is soy based, so minimize the amount you consume and make sure to purchase organic when possible. The benefit of tamari sauce is that it doesn't contain gluten as soy sauce does. At home I have low-sodium organic tamari sauce that I will sometimes carry to restaurants. However, many restaurants have tamari sauce with so many people eating a gluten-free diet. This is an occasional treat. Often these dishes taste amazing without any sauce.

MEXICAN FOOD SUGGESTIONS:
- ▶ Fajitas without tortillas and rice
- ▶ Skip the beans and opt for more guacamole and salsa. If you eat the beans, ask for pinto or black beans instead of refried beans, and eat no more than about ¼ cup.
- ▶ Swap heavy cheese sauces with salsa and guacamole.
- ▶ Order a salad topped with shrimp or chicken. Vegetarians can ask for grilled vegetables.
- ▶ Make sure salads are not served in fried tortilla shells or with tortilla strips.

We use guacamole for everything! I use it as a dip and a spread. Sometimes I just eat it plain. Avocados are not only healthy; they are satisfyingly delicious!

INDIAN FOOD SUGGESTIONS:
- ▶ Tandoori chicken can usually be prepared very simply, without heavy sauces and cheap oils.
- ▶ Try chicken or lamb tikka.
- ▶ Chicken, lamb, or vegetable kebabs make a light and satisfying meal.
- ▶ Gobi matar tamatar (cauliflower with peas and tomato) is a good vegetarian option.
- ▶ Try curry- or coconut-based sauces in place of cream. Don't assume coconut milk sauces don't contain cream.
- ▶ Avoid the heavy popular cream, cheese, and yogurt sauces. Being served over vegetables doesn't make them healthy.

The exotic aromas and taste explosions that are a natural part of Indian food are what make it a favorite for many people around the globe. But it's the spices that make it a favorite in our house. Turmeric, a staple spice used in many Indian dishes, has been shown to be protective against Alzheimer's disease, cancer, and heart disease.

ITALIAN FOOD SUGGESTIONS:
- ▶ Ask for fresh fish or poultry that isn't breaded
- ▶ Order extra steamed vegetables instead of pasta.
- ▶ Swap cream sauces for marinara.
- ▶ Cioppino (seafood stew with tomato broth) is one of our favorite dishes. Order it without the pasta and bread that is often served with it. Order a side of steamed broccoli instead.

The beauty of good Italian food is the incredible amount of garlic, basil, and oregano used in, well, almost everything. These herbs are not only delicious; they are incredibly healthy. Why ruin the amazing health benefits with a big plate of sugary pasta?

GENERAL DINING TIPS
- ▶ Ask for cut vegetables for dipping in guacamole and salsa or hummus instead of using bread.
- ▶ Sparkling water with a slice of lime and berry-flavored stevia (or chocolate) tastes like soda.
- ▶ Always skip the baked potato or mashed potatoes (unless they are sweet potatoes), and ask for an extra portion of steamed vegetables instead.
- ▶ Instead of eggs Benedict, try poached eggs with chicken or turkey, served over a bed of steamed spinach.
- ▶ Order steaks, poultry, and seafood dishes without heavy sauces (especially in Italian and French restaurants). Ask for a side of marinara sauce if you just have to have something.
- ▶ In an airport or on the go, look for a simple salad and dump a can of wild salmon that *you will always carry* on it. It's a perfect lunch. If you're vegetarian, open the bag of nuts you now have with you and ask for avocado.
- ▶ If you are inclined to have dessert, ask for fresh berries and split them with someone special. Skip the whipped cream.

Hopefully these simple tips will start to stimulate your own thought process and you can begin to formulate a strategy for eating a healthy diet in a world filled with unhealthy options. Copy this list, try adding a few of your own ideas, and keep it with you!

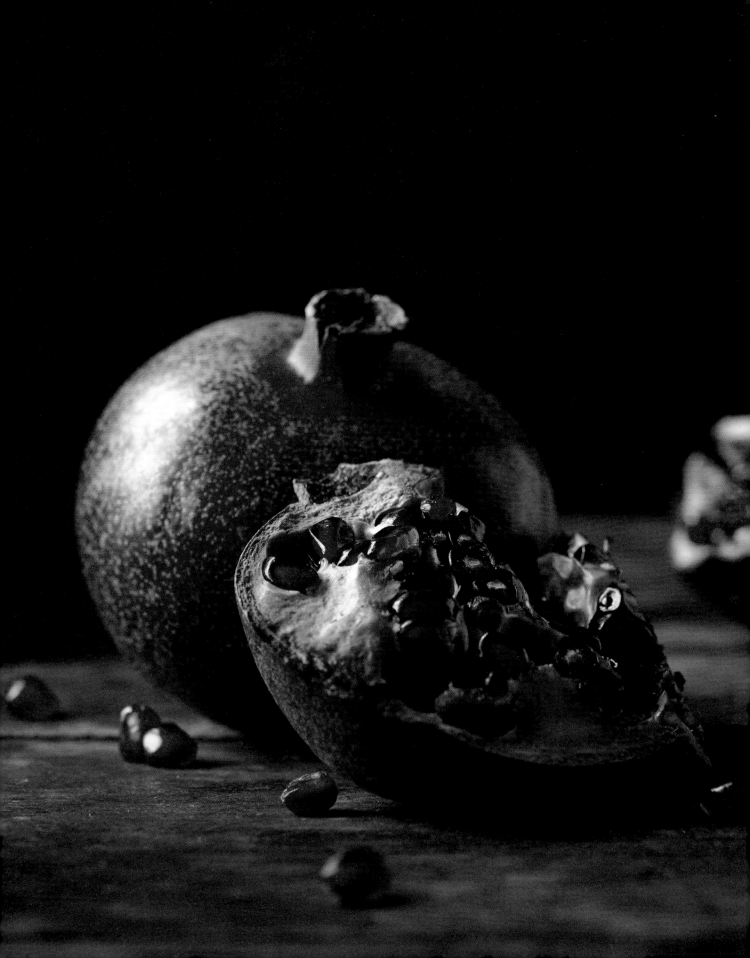

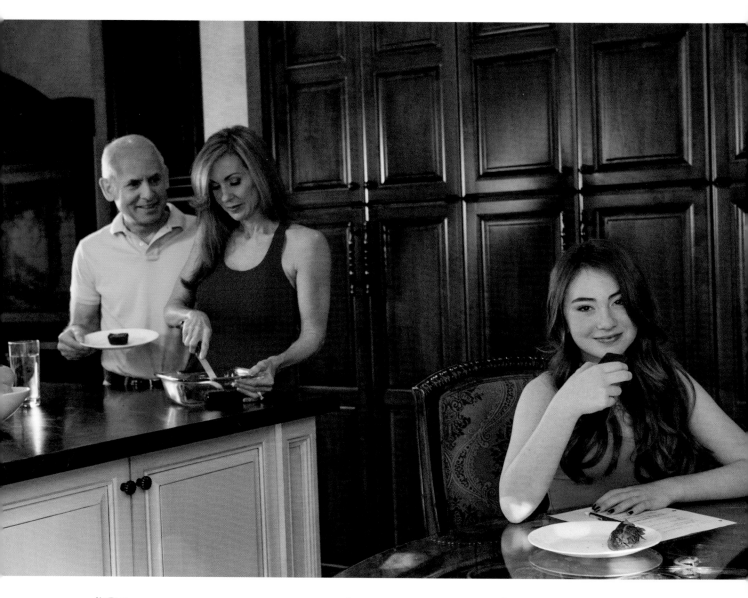

"If you are a parent, you're a warrior. We've learned with a teenager that the insignificant battles are less important than the war. Our philosophy of firm, kind and open makes life a lot more fun."

—Daniel and Tana

Junior Brain Warriors

Get Kids of All Ages Involved Early

■

First they ignore you, then they laugh at you, then they
fight you, then you win.

—GANDHI

Imagine being the mother of a young Spartan warrior going off to war. Spartans were arguably the fiercest and bravest of all warriors. Parents, especially mothers, played a significant role in this warrior culture by raising sons to think like warriors from birth. By age seven they were sent off to train. Before leaving for their first battle, a mother would tell her beloved child, "Son, come home with your shield or upon it." That meant he was to reign victorious in battle or die trying. If a Spartan came home without a shield, it was a sign that he was a deserter, something no Spartan could tolerate. This singular focus on victory made Spartans formidable opponents. We certainly don't want you teaching your junior warriors to come home upon a shield, but we honor and respect the dedication of these mothers, because it works. Children don't do what you say to do; they do what you do.

- 11 percent of children have been diagnosed with ADD.
- Childhood obesity is increasing at alarming rates.
- Obesity doubles your risk for Alzheimer's disease.
- It is estimated that one out of every three children born after the year 2000 will develop type 2 diabetes.
- Type 2 diabetes is a risk factor for Alzheimer's disease, and Alzheimer's is now referred to as type 3 diabetes.
- Type 2 diabetes is one of the most preventable diseases with simple lifestyle changes.

If you've got junior Brain Warriors in training, you *must be the change you want to see,* and you must hold your ground when it comes to a healthy brain and body! Exposure equals preference, and sugar is addictive! In other words, if you have junk food and sugar around the house, that is not only what your children will prefer; it is what they will crave.

A Brain Warrior Family: The Bowlings

Wes's testimonial is the perfect description of a family transitioning from a culture of illness-promoting food to a family determined to build a legacy of health for generations to come! He describes the process of successfully getting your family on board with your new lifestyle.

When Wes and his wife witnessed their strong, athletic eleven-year-old son, Johnny, suddenly collapse on the beach in front of them, they literally thought that he was dead. That was the wake-up call it took for the Bowling family to change everything about the way they viewed nutrition. But even after enduring endless tests and hospitalization to discover the cause of the collapse, the Bowlings were more confused than ever about what they needed to do to get their family's health back on track. They needed a change, but they were missing the specifics.

While flipping through the television stations one night, they came across our public television show *The Omni Health Revolution*. And they paid attention to the message we were sending out. The Bowlings determined they had been "poisoning" their family with the wrong food and bad habits, and they made radical and immediate changes to their nutrition. They became Brain Warriors to save their son!

This is what Wes had to say about his family's success and the improvements he has seen in their lives since they have become Brain Warriors:

"Within a week the dark areas under our kids' eyes were gone and our energy levels skyrocketed. My wife was worried that it was going to cost an arm and a leg to eat this way, but we found out that it was a whole lot cheaper. We saved a ton of money from [not] eating out, and because we were buying fresh produce, we only bought what we [planned] to eat, otherwise it would go bad. The crazy thing is, Johnny's body weight went up by almost 20 percent in a few weeks and he was taller! In July he began being active again and returned to normal form by August. The only change was eating and living clean.

"As school began in August, my kids were coming home telling my wife that they no longer get sleepy at school and that they are finding it very easy to focus on what is going on in the classroom. The grades for all four kids were twice as good as in any previous year! I also had my own improvements. The first week, I lost five pounds, and it continued to drop with very little effort. I was eating five meals a day, and pretty much stuffing myself. The only difference is that it was good stuff."

Wes is now down fifty-five pounds and going strong! Here are Wes's suggestions, in his words, as to how every family can become a Brain Warrior Family:

▶ Become a Gourmet Health Chef: My wife figured out how to cook things that were awesome tasting, gourmet-style. It took her a little more time at first. So many times people try to eat crappy, bland vegetables and a piece of chicken. There's nothing exciting about that, to hit those satisfaction buttons.

▶ Do not let your children eat the food sold to them at school. It is poison! My wife figured out how to make clean lunches that the kids would love. Now the kids have their friends asking every day to try their mom's gourmet creations.

▶ Pack bottles of water for them to take to school to drink at lunch, on the bus, and whenever else the school will let them. Make sure they drink as soon as they wake up, as soon as they get home from school, and with each meal and in the evening. It took about a month, but what my kids craved actually changed.

▶ Find some sort of activity you do on your feet instead of an exercise program, even if it's shopping for a couple of hours. It's that simple.

▶ Educate your kids and husband why the bad stuff is poison; show them what is really in it and how it's killing their body. Show the nastiest preparation process possible to them in a YouTube video. Once they associate pain and nastiness with it, they will no longer want it.

Seven Tips for Brain Warrior Families

We're the first to admit that making changes to start feeding kids a healthier diet can be challenging. And it's particularly difficult in a culture where children are constantly exposed to unhealthy foods and given powerful cues and rewards to eat these foods. For example, in 2009, the fast-food industry overall spent nearly $4.3 billion on advertising specifically designed for children between the ages of two and seventeen years old. When a clown with a billion-dollar bankroll can come into your living room and entice your children with toys for eating French fries and milk shakes, we are dealing with some strange and powerful forces that make it tough for you to serve broccoli and halibut. But that does not mean your kids are naturally inclined to prefer fast food. They aren't. No human being is.

Sure, the food industry cashes in on our predisposition for seeking out sugar, fat, and salt, and creates hyperpalatable Frankenfoods designed to pull genetic triggers that keep us craving these highly processed, chemically altered foodlike substances. Yet, there is nothing natural about these foods or the cravings they elicit. If you've bought into the idea that your kids "naturally" prefer Pop-Tarts and pizza, you are not alone. But there is hope to transform the eating habits of the fussiest young eaters.

Here are seven tips we've used with our daughter and clients with wonderful results. So get ready to say good-bye to foolish clowns with bad hair bribing your kids with cheap toys once and for all.

Tip #1: Expose Kids to Healthy Food Early

Exposure equals preference. In other words: what your children are exposed to is what they will crave for a lifetime. Why do you think the fast-food industry spends so much money advertising to kids, using such affable jesters as their mascots? They know that it's as simple as exposure and conditioning to hook in consumers for a lifetime.

This tip is especially important for young families: Don't keep unhealthy or "taboo" foods in your house. Trash the cookies, candies, ice cream, pizza, pasta, and soda. If you don't want your children eating it, don't rely on willpower to keep them away from foods that are chemically designed to hijack their taste buds.

We have a bizarre cultural concept that children require some kind of "special diet." With a few important exceptions, like allergies and avoiding nuts, shellfish, and honey until your kids are two, this simply isn't true. Somehow we bought into the idea that it's a constitutional right for children to eat junk food if they refuse everything else.

If you eat a healthy diet, feed your kids what you eat. If you don't eat healthy, your kids won't either. Lead by example and choose foods that support your biology and the growing bodies of your children: namely, fresh vegetables and fruits filled with phytonutrients, lean and pasture-raised protein, and healthy fats. Expose your kids to these foods when they're young, and they will crave them for a lifetime.

Tip #2: Play with Your Food

In our home, playing with your food is not only allowed, but encouraged! We played a game with our daughter from the time she was a toddler. We call it "Chloe's Food Game," and we've found it works with adults as well as kids.

Here's how to play: The next time you sit down to dinner, tell your children you are going to play a little game. You are going to name certain foods and they get to judge them. You can talk about the foods on your table or any others that pop into your mind. Your kids get to judge them on the following scale:

Two thumbs up = Super healthy. You and your kids could eat this food every day.

One thumb up, one thumb down = Moderately healthy. You could have this from time to time but wouldn't want to eat it often.

Two thumbs down = Terribly unhealthy and doesn't serve your body at all.

For example, if we said, "Soda," Chloe would put two thumbs down and say, "That's poison." On the other hand, if we said, "Blueberries," Chloe asked if they were organic. She knows that blueberries hold more pesticides than almost any other fruit, and pesticides have been linked to an increased incidence of ADD.

If you come up with a food you aren't sure of, go online and do some research. You will learn just as much playing this game with your kids as they do!

Tip #3: Knowing When Enough Is Enough

We're not usually big fans of the "take it a little at a time" approach when it comes to getting sugar or processed fast foods out of our diet. When counseling adults we always encourage them to "jump the canyon." Here's why: You can't cross a canyon in two small steps. "Just a little" sugar is no

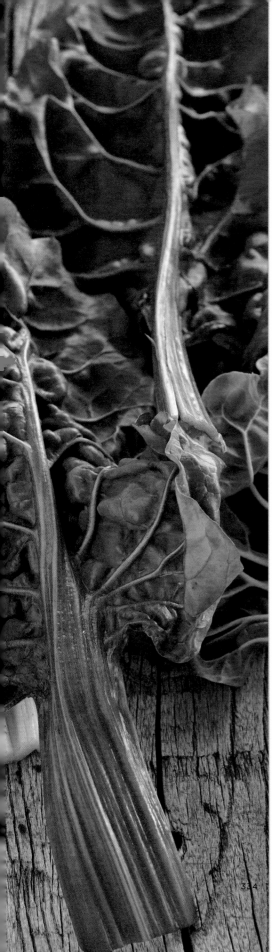

better for you than "just a little" cocaine, and, in point of fact, the sugar is probably more addictive. When you make a radical change and eliminate these foods from your diet entirely, cravings typically vanish in about three days except in cases of extreme sugar addiction. Eat "just a little" and you simply keep the cycle going needlessly.

However, there are some exceptions. Whether you are the parent of a sensitive teenager who is being exposed to cultural messages about body image for the first time or a toddler who is rebelling against eating her peas, the last thing you want to be is the food police. That is an instant signal for kids to rebel! And you run the risk of creating unhealthy relationships with food if you are constantly saying "no" and making your kids feel like food is a stress point. It's always good to give choices when possible, but try to give choices from several healthy options.

Rather than demanding your children "eat this, not that," focus on the relationship between food and health and help them draw conclusions about how they feel when they eat certain foods. Do not—we repeat, DO NOT—make this about "going on a diet." Health is about much more than weight. The last thing you want to do is give your child a body image complex and feel as if they need to "go on a diet" when really you are just aiming to teach them about lifelong healthy eating habits.

If you are in the process of changing the way you eat as a family, I suggest you pay attention to cues from your family. The younger your children, the faster you can usually make the transition. For older children, you may need to take more time and get them involved in the process. Start by getting rid of the worst stuff in their diet first and replacing it with healthier alternatives. And balance this with allowing them to keep some of their favorite foods in the house initially. The most important thing is to make it fun and get their input. Find healthy alternatives to their favorite foods. Replace, don't erase! For example, you could stop buying soda and replace it with Zevia or sparkling water with a few drops of root-beer-flavored stevia. Make Coconut Avocado Protein Pudding or fruit smoothies with protein powder. Freeze these and they become a replacement for Popsicles. Maybe your youngster loves peanut butter and jelly. You could substitute that with almond butter on coconut wraps and sliced banana. If your teenage son LOVES pasta, and you're afraid you will face World War III without it, seek out healthier alternatives like zucchini noodles, shirataki noodles, or quinoa pasta (purchase corn-free brands), which are gluten free. With a little creativity and research, you can effectively moderate much of what you feed your kids. But whatever you do, you will never be able to fully control what your kids eat, and that leads us to our next and toughest bit of advice.

Tip #4: Let Your Kids Make Their Own Food Mistakes

Your children will not make all the choices you want them to make. That's true in nutrition, just as it is in every other part of their lives. That can be a tough pill to swallow for us parents, but it's reality. You have to let your kids make some mistakes, even when it comes to food. We don't live in a glass bubble—our daughter doesn't either, and we wouldn't want her to. She's exposed to pizza, cupcakes, and candy at birthday parties, at school, even at religious functions. No matter how much this upsets us, this is simply how things are. But Chloe's strong will helps her make her own choices, and she tends not to choose unhealthy foods on a regular basis or in excess, and we believe it's because we've given her a background that allows her to make smart, well-informed choices. We never want to take her strong will away from her, because we want that strength to guide her when making tough decisions. We want her to start listening to her internal voice as she gets older and we can't be there to guide her. Even when she does make unhealthy food choices, she knows her limit. We don't nag her, but we do help her make the connection to acne, stomachaches, and brain fog when she eats junk.

You can do the same with your kids. Lead the way, expose them to healthy nutritious food in your home, and encourage them to be attentive to the way food affects their bodies. You may find they would rather have ginger-glazed salmon and kale salad than Happy Meals and sodas.

Tip #5: Create Positive Associations to Healthy Living

When Daniel and I decided to completely remove the last remnants of junk from the house, there was some squeaking and squealing from Chloe (then five years old). We were very firm about our decision, but also came up with a game to help her transition. I took her on a scavenger hunt at the local health food store. It started with a healthy snack from the restaurant. This helped create and anchor the positive associations. Then I told her that I'd give her a treat for each healthy alternative she could help find to replace the ones we were removing. The treats were as simple as a hair clip, lip gloss, or a quarter. Chloe and I found twelve alternatives! The next step was to go home and come up with some delicious recipes together. We played in the kitchen and made a big mess, had a blast, and made fun memories together. As a result of these games, Chloe is unusually confident in the kitchen for her age.

Tip #6: Create Healthy Alternatives for Kid-Favorite Recipes

According to my family, one of my gifts is transforming really healthy food to make it taste decadent. I love to rehabilitate our unhealthy favorites into delicious, nutritious recipes that often taste better than the originals. "Rehabbing" the unhealthy recipes that your kids love will give you a huge advantage in the war to protect the health of your family. If they feel deprived because Mom and Dad take all their favorite foods away, pushing a big plate of green veggies and chicken breast in front of them is likely to create mutiny. Parent to parent, there are many ways to accomplish your nutrition goals. While some of these ways may seem devious, they work and will ultimately help keep your kids healthier while also developing Brain Warrior habits.

Besides the many dessert and snack recipes, you will find many healthy versions of classic kid favorite meals including:

- ► Mac-n-Cheese becomes Mac-N-No Cheese (page 216)
- ► Chicken nuggets become Smarty-Pants Chicken Fingers (page 158)
- ► Battered coconut shrimp becomes Crafty Coconut Shrimp (page 134)
- ► Fried fish sticks become Fat Head Fish Sticks (page 133).
- ► Fettuccine Alfredo becomes Creamy Fettucine-Style Noodles (page 203).
- ► Chicken wings become Chloe's Favorite Chicken Wings (page 157).

Tip #7: Work on Ways to Collaborate and Compromise with Older Children

The younger children are when you plant the Brain Warrior's Way into their lives, the easier it will be for them to adapt. But even children raised in a healthy environment from birth will usually begin to seek independence and challenge your beliefs about healthy eating, along with many other beliefs. If you accept this as a normal part of development on the way to independence, you will enjoy the journey much more.

To thwart a battle of the wills and the resentment that children often feel as a result, we came up with a plan for our daughter that involved collaboration, compromise, and taking responsibility for outcomes. Here's an example of what such an agreement might look like:

Since we do the grocery shopping, we make the decisions about what to buy at home. Chloe can pick out whatever she wants from an approved list of foods. If we are in a restaurant, we give her freedom to choose what she wants from the menu, within reason. She may choose pasta as long as she also chooses either protein or vegetables to go with it. We will not buy soda under any circumstances, as it is too harmful to her health. However, when Chloe is at a party or sleepover with her peers, she can make her own food choices without our interference. If she goes to the mall or an amusement park with friends and wants ice cream or lemonade, she can have it—as long as she can afford it. She must pay for junk food from her allowance. The only input we give is if she feels sick or experiences consequences from her choices. We are kind and loving about it, but clear that her discomfort was likely a result of what she ate. So far, we've had very good luck with this approach. Chloe makes healthy choices about 90 percent of the time.

We don't have magic fairy dust that makes Chloe love healthy food. She is a strong-willed, normal teenager. The only magic formula is that we have been consistent with the tips we're sharing with you now. Chloe is becoming her own health advocate. She makes mistakes, but she's wiser in her early teens than we were in our thirties.

It is oddly comforting when our daughter comes home from a friend's house and another parent tells us how health-focused Chloe is, and that she has been proselytizing to the other children about making better choices. Even though she constantly pushes back at home and tests boundaries, the message is obviously getting through. One day, when Chloe was ten years old, her teacher took a picture of her lunch (that Chloe made herself) to use as an example, as she was trying to learn healthier lunch alternatives.

As children move toward adolescence, independence is a natural part of their development. This often translates to "pushing back" when being told what's for dinner. Handling older children and teens may require some patience and creativity. Look around and you will see that we live in a society that is steeped in "food issues," and our children are the victims.

We are no strangers to the exasperation teenagers can cause. Imagine being well known for the health advice you give, only to have your child taunt you by waving chocolate cake in your face, giggling. I have scars on my tongue from biting back the mom comments I desperately want to shout in these moments. Instead I have a rehearsed line ready to go. With indifference I usually say, "I'm glad those things don't look good to me any longer. That makes my stomach hurt just looking at it."

Don't give up hope even for the toughest junk-food junkies. The moment when they feel like throwing in the towel in total despair is often when we hear parents say they had miraculous breakthroughs. Eye rolls and teasing from a teenager are often normal forms of communication. It doesn't necessarily mean they aren't listening to you. It often just means they don't want you to know it. Learning how to tease back in the cryptic language of teenagers has gone a long way in our house for opening communication with my daughter and her friends. While this applies to far more than food, I always seize the opportunity to *use healthy food as a catalyst.*

By making healthy food that tastes delicious when the kids are around, I'm usually able to keep them gathered in the kitchen talking about serious life issues. Imagine my delight one day when one of Chloe's friends said to me, "I love you! This food is so good it's hard to imagine that it's good for me. I'd be so healthy if I lived here for a month. My dad is diabetic and would love this!" I made sure to send her home with healthy treats for her dad.

Shortly after that incident, Chloe came home and said, "I need you to help me eat healthier. I'm starting to feel bloated more often (Puberty!). A lot of kids are talking about using diuretic tea and stuff that makes them lose weight. I know it's not healthy. What can I do that is healthy?" She even admitted that she doesn't really like eating junk food because it makes her feel bad, but that she doesn't always want to be the weird kid eating seaweed snacks when her friends go out for something as "normal" as a pizza. We had a great strategizing session, without eye rolls! I never would have had this amazing opportunity to weigh in on the critically important issue of eating disorders and how food affects mood if I hadn't been doing my part to keep the lines of communication open.

Recommended Brand List

Many of the recipes in this book give suggestions for ingredients that may seem new to you. I've created a list of the brands I most commonly use for some of these ingredients to help with ease of shopping.

Many of these items can be found in mainstream grocery stores. Some will most commonly be found in your local health food store. By far my favorite place to shop for both convenience and cost saving is online. I always look online for anything that isn't perishable before making a trip to the grocery store.

CHOCOLATE:
Brain in Love, sugar-free, dairy-free
Brain on Joy, sugar-free, dairy-free
Lily's Chocolate Chips

CRACKERS:
Go Raw Flax Snax
Mary's Gone Crackers

GRAIN-FREE CEREAL:

On the Go Paleo

Paleo People

Steve's PaleoGoods

MEAT PRODUCTS:

Steve's PaleoGoods Grass-Fed PaleoJerky

Vital Choice Wild Salmon and Mackerel

MILKS AND CREAMERS:

365 Organic

Elmhurst Harvest

Natura

New Barn

Nutpods

NUT BUTTERS AND COCONUT PRODUCTS:

Artisana

Carrington Farms

Kelapo

Nutiva

OILS:

International Collection

La Tourangelle

Piping Rock

Vital Choice

Spectrum Naturals

Zoe

PROTEIN POWDER:

Brain M.D. Life

Vega

SWEETENERS:

SweetLeaf liquid Sweet Drops and powdered stevia packets

NuNaturals powdered stevia

Wholesome! ZERO (erythritol)

WRAPS AND BREAD REPLACEMENTS:

Green Leaf Foods Raw Wraps

The Pure Wraps Coconut Wraps

SeaSnax Seaweed Wraps

WrawP Vegan Flat Bread

"Your health decisions don't only affect you; they affect generations of you."

—Daniel and Tana

WHY DON'T KIDS LIKE GREEN FOOD?

There is scientific evidence to suggest that there is a biological reason that you may end up locked in a battle of the wills when you ask your child to eat greens! Have you noticed that your kids don't hate all vegetables? Usually it's the really green, bitter ones like spinach, kale, and sometimes broccoli (unless we camouflage the taste). Chloe loves red bell peppers, carrots, squash, cauliflower, and even broccoli—pretty much any vegetable except the leafy, dark green ones. This bothered me until I understood the reason. It turns out that taste bud receptors for bitter foods usually are not activated until around the time that people stop growing. The same qualities in bitter vegetables that make them "good for you" also slow down rapid cell growth. Of course, this is the opposite of what children are doing: they are rapidly growing! In general, around or shortly after the time that children stop growing is also the time that cancer usually becomes more of a threat, and cancer is a group of rapidly growing cells! According to recent research, children have a natural tendency to reject foods that stunt growth until they are finished growing.

There is no need to get into that battle of wills with your children over vegetables. While it is still important for your children to eat vegetables, you can accomplish the same goal with a little creativity. Flavoring foods with powerful spices to make them "taste good," providing less bitter vegetables, and offering fruit are just a few suggestions.

ENTICE YOUR CHILDREN TO LOVE VEGGIES
- Hide greens and other nutritious treats in fruit smoothies.
- Make cauliflower mashed potatoes.
- Make "creamed spinach" with almond milk.
- Add small amounts of veggies to some of their favorite foods.
- Cook veggies more in order to soften them up.
- Be creative with spices that have condensed antioxidant plant power.
- Add a little ghee to enhance the flavor.
- Sprinkle a little nutritional yeast over broccoli for a cheesy flavor.
- Combine greens with another vegetable that your children like.
- Use raw almond butter on celery sticks and on red bell peppers.
- Try chocolate- or cheesy-flavored kale chips. My daughter LOVES these.

We understand the sacrifice and dedication it takes to raise a brain-healthy family and we applaud you for being a warrior, not only for your health, but for theirs! We can't promise that it will always be easy, but we can state with great certainty that the increased health, energy, focus, and productivity your family feels as a result of your dedication will be worth the few moans and groans you may get along the way.

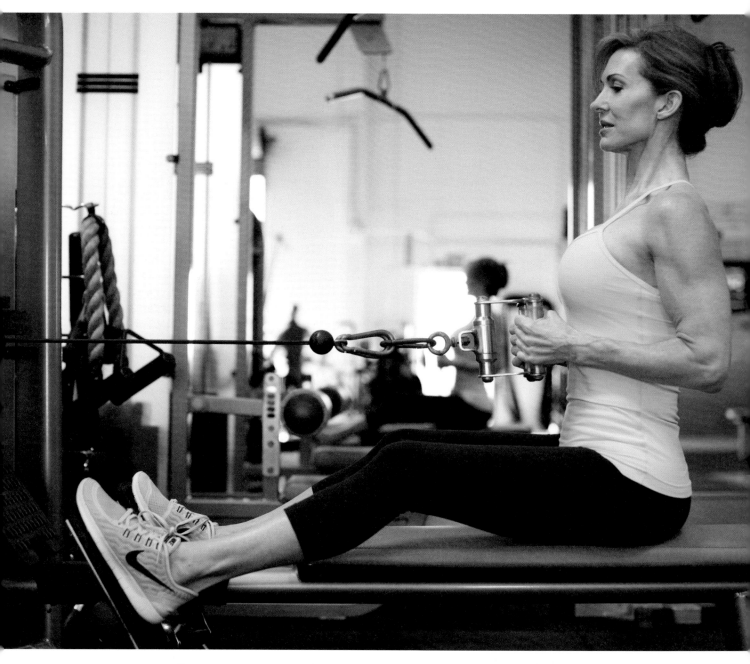

"Eat to strengthen your body and nourish
your mind. Eat to win!"

—Tana Amen

About the Authors

■

Tana Amen, RN, BSN

Tana Amen helps people realize that they are not stuck with the brain and body they have by empowering them with simple strategies that will transform them into Warriors for their health. Tana is the executive vice president of Amen Clinics, *New York Times* bestselling author of *The Omni Diet*, a highly respected health and fitness expert, and a nationally renowned speaker and media guest.

Tana and Daniel have written and hosted two national public television shows: *Healing ADD* and *The Omni Health Revolution*. Working side by side, they are creating an army of people dedicated to transforming the health of their brains and bodies using the tips and strategies they've created called "The Brain Warrior's Way."

Besides being a guest on *The Doctors*, the *Today* show, *Good Day New York*, *Extra*, *The Joy Behar Show*, and others, Tana has given presentations at the American Academy of Anti-Aging Medicine, Saddleback Church, High Performance Academy, SuperheroYou, the Institute for the Advancement of Human Behavior, the Omega Institute, the Kripalu Center, Beacon House, Salvation Army Adult Rehabilitation Center, and many other wellness-focused organizations.

After graduating magna cum laude from the Loma Linda University School of Nursing, Tana spent years working at Loma Linda's level A trauma unit as a neurosurgical intensive care nurse, taking care of some of the sickest patients in the hospital. There she learned firsthand the value of diet and nutrition on brain health. Tana is the author of six highly successful books, including: *The Omni Diet*; *Healing ADD Through Food*; *Change Your Brain, Change Your Body Cookbook*; *Get Healthy with the Brain Doctor's Wife*; *Eat Healthy with the Brain Doctor's Wife*; and *Live Longer with the Brain Doctor's Wife*.

In addition to working with her husband at Amen Clinics, Tana was a nutrition consultant, coach, and part of the team, which included psychiatrist Dr. Daniel Amen, functional medicine specialist Dr. Mark Hyman, and heart surgeon Dr. Mehmet Oz, that helped create the wildly popular Daniel Plan (www.danielplan.com) for Saddleback Church at the request of Pastor Rick Warren.

Tana hosts a unique tribe of "Brain Warriors" in the community started by the Amens, Brain Fit Life (www.mybrainfitlife.com), where she shares healthy eating tips and lifestyle strategies. She has also played an important part in Dr. Amen's astonishingly successful PBS specials, which have aired more than 80,000 times across North America and have raised more than $65 million for public television.

Tana is passionate about martial arts and has a black belt in Kenpo karate and tae kwon do. Being a mother and wife is Tana's first passion. Keeping her family and friends focused on fitness and health is a primary value for her. Tana believes that everyone can optimize his or her health by using the Brain Warrior's Way.

Daniel G. Amen, MD

Daniel Amen believes that brain health is central to all health and success. When your brain works right, he says, you work right; and when your brain is troubled, you are much more likely to have trouble in your life. His work is dedicated to helping people have better brains and better lives.

The Washington Post wrote that Dr. Amen is the most popular psychiatrist in America, and Sharecare named him the Web's number one most influential expert on and advocate for mental health.

Dr. Amen is a physician, double board-certified psychiatrist, and ten-time *New York Times* bestselling author. He is the founder of Amen Clinics in Costa Mesa and San Francisco, California; Bellevue, Washington; Reston, Virginia; Atlanta, Georgia; and New York, New York. Amen Clinics have the world's largest database of functional brain scans relating to behavior, totaling more than 125,000 scans on patients from 111 countries.

He is a Distinguished Fellow of the American Psychiatric Association, the highest award given to members, and is the lead researcher on the world's largest brain imaging and rehabilitation study on professional football players. His research has not only demonstrated high levels of brain damage in players, but he has also shown the possibility of significant recovery for many with the principles that underlie his work.

Together with Pastor Rick Warren and Dr. Mark Hyman, Dr. Amen is also one of the chief architects on Saddleback Church's Daniel Plan, a program to get the world healthy through religious organizations.

Dr. Amen has written, produced, and hosted ten popular shows about the brain, which have aired more than 100,000 times across North America.

Dr. Amen is the author or coauthor of seventy professional articles, seven book chapters, and over thirty books, including the number one *New York Times* bestsellers *The Daniel Plan* and *Change Your Brain, Change Your Life*; *Magnificent Mind at Any Age*; *Change Your Brain, Change Your Body*; *Use Your Brain to Change Your Age*; *Unleash the Power of the Female Brain*; and *Healing ADD*.

Dr. Amen's published scientific articles have appeared in the prestigious journals of Nature's *Molecular Psychiatry*, *PLOS ONE*, Nature's *Translational Psychiatry*, Nature's *International Journal of Obesity*, *The Journal of Neuropsychiatry and Clinical Neurosciences*, *Minerva Psichiatrica*, *Journal of Neurotrauma*, *The American Journal of Psychiatry*, *Nuclear Medicine Communications*, *Neurological Research*, *Journal of the American Academy of Child and Adolescent Psychiatry*, *Primary Psychiatry*, *Military Medicine*, and *General Hospital Psychiatry*. His research on post-traumatic stress disorder and traumatic brain injury was recognized by *Discover* magazine as one of the top 100 Stories in Science in 2015.

Dr. Amen has appeared in movies, including *After the Last Round* and *The Crash Reel*, and has appeared in Emmy-winning shows, such as *The Truth about Drinking* and *The Dr. Oz Show*. He was a consultant on the movie *Concussion*, written and directed by Peter Landesman, starring Will Smith. He has also spoken for the National Security Agency (NSA), the National Science Foundation (NSF), Harvard's Learning and the Brain Conference, the U.S. Department of the Interior, the National Council of Juvenile and Family Court Judges and the Supreme Courts of Delaware, Ohio, and Wyoming. Dr. Amen's work has been featured in *Newsweek*, *Time*, *The Huffington Post*, *ABC World News*, *20/20*, the BBC, *The Telegraph*, *Parade* magazine, *The New York Times*, *The New York Times Magazine*, *The Washington Post*, *The Los Angeles Times*, *Men's Health*, and *Cosmopolitan.*

Dr. Amen is married to Tana, is the father of four children, and grandfather to Elias, Emmy, Liam, and Louie. He collects penguins and is an avid table tennis player.

"Develop an indomitable will! Never allow the limitations of others to define your strength, ability, and especially your health."

—Tana Amen

Gratitude and Appreciation

∎

So many people have been involved in the process of creating this book and helping us create brain health warriors. We know it takes a village, and a strong tribe, to accomplish great things. We are grateful for and appreciate:

The tens of thousands of patients and families who have believed in our work, who allowed the staff at Amen Clinics and me to help them have better brains and better lives.

The amazing staff at Amen Clinics. As we write this, we currently serve 4,000 patient visits a month, making us one of the most active private mental and brain health centers in the world. Our professionals work hard every day serving our patients. Special appreciation to our fearless CEO, Terry Weber, who helps our organization run smoothly, as well as Tana's brand leader, Jasmine Patterson, who is a constant source of energy and creativity. Many thanks to CJ Ramos for her contribution to the beautiful cover design. Additionally, we'd like to acknowledge our dedicated and talented marketing and social media team. It is this hardworking team that creates attention and exposure to the work we so dearly love, so that others may benefit.

EJ Armstrong and her team at Armstrong Photography were an absolute pleasure to work with. Their professionalism and creativity helped give the food photos stunning visual expression and character.

Special thanks to Lauren Hillary for her wonderful work on additional lifestyle and family photos.

Carina Lindgren, makeup artist, and Victor Paul, hair stylist, are also greatly appreciated for their talent in the many projects involving professional hair and makeup services.

Rebecca Club, founder of Whole Health Everyday, and chefs Robyn Larson and Sarah Guiles were instrumental in collaborating to create dozens of simple, nutritious, and delicious recipes that meet Brain Warrior standards and will help you in the journey to feeling strong and healthy.

Our professional colleagues who believed in us and sent us their patients to evaluate, especially Earl Henslin, Mark Laaser, Daniel McQuoid, David Jarvis, Jane Massengill, Jennifer Lendl, Sheila Krystal, Rick Lavine, David Smith, Rick Gilbert, Mark Kosins, Leon and Linda Webber, Matt Stubblefield, Mark Hyman, Steve Lawrence, Jerry Kartzinel, Marcello Urban, Jack Felton, Peg Kay, Glen Havens, Rick Sponaugle, Charles Parker, Orlando Vargas and our friends at the House of Freedom and the Crosby Center, Terrina Picarello, Russ Talbott and Talbott Recovery, Bruce Rind, Raphael Stricker, Curt Rouanzoin, Steve Eggleston, Darren and Jill CdeBaca, Bart Main, Barry Jay, Thomas Morell, Stephen Cobb, Paula Jo Husack, Heidi Kunzli at Privé Swiss, Jan Hackelman, Connie Hornyak, Michael Sampley, Susie Graff, Rogério Rita, Begoña Quintana, Fabiola Albani, and many others.

Our Berkley editorial team: Thomas Colgan and Allison Janice, who believed in this book and helped make it possible.

Our friends and colleagues at public television stations across the country, including my mentors and friends Alan Foster, Alicia Steele, Kurt Mendelsohn, Greg Sherwood, Camille Dixon, Stacey Wiggins, Maura Phinney, Henry Broderson, Karen Nowak, Jackie Boyer, Jerry Liwanag, Suzanna Fiske, BaBette Davidson, Claire O'Connor Solomon, Duane Huey, and countless others. Public television is a treasure and I am grateful to be able to partner with stations to bring our message of hope and healing to millions.

Our family, who have lived through our obsession with everything Brain Warriors Way, especially our children Antony, Breanne, Kaitlyn, and Chloe, our grandchildren, and our parents, Mary Meeks (Tana's mom) and Louis and Dorie Amen. We know that many times you were tired of listening about the brain, but nonetheless gave us unending support.

Resources

∎

For ongoing recipes, brain health tips and lifestyle strategies, follow Tana Amen and Dr. Daniel Amen on social media and sign up for our free newsletters:

Facebook: Tana Amen BSN, RN https://www.facebook.com/TanaAmenBSNRN/

Dr. Daniel Amen https://www.facebook.com/drdanielamen/

Instagram: @TanaAmen

@docamen

Newsletters: Tana's Pantry http://www.amenlifestyle.com

Brain in the News http://danielamenmd.amenclinics.com/blog/

Amen Clinics, Inc.

www.amenclinics.com

Amen Clinics, Inc. (ACI) was established in 1989 by Daniel G. Amen, MD. We specialize in innovative diagnosis and treatment planning for a wide variety of behavioral, learning, emotional, cognitive, and weight issues for children, teenagers, and adults. ACI has an international reputation for evaluating brain-behavior problems, such as ADD, depression, anxiety, school failure, brain trauma, obsessive-compulsive disorders, aggressiveness, marital conflict, cognitive decline, brain toxicity from drugs or alcohol, and obesity. In addition, we work with people to optimize brain function and decrease the risk for Alzheimer's disease and other age-related issues.

Brain SPECT imaging is performed in the clinics. ACI has the world's largest database of brain scans for emotional, cognitive, and behavioral problems. ACI welcomes referrals from physicians, psychologists, social workers, marriage and family therapists, drug and alcohol counselors, and individual patients and families.

Our toll-free number is (888) 546-2700.

Amen Clinics Orange County, California
3150 Bristol St., Suite 400
Costa Mesa, CA 92626

Amen Clinics San Francisco
350 Wiget Lane, Suite 100
Walnut Creek, CA 95498

Amen Clinics Northwest
616 120th Ave. NE, Suite C100
Bellevue, WA 98005

Amen Clinics Washington, DC
10701 Parkridge Blvd., Suite 110
Reston, VA 20191

Amen Clinics New York
16 East 40th St., 9th Floor
New York, NY 10016
(888) 564-2700

Amen Clinics Atlanta
5901-C Peachtree Dunwoody Road, NE, Suite 65
Atlanta, Georgia 30328
(888) 564-2700

Amenclinics.com is an educational, interactive website geared toward mental health and medical professionals, educators, students, and the general public. It contains a wealth of information and resources to help you learn about and optimize your brain. The site contains more than three hundred color brain SPECT images, thousands of scientific abstracts on brain SPECT imaging for psychiatry, a free brain health audit, and much, much more.

Brain Fit Life

www.mybrainfitlife.com

Based on Dr. Amen's thirty-five years as a clinical psychiatrist, he and his wife Tana have developed a sophisticated online community to help you feel smarter, happier, and younger. It includes:

- ▶ Detailed questionnaires, to help you know your BRAIN TYPE and personalize a program to your own needs
- ▶ Webneuro, a sophisticated neuropsychological test, to assess your brain
- ▶ Based on Webneuro results, targeted brain exercises in the form of fun games to strengthen your vulnerable areas
- ▶ Exclusive, award-winning 24/7 BRAIN GYM MEMBERSHIP
- ▶ Hundreds of brain-healthy recipes, tips, shopping lists, and menu plans
- ▶ Daily tips that can be sent via text messages to help you remember your supplements and stay on track
- ▶ Relaxation room to help you eliminate stress and overcome negative thinking patterns
- ▶ Hypnosis audios for sleep, anxiety, peak performance and overcoming weight issues and pain
- ▶ Amazing brain-healthy music

BrainMD Health

www.brainmdhealth.com

See for the highest-quality brain-healthy supplements, courses, books, and information products.

Index